RAPID REVIEW SERIES

PHARMACOLOGY

Visit our website at **www.mosby.com**

RAPID REVIEW SERIES

Series Editor
Edward F. Goljan, MD

PHARMACOLOGY

Thomas L. Pazdernik, PhD
Professor
Pharmacology, Toxicology, and Therapeutics
University of Kansas Medical Center
Kansas City, Kansas

Laszlo Kerecsen, MD
Professor
Department of Pharmacology
Arizona College of Osteopathic Medicine
Midwestern University
Glendale, Arizona

Mrugeshkumar K. Shah, MD, MPH
Chief Resident
Department of Physical Medicine & Rehabilitation
Harvard Medical School / Spaulding Rehabilitation Hospital
Boston, Massachusetts

Mosby
An Imprint of Elsevier Science
St. Louis London Philadelphia Sydney Toronto

Mosby
An Imprint of Elsevier Science

The Curtis Center
Independence Square West
Philadelphia, PA 19106

NOTICE

Pharmacology is an ever-changing field. Standard safety precautions must be followed, but as new research and clinical experience broaden our knowledge, changes in treatment and drug therapy may become necessary or appropriate. Readers are advised to check the most current product information provided by the manufacturer of each drug to be administered to verify the recommended dose, the method and duration of administration, and contraindications. It is the responsibility of the licensed prescriber, relying on experience and knowledge of the patient, to determine dosages and the best treatment for each individual patient. Neither the publisher nor the editor assumes any liability for any injury and/or damage to persons or property arising from this publication.

The Publisher

International Standard Book Number 0-323-00838-0

Acquisitions Editor: Jason Malley
Managing Editor: Susan Kelly
Developmental Editors: Martha Cushman, Mary Durkin, Donna Frassetto, Sharon Maddox
Publishing Services Manager: Patricia Tannian
Project Manager: Richard Hund
Senior Designer: Kathi Gosche
Cover Designer: Melissa Walter
Illustrator: Matt Chansky

GW/FF

Printed in the United States of America

Last digit is the print number: 9 8 7 6 5 4 3 2 1

To my wife, Betty; my daughter Nancy and her husband, Billy;
my daughter Lisa and her husband, Chris; and my triplet grandbabies,
Cassidy Rae, Thomas Pazdernik, and Isabel Mari. –TLP

To Gabor and Tamas, my sons. –LK

To my wife, Stephanie, for her patience and support; to my parents and
sister for their love, inspiration, and wisdom. –MKS

Preface

The *Rapid Review Series* is designed for today's busy medical student who has completed basic sciences courses and has only a limited amount of time to prepare for the United States Medical Licensing Examination (USMLE) Step 1. With a commitment to meeting the needs of these students, we conducted numerous focus groups throughout the United States, trying to learn what would better prepare students for the Step 1 examination. Each book in the *Rapid Review Series* offers a visually integrated approach to review and is packaged with a CD-ROM to help students practice for the actual USMLE Step 1.

Special Features

BOOK

- **Target topics:** summary of major topics discussed in the chapter
- **Two-color, easy-to-follow outline:** concisely organized need-to-know information integrating basic science and clinical correlations
- **High-yield margin notes**: recall topics most likely tested on Step 1
- **Visual elements**: computer-generated two-color schematics, summary tables, and clinical boxes
- **Bold and color text**: highlights key words and phrases
- **Practice examinations**: two sets of 50 multiple-choice, clinically oriented questions in current USMLE Step 1 format, including complete discussions (rationales) for all options
- **Table of normal laboratory values**

CD-ROM

- **Full-color: 500 clinically oriented multiple-choice questions** in current USMLE Step 1 format and content
- **Test mode:** 60-minute timed test of 50-question block by topic, system, or random selection
- **Tutorial (review) mode:** customize your review (questions and discussions) by science, system, or random selection with immediate feedback
- **Bookmark capability**
- **Table of common laboratory values**
- **Scoring function:** instant statistical analysis showing your strengths and weaknesses; print capability

Acknowledgment of Reviewers

The publisher wishes to express sincere thanks to the medical students who provided many useful comments and helpful suggestions for improving both the text and the questions for the book and the CD-ROM. Our publishing program will continue to benefit from the combined insight and experience provided by your reviews. For always encouraging us to focus on our target, the USMLE Step 1, we thank the following:

Patricia C. Daniel, PhD
Kansas University Medical Center

Steven J. Engman
Loyola University of Chicago
Stritch School of Medicine

Omar A. Khan
University of Vermont College of Medicine

Michael W. Lawlor
Loyola University of Chicago
Stritch School of Medicine

Lillian Liang
Jefferson Medical College

Erica L. Magers
Michigan State University College of Human Medicine

Acknowledgments

The authors wish to acknowledge Susan Kelly, Managing Editor, for her persistence and expertise in completing this project. We also thank Mary Durkin and Martha Cushman for editing the text; Donna Frassetto and Sharon Maddox for editing the questions; and Matt Chansky for his excellent illustrations. We give a special thanks to Tibor Rozman, MD, for his contributions to the development of clinically relevant questions and to Tamas Kerecsen for processing the questions. We also thank the faculty of the Department of Pharmacology, Toxicology and Therapeutics at the University of Kansas Medical Center and the faculty of the Department of Pharmacology at Arizona College of Osteopathic Medicine, Midwestern University, for their superb contributions to the development of materials for our teaching programs. Finally, we thank the numerous medical students who, over the years, have been our inspiration for developing teaching materials.

Thomas L. Pazdernik, PhD
Laszlo Kerecsen, MD
Mrugeshkumar K. Shah, MD, MPH

Table of Contents

SECTION I

Principles of Pharmacology

1

Pharmacokinetics

Target Topics

- Drug absorption
- Drug distribution
- Drug metabolism
- Drug excretion
- Drug kinetic processes

I. Definition

- **Pharmacokinetics** is the **fate** of drugs within the body.
- It involves **a**bsorption, **d**istribution, **m**etabolism, and **e**xcretion (ADME) (Figure 1-1).

Pharmacokinetics: Absorption, Distribution, Metabolism, Excretion (ADME)

II. Absorption

- Absorption is the **uptake** of a drug by the body (i.e., entry into the body).

A. Processes of absorption

1. Passive diffusion

a. Characteristics

(1) Does *not* make use of a carrier

(2) Not saturable

(3) Low structural specificity

(4) Driven by concentration gradient

b. Aqueous diffusion: passage through central pores in cell membranes

- Possible for low-molecular-weight substances

c. Lipid diffusion: direct passage through lipid bilayer

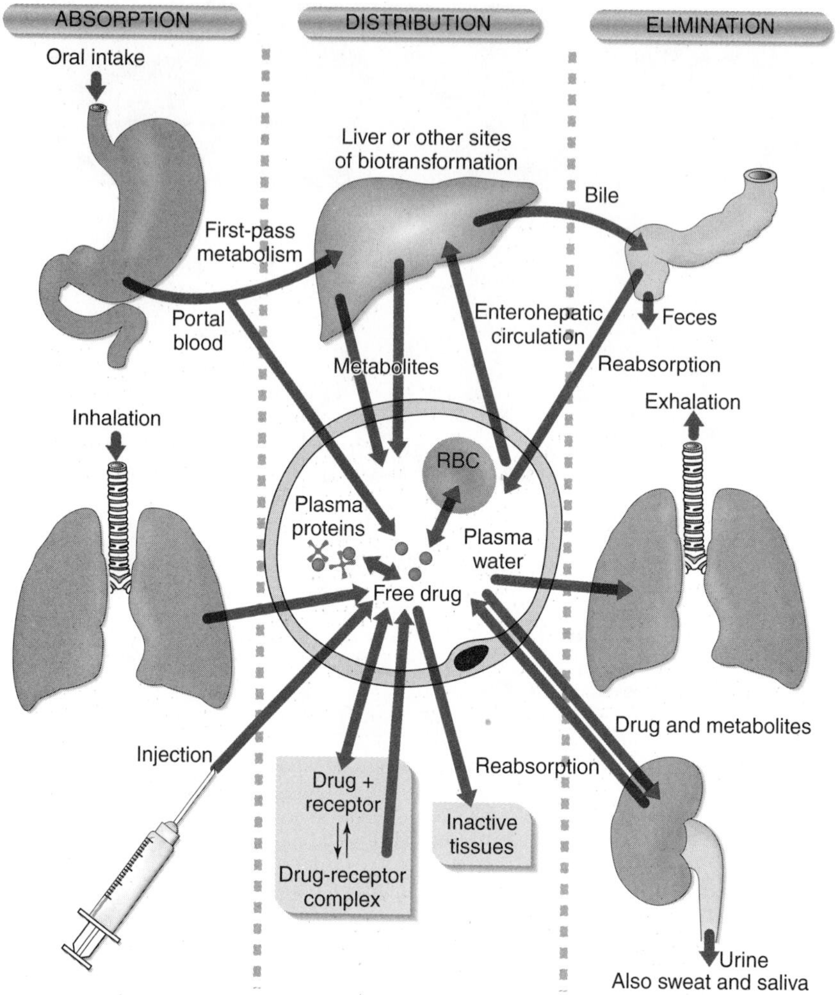

Figure 1-1 Schematic representation of the fate of a drug in the body (pharmacokinetics). *Green circles* indicate passage of drug through the body (intake to output). *RBC,* Red blood cell.

- Facilitated by increased degree of lipid solubility
- Driven by a concentration gradient (nonionized forms move most easily)

(1) **Lipid solubility** is the most important limiting factor for drug permeation; a large number of lipid barriers separate body compartments.

(2) **Lipid:aqueous partition coefficient** determines how readily a drug molecule moves between lipid and aqueous media.

2. Active transport

a. Characteristics

(1) Carrier-mediated

(2) Structural selectivity

(3) Competition by similar molecules

(4) Energy-dependent
(5) Saturable
(6) Movement occurs against a concentration or electrochemical gradient
(7) Rapid

b. **Sites of active transport:** neuronal membranes, choroid plexus, renal tubular cells, hepatocytes

3. **Facilitated diffusion**
   - Carrier-mediated process that does *not* require energy
   - Involves movement along a concentration or electrochemical gradient
4. **Pinocytosis**
   - Process in which a cell engulfs extracellular material within membrane vesicles
   - Used by exceptionally large molecules (molecular weight > 1000), such as **iron-transferrin complex** and **vitamin B_{12}–intrinsic factor complex**

B. Factors that affect absorption

1. **Solubility**
   a. Drugs in **aqueous solutions mix more readily** with the aqueous phase at absorptive sites, so they are absorbed more rapidly than those in oily solutions.
   b. Drugs in **suspension or solid form are dependent on the rate of dissolution** before they can mix with the aqueous phase at absorptive sites.
2. **Concentration**
   - Drugs in **highly concentrated solutions** are absorbed more readily than those in dilute concentrations.
3. **Blood flow**
   - **Greater blood flow** means **higher rates of drug absorption** (e.g., absorption is greater in muscle tissue than in subcutaneous sites).
4. **Absorbing surface**
   - **Organs with large surface areas,** such as the lungs and intestines, have **more rapid drug absorption** (e.g., absorption is greater in the intestine than in the stomach).
5. **Contact time**
   - The greater the time, the greater the amount of drug absorbed.
6. **pH**
   - For weak acids and weak bases, the pH determines the relative amount of drug in ionized or nonionized form, which in turn affects solubility.

   a. **Weak organic acids** donate a proton to form anions (Figure 1-2), as shown in the following equation:

$$HA \leftrightarrow H^+ + A^-$$

where:

HA = weak acid
H^+ = proton
A^- = anion

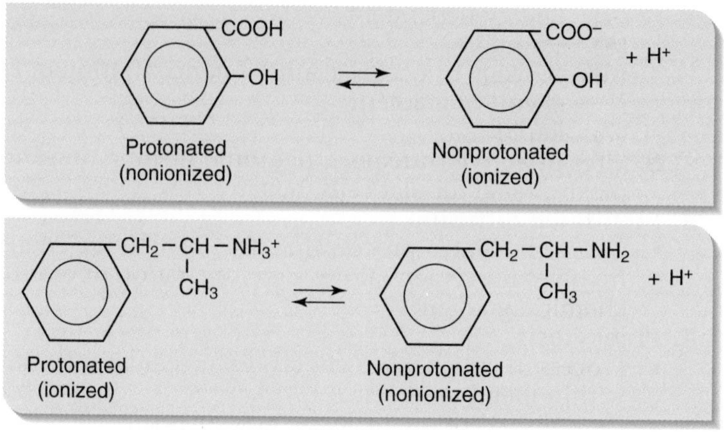

Figure 1-2 Examples of the ionization of a weak organic acid (salicylate; *top*) and a weak organic base (amphetamine; *bottom*).

b. Weak organic bases accept a proton to form cations (see Figure 1-2), as shown in the following equation:

$$HB^+ \leftrightarrow B + H^+$$

where:

B = weak base
H^+ = proton
HB^+ = cation

Weak organic acids pass through membranes best in acidic environments; weak organic bases pass through membranes best in basic environments.

c. Only the nonionized form of a drug can readily cross cell membranes.

d. The **ratio of ionized versus nonionized forms** is a function of **pK_a** (measure of drug acidity) and the pH of the environment. When pH = pK_a, a compound is 50% ionized and 50% nonionized.

- The **Henderson-Hasselbalch equation** can be used to determine the ratio of the nonionized form to the ionized form.

$$\log \frac{[\text{protonated form}]}{[\text{unprotonated form}]} = pK_a - pH$$

Bioavailability: depends on the extent of absorption

Sublingual nitroglycerin avoids first-pass metabolism, promoting rapid absorption.

III. Bioavailability

- Bioavailability is the relative **amount of** the administered **drug that reaches the general circulation.**
- Several factors influence bioavailability.

A. First-pass metabolism

- Enzymes in the intestinal flora, intestinal mucosa, and liver metabolize drugs before they reach the general circulation, significantly decreasing systemic bioavailability.

B. Drug formulation

- Bioavailability after oral administration is affected by the **extent of disintegration** of a particular drug formulation.

TABLE 1-1 Routes of Administration

Route	Advantages	Disadvantages
Enteral		
Oral	Most convenient Produces slow, uniform absorption Relatively safe Economical	Poor absorption of large and charged particles Destruction of drug by enzymes or low pH (e.g., peptides, proteins, penicillins) Drugs bind or complex with gastrointestinal contents (e.g., calcium binds to tetracycline) Cannot be used for drugs that irritate the intestine
Rectal	Limited first-pass metabolism Useful when oral route precluded	Absorption often irregular and incomplete May cause irritation to rectal mucosa
Sublingual/buccal	Rapid absorption Avoids first-pass metabolism	Absorption of only small amounts (e.g., nitroglycerin)
Parenteral		
Intravenous	Most direct route Bypasses barriers to absorption (immediate effect) Suitable for large volumes Dosage easily adjusted	Increased risk of adverse effects from high concentration immediately after injection Not suitable for oily substances or suspensions
Intramuscular	Quickly and easily administered Possible rapid absorption May use as depot Suitable for oily substances and suspensions	Painful Bleeding May lead to nerve injury
Subcutaneous	Quickly and easily administered Fairly rapid absorption Suitable for suspensions and pellets	Painful Large amounts cannot be given
Inhalation	Used for volatile compounds (e.g., halothane and amyl nitrite) and drugs that can be administered by aerosol (e.g., albuterol) Rapid absorption due to large surface area of alveolar membranes and high blood flow through lungs Aerosol delivers drug directly to site of action and may minimize systemic side effects	Variable systemic distribution
Topical	Application to specific surface (skin, eye, nose, vagina) allows local effects	May irritate surface
Transdermal	Allows controlled permeation through skin (e.g., nicotine, estrogen, testosterone, fentanyl, scopolamine, clonidine)	May irritate surface

TABLE 1-2 Body Compartments in Which Drugs May Distribute

Compartment	Volume (L/kg)	Liters in 70-kg Human	Drug Type
Plasma water	0.045	3	Strongly plasma–protein bound drugs and very large drugs (e.g., heparin)
Extracellular body water	0.20	14	Large water-soluble drugs (e.g., mannitol)
Total body water	0.60	42	Small water-soluble drugs (e.g., ethanol)
Tissue	> 0.70	> 49	Drugs that avidly bind to tissue (e.g., chloroquine; 115 L/kg)

Bioequivalence: depends on both rate and extent of absorption

C. Route of administration (Table 1-1)

D. Bioequivalence

- Two drug formulations with the same bioavailability (extent of absorption) and rate of absorption are **bioequivalent.**

IV. Distribution

- Distribution is the **spread of a drug** throughout the body.
- Drugs may distribute into certain body compartments (Table 1-2).

A. Apparent volume of distribution (V_d): space in the body into which the drug appears to disseminate

1. The V_d is calculated according to the following equation:

$$V_d = \frac{\text{Amount of drug in body}}{C_0}$$

where:

C_0 = **concentration of drug** in plasma at time 0 after equilibration.

2. A **large V_d** means that a drug is concentrated in **tissues.**

3. A **small V_d** means that a drug is in the **extracellular fluid or plasma;** that is, the V_d is inversely related to plasma drug concentration.

B. Factors that affect distribution: plasma protein and tissue binding, gender, age, amount of body fat, relative blood flow, size, and lipid solubility

1. Plasma protein binding

a. Drugs with high plasma protein binding remain in plasma; thus, they have a low V_d and a prolonged half-life.

b. Binding acts as a **drug reservoir,** slowing onset and prolonging duration of action.

c. Many drugs bind **reversibly** with one or more plasma proteins (e.g., albumin) in the vascular compartment.

TABLE 1-3 Sites of Drug Concentration

Site	Characteristics
Fat	Stores lipid-soluble drugs
Tissue	May represent sizable reservoir, depending on mass, as with muscle Several drugs accumulate in liver
Bone	Tetracyclines are deposited in calcium-rich regions (bones, teeth)
Transcellular reservoirs	Gastrointestinal tract serves as transcellular reservoir for drugs that are slowly absorbed or that are undergoing enterohepatic circulation

d. Disease states (e.g., liver disease, which affects albumin concentration) or drugs that alter protein binding influence the concentration of other drugs.

2. Sites of drug concentration (Table 1-3)

a. Redistribution

(1) Intravenous thiopental is initially distributed to areas of highest blood flow, such as the brain, liver, and kidneys.

(2) The drug is then redistributed to and stored in muscle and adipose tissue.

b. Ion trapping

(1) **Weak organic acids** are trapped in **basic** environments.

(2) **Weak organic bases** are trapped in **acidic** environments.

c. Sites of drug exclusion (places where it is difficult for drugs to enter)

- Cerebrospinal, ocular, lymph, pleural, and fetal fluids

V. Biotransformation or Metabolism

- The primary site of biotransformation or metabolism is the **liver,** and the primary goal is **drug inactivation.**

Diseases that affect the liver influence drug metabolism.

A. Products of drug metabolism

- Are usually less active pharmacologically
- However, products are sometimes **prodrugs,** in which the drug form is inactive and the metabolite is active.

B. Phase I biotransformation (oxidation, reduction, hydrolysis)

1. The products are usually more **polar metabolites,** resulting from introducing or unmasking a function group (–OH, $-NH_2$, –SH, $-COO^-$).

2. The process involves **enzymes located in the smooth endoplasmic reticulum.**

3. Oxidation usually occurs via a **cytochrome P450 system.**

C. Phase II biotransformation

- Involves **conjugation,** in which an endogenous substance, such as glucuronic acid, combines with a phase I metabolite to form a conjugate with high polarity

Conjugation reactions usually make drugs more water soluble and more excretable.

TABLE 1-4 Genetic Polymorphisms and Drug Metabolism

Predisposing Factor	Drug	Clinical Effect
G6PD deficiency	Primaquine, sulfonamides	Acute hemolytic anemia
Slow *N*-acetylation	Isoniazid	Peripheral neuropathy
Slow *N*-acetylation	Hydralazine	Lupus syndrome
Slow ester hydrolysis	Succinylcholine	Prolonged apnea
Slow oxidation	Tolbutamide	Cardiotoxicity
Slow acetaldehyde oxidation	Ethanol	Facial flushing

G6PD, Glucose-6-phosphate dehydrogenase.

Methylation and acetylation reactions often make drugs less water soluble.

1. **Glucuronidation**
   - A major route of metabolism for drugs and endogenous compounds (steroids, bilirubin)
   - Occurs in the **endoplasmic reticulum**
2. **Sulfation**
   - A major route of drug metabolism
   - Occurs in the **cytoplasm**
3. **Methylation and acetylation reactions**
   - Involve the **conjugation of drugs** (by transferases) with other substances (e.g., methyl, acetyl) to metabolites, thereby **decreasing drug activity**

D. Drug interactions
- May occur as a result of changes to the cytochrome P450 enzyme system

1. **Inducers of cytochrome P450**
   - Hasten metabolism of drugs metabolized in the liver
   - **Examples:** phenobarbital, phenytoin, rifampin, carbamazepine
2. **Inhibitors of cytochrome P450**
   - Decreases metabolism of drugs metabolized in the liver
   - **Examples:** cimetidine, ketoconazole, erythromycin

E. Genetic polymorphisms
- Influence the metabolism of a drug, thereby altering its effects (Table 1-4)

F. Reactive metabolite intermediates
- Are responsible for mutagenic, carcinogenic, and teratogenic effects, as well as specific organ-directed toxicity
- **Examples of resulting conditions:** acetaminophen-induced hepatotoxicity, aflatoxin-induced tumors, cyclophosphamide-induced cystitis

A drug with a larger V_d is eliminated more slowly than one with a smaller V_d.

VI. Excretion
- Excretion is the amount of drug and drug metabolites excreted by any process per unit time.

A. Excretion processes in kidney

1. **Glomerular filtration rate**
   - Depends on the **size, charge,** and **protein binding** of a particular drug
   - Is lower for highly protein-bound drugs

- Drugs that are *not* protein bound or *not* reabsorbed are eliminated at a rate equal to the creatinine clearance rate (125 mL/min).

2. Tubular secretion
- Occurs in the **middle segment of the proximal convoluted tubule**
- Provides **transporters for anions** (e.g., salicylates) and **cations** (e.g., pyridostigmine)
- Can be used to increase drug concentration by use of another drug that competes for the transporter (e.g., probenecid inhibits penicillin secretion)
- Has **a rate that approaches renal plasma flow (660 mL/min)**

a. Characteristics of tubular secretion
(1) Competition for the transporter
(2) Saturation of the transporter
(3) Unaffected by plasma protein binding

b. Examples of drugs that undergo tubular secretion: penicillin, salicylates, thiazide diuretics, uric acid

3. Passive tubular reabsorption

a. Uncharged drugs can be reabsorbed into the systemic circulation in the distal tubule.

b. Ion trapping
- Trapping of the ionized form of drugs in the urine

(1) With **weak acids** (phenobarbital, methotrexate, aspirin), alkalinization of urine (sodium bicarbonate) increases renal excretion.
(2) With **weak bases** (amphetamine), acidification of urine (ammonium chloride) increases renal excretion.

B. Excretion processes in the liver

1. Large polar compounds (molecular weight > 325) may be actively secreted into bile.
- Separate transporters for anions (e.g., glucuronide conjugates), neutral molecules (e.g., ouabain), and cations (e.g., tubocurarine)

2. These large drugs often undergo **enterohepatic recycling,** in which drugs secreted in the bile are again reabsorbed in the small intestine.
- The enterohepatic cycle can be interrupted by agents that bind drugs in the intestine (e.g., charcoal, cholestyramine).

C. Other sites of excretion
- **Example:** excretion of gaseous anesthetics by the **lungs**

VII. Kinetic Processes

- The therapeutic utility of a drug depends on the rate and extent of **input, distribution,** and **loss.**

A. Clearance kinetics

1. Clearance
- The volume of plasma from which a substance is removed per unit time

- To calculate clearance, **divide the rate of drug elimination by the plasma concentration of the drug.**

2. **Total body clearance**
   - Is calculated using the following equation:

$$Cl = V_d \times K_{el}$$

where:

V_d = **volume of distribution**
K_{el} = **elimination rate constant**

3. **Renal clearance**
   - Is calculated using the following equation:

$$Cl_r = \frac{U \times C_{ur}}{C_p}$$

where:

U = **urine flow** (mL/min)
C_{ur} = **urine concentration of a drug**
C_p = **plasma concentration of a drug**

B. Elimination kinetics

1. **Zero-order kinetics**
   - The elimination of a constant amount of drug per unit time
   - **Examples:** ethanol, heparin, phenytoin (at high doses)

   a. **Important characteristics of zero-order kinetics**
      (1) **Rate** is independent of drug concentration.
      (2) **Elimination pseudo–half-life** is proportional to drug concentration.
      (3) Small increase in dose can produce larger increase in concentration.
      (4) Process only occurs when enzymes or transporters are saturated.

   b. Graphically, plasma drug concentration versus time yields a straight line (Figure 1-3, *A*).

2. **First-order kinetics**
   - The elimination of a constant percentage of drug per unit time
   - **Examples:** most drugs (unless given at very high concentrations)

   a. **Important characteristics of first-order kinetics**
      (1) **Rate of elimination is proportional** to drug concentration.
      (2) **Drug concentration changes by some constant fraction** per unit time (i.e., 0.1/h).
      (3) **Half-life** ($t_{1/2}$) is **constant** (i.e., independent of dose).

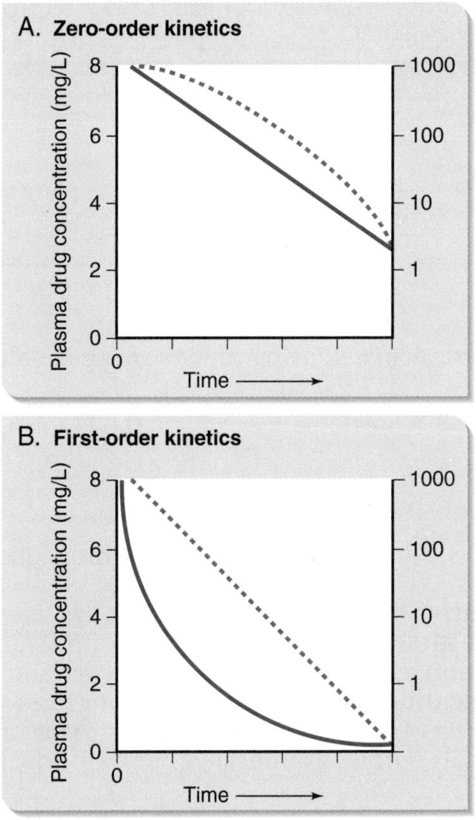

Figure 1-3 Kinetic order of drug disappearance from the plasma. Note that the scale on the left x-axis **(A)** is arithmetic, yielding a relationship shown by the *solid line,* and the scale on the right x-axis **(B)** is logarithmic, yielding a relationship shown by the *dashed line.*

b. Graphically, a semilogarithmic plot of plasma drug concentration versus time yields a straight line (see Figure 1-3, *B*).

c. Elimination rate constant (K_{el})

- **Sum of all rate constants** due to metabolism and excretion

$$K_{el} = K_m + K_{ex}$$

where:

K_m = **metabolic rate constant**
K_{ex} = **excretion rate constant**
K_{el} = **elimination rate constant**

d. Biologic or elimination half-life

- **Time required for drug concentration to drop by one-half;** independent of dose.

TABLE 1-5 Number of Half-Lives ($t_{1/2}$) Required to Reach Steady-State Concentration (C_{ss})

% C_{ss}	Number of $t_{1/2}$
50.0	1
75.0	2
87.5	3
93.8	4
98.0	5

- Is calculated using the following equation:

$$t_{1/2} = \frac{0.693}{K_{el}}$$

where:

K_{el} = elimination rate constant

3. **Repetitive dosing kinetics**
   - The **attainment of steady state** of plasma drug concentration of a drug following first-order kinetics when a fixed drug dose is given at constant time interval

   a. **Concentration at steady state** (C_{ss}) occurs when input equals output, as indicated by the following equation:

$$C_{ss} = \frac{\text{Input}}{\text{Output}} = \frac{F \times D/\tau}{Cl}$$

where:

F = bioavailability
D = dose
τ = dosing interval
Cl = clearance

   b. The time required to reach the **steady-state condition** is $t_{1/2} \times 4\frac{1}{2} - 5$ (Table 1-5).

   c. The **loading dose** necessary to reach the **steady-state condition** immediately can be calculated using the following equation:

$$LD = 1.44\ C_{ss} \times \frac{V_d}{F}$$

where:

LD = loading dose
C_{ss} = concentration at steady state
V_d = volume of distribution
F = bioavailability

2

Pharmacodynamics

Target Topics

- Dose-response relationships
- Drug receptors and their signaling mechanisms
- Drug agonists
- Drug antagonists
- Pharmacodynamically altered responses

I. Definition

- **Pharmacodynamics** is the **biochemical** and **physiologic effects** of drugs on the body.

II. Dose-Response Relationships

A. These relationships are usually expressed as a **log dose-response (LDR) curve.**

B. Properties of LDR curves

- LDR curves are typically **S-shaped.**
- A steep slope in the midportion of the "S" indicates that a small increase in dosage will produce a large response.

1. Graded response (Figure 2-1): response in one subject or test system

- **Median effective concentration (EC_{50}):** concentration that corresponds to 50% of the maximal response

2. All-or-none (quantal) response: number of individuals within a group responding to a given dose

- The endpoint is set, and an individual is either a **responder** or a **nonresponder.**

a. This response is expressed as a normal histogram or cumulative distribution profile (Figure 2-2).

- The normal histogram is usually bell-shaped.

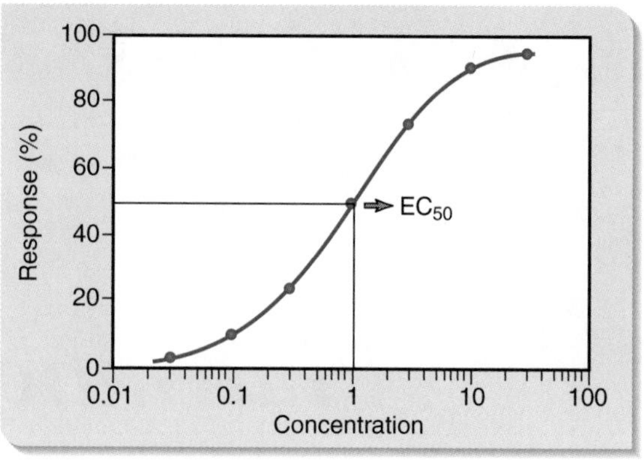

Figure 2-1 Log dose-response curve for an agonist-induced response. The median effective concentration (EC_{50}) is the concentration that results in a 50% maximal response.

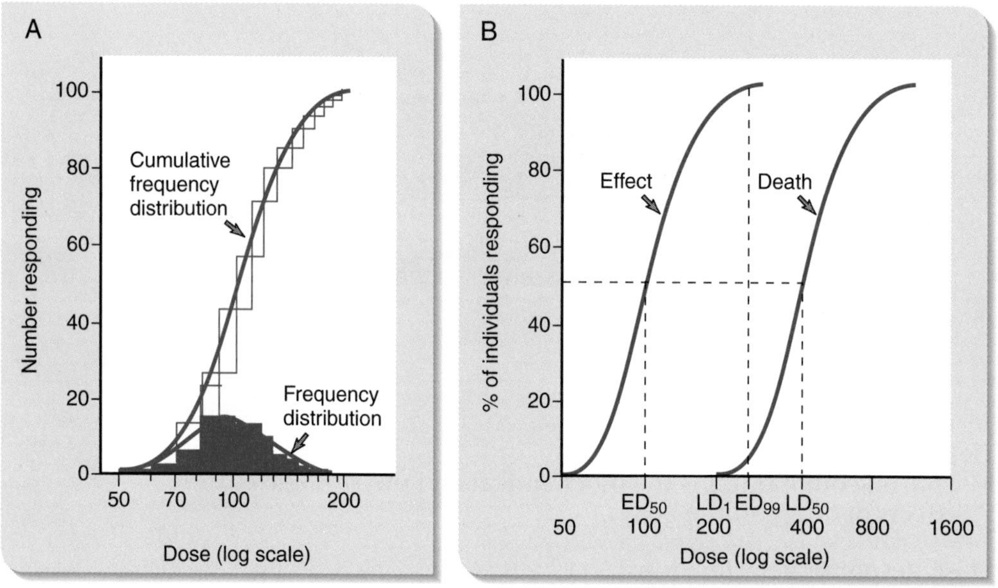

Figure 2-2 **A,** Cumulative frequency distribution and frequency distribution curves for a drug using a logarithmic dose scale. **B,** Cumulative frequency distribution curves for the therapeutic and lethal effects of a drug using a logarithmic dose scale.

b. **Median effective dose (ED_{50}):** dose to which 50% of subjects respond

c. The **therapeutic index (TI)** and the **margin of safety (MS)** are based on quantal responses.
   - **TI:** ratio of the lethal dose in 50% of the population (LD_{50}) divided by the effective dose for 50% of the population (ED_{50}), or

$$TI = \frac{LD_{50}}{ED_{50}}$$

- **MS:** ratio of the lethal dose for 1% of the population (LD_1) divided by the effective dose for 99% of the population (LD_{99}), or

$$MS = \frac{LD_1}{ED_{99}}$$

III. Drug Receptors

- Drug receptors are biologic components on the surface of or within cells that bind with drugs, resulting in molecular changes that produce a certain response.

A. Types of receptors and their signaling mechanisms (Table 2-1)

1. **Membrane receptors** are coupled with a G protein, an ion channel, or an enzyme.
   a. **Receptor-linked enzymes**
   b. **Ligand-gated channels**
      (1) Signals cross membranes due to changes in ion conductance and alter the electrical potential of cells.
      (2) The speed of the response is rapid.
   c. **G protein–coupled receptors**
      - These receptors are a superfamily of diverse **guanosine triphosphate** (GTP)–binding proteins that couple to "serpentine" transmembrane receptors (Figure 2-3).
2. **Intracellular receptors** (inside cells)
   - Cytoplasmic guanylyl cyclase (activated by nitric oxide)
   a. **Ligand-responsive transcription factors:** alter gene expression and protein synthesis
   b. **Other intracellular sites** can serve as targets for drug molecules crossing cell membranes (e.g., structural proteins, DNA, RNA).
   c. **Drugs using these mechanisms:** steroids, lipid-soluble drugs, nitric oxide

B. Degree of receptor binding

1. Drug molecules bind to receptors at a rate that is dependent on drug concentration.
2. The **dissociation constant** ($K_D = k_{-1}/k_1$) of the drug-receptor complex is inversely related to the affinity of the drug for the receptor.
   - A drug with a K_D of 10^{-7} M has a higher affinity than a drug with a K_D of 10^{-6} M.
   - k_1 is the **rate of onset**, and k_{-1} is the **rate of offset** for receptor occupancy.
3. The intensity of response is proportional to the number of receptors occupied.

C. Terms used to describe drug-receptor interactions

1. **Affinity**
   - **Propensity** of a drug to **bind** with a given receptor
2. **Potency**
   - **Comparative expression** that relates the dose required to produce a particular effect of a given intensity relative to a standard reference (Figure 2-4)

TABLE 2-1 Drug Receptors and Mechanisms of Signal Transduction

Receptor	Ligand	Mechanism	Time
G Protein–coupled Receptors			
α_1-Adrenergic receptors	Phenylephrine (agonist) Prazosin (antagonist)	Activation of phospholipase C	sec
α_2-Adrenergic receptors	Clonidine (agonist) Yohimbine (antagonist)	Inhibition of adenylyl cyclase	sec
β-Adrenergic receptors	Isoproterenol (agonist) Propranolol (antagonist)	Stimulation of adenylyl cyclase	sec
Muscarinic receptors	Pilocarpine (agonist) Atropine (antagonist)	Activation of phospholipase C	sec
Ligand-gated Ion Channels			
$GABA_A$ receptors	Benzodiazepines (agonists) Flumazenil (antagonist)	Chloride flux	msec
Nicotinic ACh receptors	Nicotine (agonist) Tubocurarine (antagonist)	Sodium flux	msec
Membrane-bound Enzymes			
Insulin receptors	Insulin	Activation of tyrosine kinase	min
Cytokine receptors	Interleukin-2	Activation of tyrosine kinase	min
Cytoplasmic Receptors			
Cytoplasmic guanylyl cyclase	Nitroglycerin	Activation of guanylyl cyclase	min
Nuclear Receptors			
Steroid receptors	Adrenal and gonadal steroids	Activation of gene transcription	h
Thyroid hormone receptors	Thyroxine	Activation of gene transcription	h

ACh, Acetylcholine; *GABA,* γ-aminobutyric acid.

3. **Efficacy (intrinsic activity)**
   - **Maximal response** resulting from binding of drug to its receptor (see Figure 2-4)
4. **Agonist**
   - Drug that **stimulates a receptor,** provoking a **biologic response**
5. **Partial agonist**
   - Drug that provokes a **submaximal response**
   - In Figure 2-4, drug C is a partial agonist.

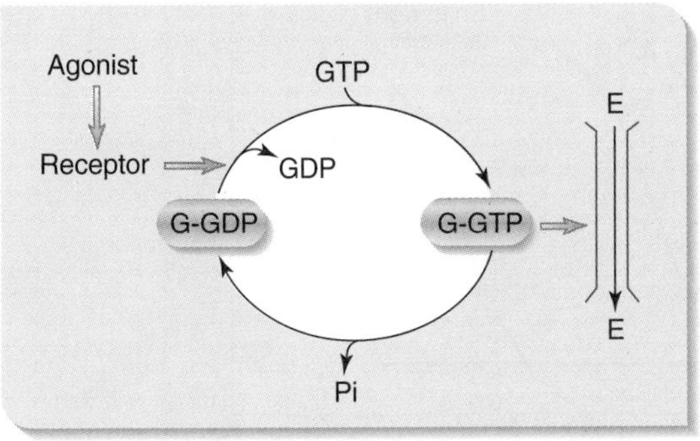

Figure 2-3 The guanine nucleotide–dependent activation-inactivation cycle of G proteins. The agonist activates the receptor, releasing GDP from the G protein and allowing GTP to bind to the G protein. The G protein, in its G-GTP state, regulates activity of an effector enzyme or ion channel *(E)*. The signal is terminated by the hydrolysis of GTP, yielding GDP bound to the G protein. *GDP,* Guanosine diphosphate; *GTP,* guanosine triphosphate; *Pi,* inorganic phosphate.

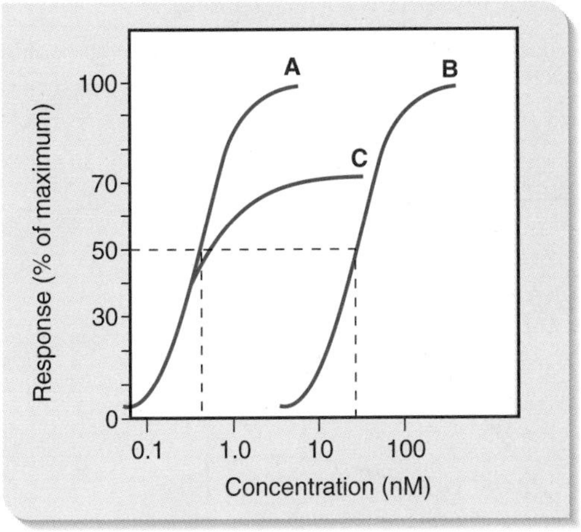

Figure 2-4 Dose-response curves of three agonists with differing potency and efficacy. Agonists A and B have the same efficacy but different potency; A is more potent than B. Agonists A and C have the same potency but different efficacy; A is more efficacious than C.

6. Antagonist
- Drug that interacts with a receptor but does not result in a biologic response (no intrinsic activity)

a. Competitive antagonist (Figure 2-5)
- Binds reversibly to the same receptor site as an agonist

(1) Effect can be overcome by increasing the dose of the agonist **(reversible effect).**

(2) A fixed dose of a competitive antagonist causes the **dose-response curve** of an agonist to make a parallel **shift to the right.**

(3) A partial agonist may act as a competitive inhibitor to a full agonist.

b. Noncompetitive antagonist (Figure 2-6)
- Binds irreversibly to the receptor site for the agonist.

(1) Its effects cannot be overcome completely by increasing the concentration of the agonist.

(2) A fixed dose of a noncompetitive antagonist causes a nonparallel, **downward shift** of the **dose-response curve** of the agonist **to the right.**

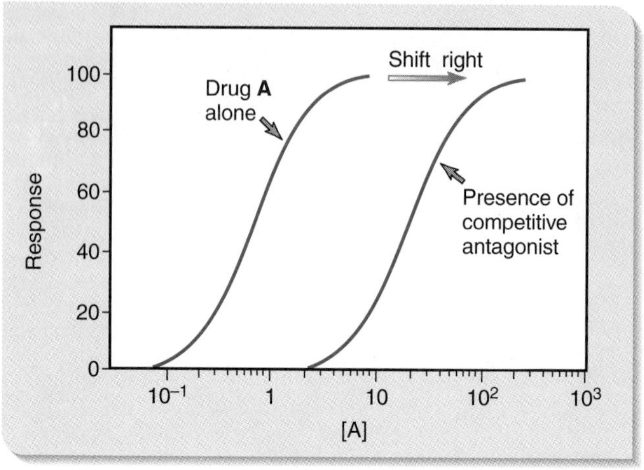

Figure 2-5 Competitive antagonism. The dose-response curve for drug A shifts to the right in the presence of a fixed dose of a competitive antagonist.

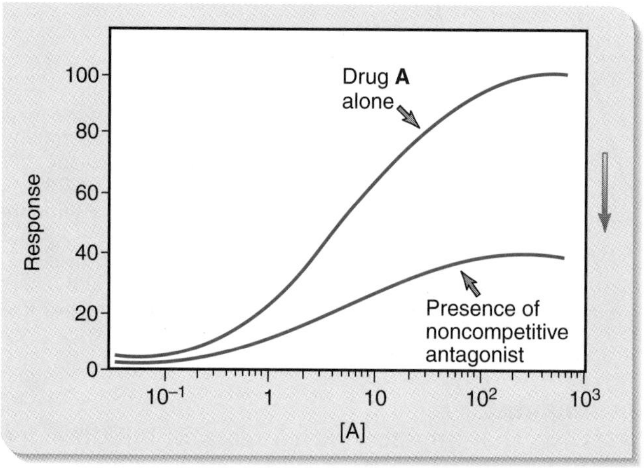

Figure 2-6 Noncompetitive antagonism. The dose-response curve for drug A shifts to the right and downward in the presence of a fixed dose of a noncompetitive antagonist.

IV. Pharmacodynamically Altered Responses

A. Decreased drug activity

1. Antagonism resulting from drug interactions

a. Physiologic (functional) antagonism

- This response occurs when two agonists with opposing physiologic effects are administered together.
- **Examples: histamine** (vasodilation), **norepinephrine** (vasoconstriction)

b. Competitive antagonism

- This response occurs when a receptor antagonist is administered with an agonist.

- **Examples**
  - **(1) Naloxone**, when blocking the effects of morphine
  - **(2) Atropine**, when blocking the effects of acetylcholine (ACh) at a muscarinic receptor

2. Tolerance: diminished response to the same dose of a drug over time

3. Mechanisms of tolerance

a. Desensitization

- Rapid process involving **continuous exposure** to a drug, altering the receptor so that it **cannot produce a response**
- Continuous exposure to β-adrenergic agonist (e.g., use of albuterol in asthma) results in **decreased responsiveness.**

b. Down-regulation: decrease in number of receptors caused by high doses of agonists over prolonged periods

Continuous use of β-adrenergic agonists involves both desensitization and down-regulation.

c. Tachyphylaxis: rapid development of tolerance

(1) Indirect-acting amines (e.g., tyramine, amphetamine) exert effects by releasing monoamines.

(2) Several doses given over a short time deplete the monoamine pool, reducing the response to successive doses.

B. Increased drug activity

1. Supersensitivity or hyperactivity

- Enhanced response to a drug may be due to an **increase in the number of receptors (up-regulation).**
- Antagonists cause up-regulation of receptors.

2. Potentiation

- Enhancement of the effect of one drug, which has no effect by itself, when combined with a second drug (e.g., 0 + 5 = 20, not 5)
- Produces a **shift** of the **dose-response curve to the left**

3. Synergism

- Production of a greater response than of two drugs that act individually (e.g., 2 + 5 = 15, not 7)

C. Dependence

Drugs that may lead to dependence: alcohol, barbiturates, narcotic analgesics

1. Physical dependence

- Repeated use produces an altered or adaptive physiologic state if the drug is not present.

2. Psychological dependence: compulsive drug-seeking behavior

- Individuals use a drug repeatedly for personal satisfaction.

3. Substance dependence (addiction)

- Individuals continue substance use despite significant substance-related problems.

SECTION II

Drugs That Affect the Autonomic Nervous System and the Neuromuscular Junction

3

Introduction to Autonomic and Neuromuscular Pharmacology

Target Topics

- Parasympathetic nervous system
- Sympathetic nervous system
- Neurochemistry of the autonomic nervous system
- Drugs that affect the cholinergic system
- Drugs that affect the adrenergic system
- Physiologic aspects of autonomic nerve activity

I. Divisions of the Efferent Autonomic Nervous System (ANS) (Figure 3-1)

A. Parasympathetic nervous system: craniosacral division of the ANS

1. **Origin:** midbrain, medulla oblongata, sacral cord
2. **Nerve fibers:** long preganglionic nerve fibers, short postganglionic nerve fibers

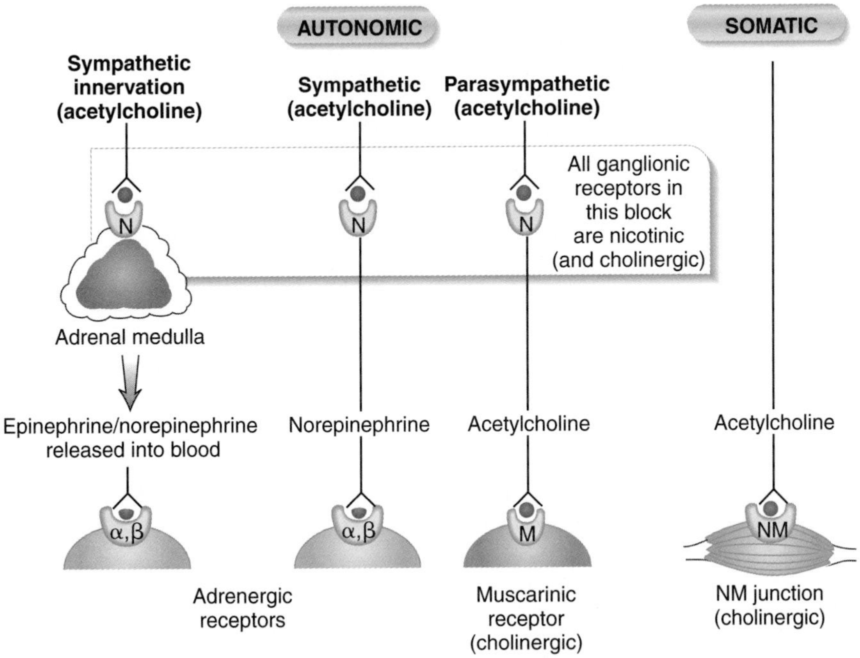

Figure 3-1 Schematic representation of sympathetic, parasympathetic, and somatic efferent neurons. *α*, α-Adrenoreceptor; *β*, β-adrenoreceptor; *M*, muscarinic receptor; *N*, nicotinic receptor; *NM*, neuromuscular.

3. **Neurotransmitter**
   - **Acetylcholine (ACh)** is the neurotransmitter both at the ganglia (stimulates **nicotinic** receptors) and at the neuroeffector junction (stimulates **muscarinic** receptors).
4. **Associated processes:** digestion, conservation of energy, maintenance of organ function

B. Sympathetic nervous system: thoracolumbar division of the ANS

1. **Origin:** thoracic and upper lumbar regions of spinal cord
2. **Nerve fibers**
   - **a.** Short preganglionic nerve fibers, which synapse in the paravertebral ganglionic chain
   - **b.** Long postganglionic nerve fibers
3. **Neurotransmitters**
   - **a. ACh** is the neurotransmitter at the ganglia (stimulates **nicotinic** receptors).
   - **b. Norepinephrine** is usually the neurotransmitter at the neuroeffector junction (stimulates **α** or **β** receptors).
     - ACh is a neurotransmitter found in most sweat glands and in some skeletal muscle vessels.
4. **Associated processes:** mobilizing the body's resources to respond to fear and anxiety ("fight-or-flight" response)

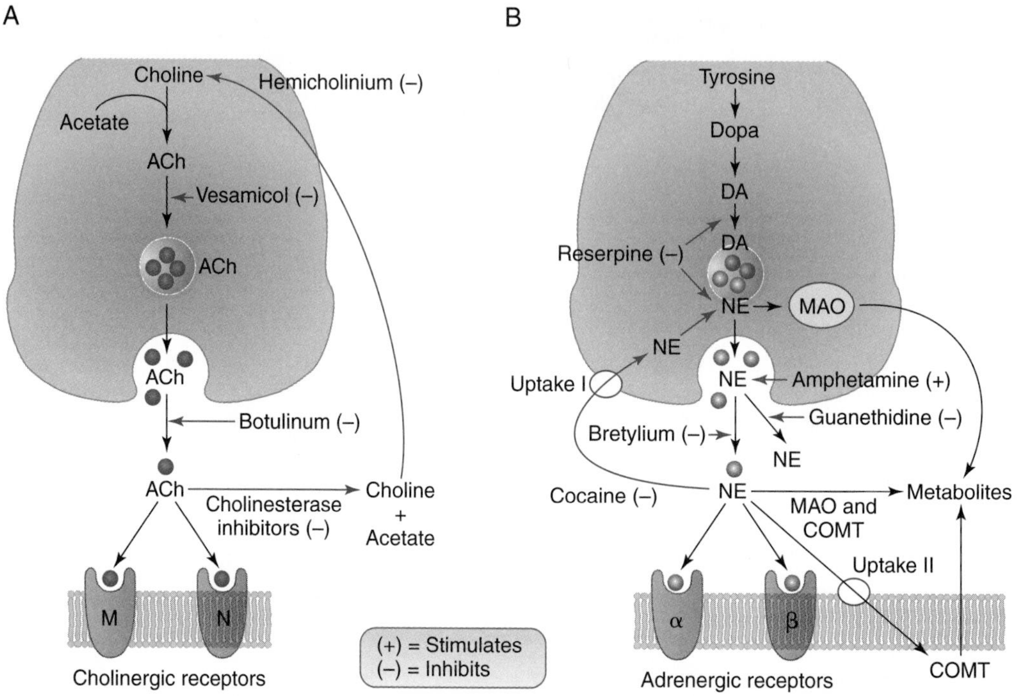

Figure 3-2 Cholinergic and adrenergic neurotransmission and sites of drug action. **A,** Illustration of the synthesis, storage, release, inactivation, and postsynaptic receptor activation of cholinergic neurotransmission. **B,** Illustration of the synthesis, storage, release, termination of action, and postsynaptic action of adrenergic neurotransmission. Uptake I is a transporter that transports NE into the presynaptic neuron. Uptake II is a transporter that transports NE into the postsynaptic neuron. *α,* α-Adrenoreceptor; *β,* β-adrenoreceptor; *ACh,* acetylcholine; *COMT,* catechol-*O*-methyltransferase; *DA,* dopamine; *M,* muscarinic receptor; *MAO,* monoamine oxidase; *N,* nicotinic receptor; *NE,* norepinephrine.

II. Neurochemistry of the Autonomic Nervous System

A. Cholinergic pathways

1. **Cholinergic fibers**
   a. **Synthesis, storage, and release** (Figure 3-2, *A*)
   b. **Receptor activation and signal transduction**
      - ACh activates nicotinic or muscarinic receptors (Table 3-1).
   c. **Inactivation**
      (1) Occurs by **acetylcholinesterase (AChE)** in the synapse
      (2) Occurs by **pseudocholinesterase** in the blood and liver
2. **Drugs that affect cholinergic pathways** (Table 3-2)
   a. **Botulinum toxin**
      (1) **Mechanism of action:** blocks release of ACh, inhibiting neurotransmitter transmission
      (2) **Uses**
         (a) Localized **spasms** of **ocular** and **facial muscles**
         (b) **Lower esophageal sphincter** spasm in **achalasia**

TABLE 3-1 Properties of Cholinergic Receptors

Type of Receptor	Principal Locations	Mechanism of Signal Transduction	Effects
Muscarinic			
M_1	Autonomic ganglia Presynaptic nerve terminals CNS neurons	Increased IP_3 and DAG Increased intracellular calcium	Modulation of neurotransmission
M_2	Cardiac tissue (sinoatrial and atrioventricular nodes) Nerves	Increased potassium efflux Inhibition of cAMP	Slowing of heart rate and conduction
M_3	Smooth muscles and glands	Increased IP_3 and DAG Increased intracellular calcium	Contraction of smooth muscles Stimulation of glandular secretions
	Endothelium	Increased nitric oxide formation	Nitric oxide vasodilation
	Vascular smooth muscle	Increased cGMP (from nitric oxide)	
Nicotinic			
N_M (muscle type)	Skeletal neuromuscular junctions	Increased sodium influx	Muscle contraction
N_N (neuron type)	Postganglionic cell body Dendrites	Increased sodium influx	Excitation of postganglionic neurons

cAMP, Cyclic adenosine monophosphate; *cGMP,* cyclic guanosine monophosphate; *CNS,* central nervous system; *DAG,* diacylglycerol; *IP_3,* inositol triphosphate.

TABLE 3-2 Drugs that Affect Autonomic Neurotransmission

Mechanism	Drugs that Affect Cholinergic Neurotransmission	Drugs that Affect Adrenergic Neurotransmission
Inhibit synthesis of neurotransmitter	Hemicholinium*	Metyrosine
Prevent vesicular storage of neurotransmitter	Vesamicol*	Reserpine
Inhibit release of neurotransmitter	Botulinum toxin	Bretylium Guanethidine
Stimulate release of neurotransmitter	Black widow spider venom*	Amphetamine Tyramine
Inhibit reuptake of neurotransmitter	—	Tricyclic antidepressants Cocaine
Inhibit metabolism of neurotransmitter	Cholinesterase inhibitors (physostigmine, neostigmine)	Monoamine oxidase inhibitors (tranylcypromine)
Activate postsynaptic receptors	Acetylcholine (M, N) Bethanechol (M) Pilocarpine (M)	Albuterol (β_2) Dobutamine (β_1) Epinephrine (α, β)
Block postsynaptic receptors	Atropine (muscarinic receptors) and tubocurarine (nicotinic receptors)	Phentolamine (α-adrenergic receptors) and propranolol (β-adrenergic receptors)

M, Muscarinic receptor; *N,* nicotinic receptor.
*Used experimentally but not therapeutically.

TABLE 3-3 Properties of Adrenergic Receptors

Type of Receptor	Mechanism of Signal Transduction	Effects
α_1	Increased IP_3 and DAG	Contraction of smooth muscles
α_2	Decreased cAMP	Inhibited norepinephrine release Decrease in aqueous humor secretion Decrease in insulin secretion Mediation of platelet aggregation and mediation of CNS effects
β_1	Increased cAMP	Increase in secretion of renin Increase in heart rate, contractility, and conduction
β_2	Increased cAMP	Glycogenolysis Relaxation of smooth muscles Uptake of potassium in smooth muscles
β_3	Increased cAMP	Lipolysis

cAMP, Cyclic adenosine monophosphate; *CNS,* central nervous system; *DAG,* diacylglycerol; *IP_3,* inositol triphosphate.

(c) **Spasticity** resulting from **central nervous system (CNS) disorders**

b. **Cholinesterase inhibitors**
  (1) **Mechanism of action:** prevent breakdown of ACh
  (2) **Examples:** indirect-acting cholinergic receptor agonists (e.g., neostigmine, physostigmine)

c. **Cholinergic receptor antagonists**
  (1) **Muscarinic receptor antagonists** such as **atropine**
  (2) **Nicotinic receptor antagonists** such as the ganglionic blocker **trimethaphan** and the neuromuscular blocker **tubocurarine**

B. Adrenergic pathways

1. Adrenergic fibers

a. **Synthesis, storage, and release** (Figure 3-2, *B*)

b. **Receptor activation and signal transduction**
  - Norepinephrine or epinephrine binds to α or β receptors on postsynaptic effector cells (Table 3-3).

c. **Termination of action: reuptake**
  - Reuptake by active transport (uptake I) is the primary mechanism for removal of norepinephrine from the synaptic cleft.
  (1) **Monoamine oxidase (MAO)** is an enzyme located in the mitochondria of presynaptic adrenergic neuron and liver.
  (2) **Catechol-*O*-methyltransferase (COMT)** is an enzyme located in the cytoplasm of autonomic effector cells and liver.

2. Drugs that affect adrenergic pathways (see Figure 3-2 and Table 3-2)

a. **Guanethidine**
  - Uptake involves active transport into the peripheral adrenergic neuron by the norepinephrine reuptake system (uptake I).

(1) **Mechanism of action**
  (a) Guanethidine eventually depletes the nerve endings of norepinephrine by replacing norepinephrine in the storage granules.
  (b) Its uptake is blocked by reuptake inhibitors (e.g., cocaine, tricyclic antidepressants).
(2) **Use:** hypertension (occasional)

b. Reserpine
(1) **Mechanism of action**
  (a) Depletes storage granules of catecholamines by binding to granules and preventing uptake and storage of norepinephrine
  (b) Acts centrally to produce **sedation, depression,** and **parkinsonian symptoms** (due to depletion of norepinephrine, serotonin, and dopamine)
(2) **Use:** mild hypertension (occasional)
(3) **Adverse effects:** pseudoparkinsonism

c. Adrenergic receptor antagonist
(1) May be nonselective or selective for either α or β receptors
(2) May be selective for a particular subtype of α or β receptor (see Chapter 5)

III. Physiologic Considerations

A. Dual innervation
- Most visceral organs are innervated by both the sympathetic and parasympathetic nervous systems.

B. Physiologic effects of autonomic nerve activity (Table 3-4)
- **α Responses:** usually **excitatory** (contraction of smooth muscle)
- **β_1 Responses:** located in the **heart** and are **excitatory**
- **β_2 Responses:** usually are **inhibitory** (relaxation of smooth muscle)

1. Adrenal medulla
  a. This modified sympathetic ganglion releases epinephrine and norepinephrine.
  b. These circulating hormones can affect **α and β responses** throughout the body.

2. Heart
  a. Sympathetic effects **increase** cardiac output.
    (1) Positive chronotropic effect (increased heart rate)
    (2) Positive inotropic effect (increased force of contraction)
    (3) Positive dromotropic effect (increased speed of conduction of excitation)
  b. Parasympathetic effects **decrease** heart rate and cardiac output.
    (1) Negative chronotropic effect (decreased heart rate)
    (2) Negative inotropic effect (decreased force of contraction)

TABLE 3-4 Direct Effects of Autonomic Nerve Activity on Body Systems

Organ/Tissue	Action	Receptor	Action	Receptor
Eye	***Sympathetic Response***		***Parasympathetic Response***	
Iris				
Radial muscle	Contracts (mydriasis)	α_1	—	—
Circular muscle	—	—	Contracts	M_3
Ciliary muscle	Relaxes for far vision	β_2	Contracts	M_3
Heart				
Sinoatrial node	Accelerates	$\beta_1 > \beta_2$	Decelerates	M_2
Ectopic pacemakers	Accelerates	$\beta_1 > \beta_2$	—	—
Contractility	Increases	$\beta_1 > \beta_2$	Decreases (atria)	M_2
Arterioles				
Coronary	Dilation	β_2	Dilation	M
	Constriction	$\alpha_1 > \alpha_2$	—	—
Skin and mucosa	Constriction	$\alpha_1 > \alpha_2$	Dilation	M
Skeletal muscle	Constriction	$\alpha_1 > \alpha_2$	Dilation	M*
	Dilation	β_2, M†	—	—
Splanchnic	Constriction	$\alpha_1 > \alpha_2$	Dilation	M*
Renal and mesenteric	Dilation	Dopamine, β_2	—	—
	Constriction	$\alpha_1 > \alpha_2$	—	—
Veins				
Systemic	Dilation	β_2	—	—
	Constriction	$\alpha_1 > \alpha_2$	—	—
Bronchiolar Muscle	Relaxes	β_2	Contracts	M
GI Tract				
Smooth muscle				
Walls	Relaxes	α_2, β_2	Contracts	M
Sphincters	Contracts	α_1	Relaxes	M
Secretion	Inhibits	α_2	Increases	M
Genitourinary Smooth Muscle				
Bladder wall	Relaxes	β_2	Contracts	M
Sphincter	Contracts	α_1	Relaxes	M
Uterus, pregnant	Relaxes	β_2	—	—
	Contracts	α_1	—	—
Penis, seminal vesicles	Ejaculation	α_2	Erection	M
Skin				
Pilomotor smooth muscle	Contracts	α_1	—	—
Sweat glands				
Thermoregulatory	Increases	M	—	—
Apocrine (stress)	Increases	α_1	—	—
Muscle Functions	Promotes K^+ Uptake	β_2	—	—
Liver	Gluconeogenesis	α, β_2	—	—
	Glycogenolysis	α_1, β_2	—	—
Fat cells	Lipolysis	β_3	—	—
Kidney	Renin release	β_1, α_1‡	—	—
	Sodium reabsorption	α_1	—	—

GI, gastrointestinal; *M,* muscarinic.

*The endothelium of most blood vessels releases endothelium-derived releasing factor, which causes vasodilation in response to muscarinic stimuli. However, these muscarinic receptors are not innervated and respond only to *circulating* muscarinic agonists.

†Vascular smooth muscle has sympathetic cholinergic dilator fibers.

‡α_1 inhibits; β_1 stimulates.

- Exogenous ACh only (no vagal innervation of the ventricular muscle)

(3) Negative dromotropic effect (decreased velocity of conduction of excitation)

3. Blood pressure

- The overall effects of autonomic drugs on blood pressure are complex and are determined by at least four parameters.

a. Direct effects on the heart

(1) **β_1 Stimulation** leads to an **increased heart rate,** and increased force means **increased blood pressure.**

(2) **Muscarinic stimulation** leads to a **decreased heart rate,** and decreased force means **decreased blood pressure.**

b. Vascular effects

(1) **Muscarinic** stimulation results in **dilation,** which decreases blood pressure.

(2) **α Stimulation** results in **constriction,** which increases blood pressure.

(3) **β_2 Stimulation** results in **dilation,** which decreases blood pressure.

c. Redistribution of blood

(1) With increased sympathetic activity, the blood is shunted away from organs and tissues such as the skin, gastrointestinal tract, and glands and toward the heart and voluntary (e.g., skeletal) muscles.

(2) This process occurs as a result of a **predominance of β_2 vasodilation** rather than α_1 constriction at these sites.

d. Reflex phenomena

(1) A **decrease in blood pressure,** sensed by baroreceptors in the carotid sinus and aortic arch, causes **reflex tachycardia.**

(2) An **increase in blood pressure** causes **reflex bradycardia.**

4 Cholinergic Drugs

Target Topics

- Muscarinic receptor agonists
- Cholinesterase inhibitors
- Ganglionic stimulants
- Muscarinic receptor antagonists
- Nicotinic receptor antagonists

I. Cholinoreceptor Agonists

A. Muscarinic receptor agonists (Box 4-1)

- Physiologic effects (Table 4-1)

1. Pharmacokinetics

a. Choline esters: quaternary ammonium compounds
- Do *not* readily cross the blood-brain barrier
- Inactivated by acetylcholinesterase (AChE) or pseudocholinesterase

b. Plant alkaloids
- **Pilocarpine**, a tertiary amine, can enter the central nervous system (CNS).

2. Mechanism of action: directly stimulate muscarinic receptors

3. Uses

a. Bethanechol, which selectively acts on smooth muscle of the gastrointestinal tract and the urinary bladder, is used in:

(1) **Urinary retention** in the absence of obstruction
(2) **Postoperative ileus**
(3) **Gastric atony and retention** after bilateral vagotomy

b. Pilocarpine

(1) **Glaucoma** (ophthalmic preparation)

BOX 4-1 Muscarinic and Nicotinic Receptor Agonists

Choline Esters
Acetylcholine (M, N)
Bethanechol (M)
Carbachol (M)

Plant Alkaloids
Muscarine (M)
Nicotine (N)
Pilocarpine (M)

M, Muscarinic; *N*, nicotinic.

TABLE 4-1 Effects of Muscarinic Receptor Agonists

Organ/Organ System	Effects
Cardiovascular	Hypotension from direct vasodilation Bradycardia at high doses Slowed conduction and prolonged refractory period of atrioventricular node
Gastrointestinal	Increased tone and increased contractile activity of gut Increased acid secretion Nausea, vomiting, cramps, and diarrhea
Genitourinary	Involuntary urination from increased bladder motility and relaxation of sphincter Penile erection
Eye	Miosis: contraction of sphincter muscle, resulting in reduced intraocular pressure Contraction of ciliary muscle; accommodated for near vision
Respiratory system	Bronchoconstriction
Glands	Increased secretory activity, resulting in increased salivation, lacrimation, and sweating

(2) **Xerostomia** (dry mouth): given orally to stimulate salivary gland secretion

4. **Adverse effects:** nausea, vomiting, diarrhea, salivation
   a. Due to overstimulation of parasympathetic effector organs
   b. **Treatment of overdose**
      (1) **Atropine** to counteract muscarinic effects
      (2) **Epinephrine** to overcome severe cardiovascular reactions or bronchoconstriction

Overstimulation of muscarinic receptors leads to DUMBELS: Defecation, Urination, Miosis, Bronchoconstriction, Emesis, Lacrimation, Salivation

B. **Cholinesterase inhibitors** (Box 4-2; see Figure 3-2, *A*)
   1. **Pharmacokinetics**
      a. **Edrophonium** is rapid and short-acting (i.e., effects last only about 10 minutes after injection).
      b. **Physostigmine** crosses the blood-brain barrier.
   2. **Mechanism of action**
      - **Bind to and inhibit AChE**, increasing the concentration of acetylcholine (ACh) in the synaptic cleft
      - **Stimulate responses at** the muscarinic receptors as well as at the neuromuscular junction

BOX 4-2 Cholinesterase Inhibitors

Reversible Inhibitors
Donepezil
Edrophonium
Neostigmine
Physostigmine
Pyridostigmine
Tacrine

Irreversible Inhibitors
Echothiophate
Isoflurophate
Malathion
Sarin

a. **Reversible inhibitors** (carbamates)
b. **Irreversible inhibitors** (organophosphates)
   - The phosphoryl group is not readily cleaved from the cholinesterase, but the enzyme can be reactivated by the early use of **pralidoxime.**

3. Uses
   a. **Alzheimer's disease:** donepezil, tacrine
   b. **Paralytic ileus and urine retention:** neostigmine
   c. **Glaucoma:** physostigmine, echothiophate
   d. **Myasthenia gravis:** edrophonium (short-acting; diagnosis only), pyridostigmine (treatment)

Drugs used in the management of myasthenia gravis: neostigmine, pyridostigmine, edrophonium

   e. **Insecticides and chemical warfare:** organophosphates used as insecticides and as components in nerve gases (sarin)
4. **Adverse effects:** nausea, vomiting, diarrhea, salivation, lacrimation, constricted pupils
   a. Due to overstimulation of parasympathetic effector organs
   b. **Treatment**
      (1) **Atropine** to counteract muscarinic effects
      (2) **Pralidoxime** to reactivate enzyme if toxicity due to an organophosphate
      (3) **Supportive therapy** (check and support vital signs)

C. **Ganglionic stimulants**
- Effects depend on the predominant autonomic tone at the organ system being assessed.

1. ACh
   - Much higher levels of ACh are required to stimulate nicotinic receptors in ganglia than muscarinic receptors at the neuroeffector junction.
2. **Nicotine**
   - Stimulates the ganglia at low doses and blocks the ganglia at higher doses by persistent depolarization of nicotinic receptors and secondary desensitization of receptors

BOX 4-3 Muscarinic Receptor Antagonists

Belladonna Alkaloids
Atropine
Hyoscyamine
Scopolamine

Synthetic Muscarinic Antagonists
Benztropine
Homatropine
Ipratropium
Oxybutynin
Trihexyphenidyl
Tropicamide

3. **Cholinesterase inhibitors**
   - Increase the concentration of ACh at the ganglia

II. Cholinoreceptor Antagonists

A. **Muscarinic receptor antagonists** (Box 4-3)
- Belladonna alkaloids
- Synthetic muscarinic antagonists
- Other classes of drugs with atropine-like effects, such as antihistamines, antipsychotics, antidepressants, and antiparkinsonian drugs

1. **Mechanism of action:** competitive inhibition of ACh at the muscarinic receptor
2. Uses
   a. **Chronic obstructive pulmonary disease (COPD)** (ipratropium)
   b. **Bradycardia** (atropine)
   c. **Motion sickness** (scopolamine)
   d. **Parkinson's disease** (benztropine, trihexyphenidyl)
   e. **Bladder or bowel spasms and incontinence** (oxybutynin)
   f. **Ophthalmic uses:** facilitation of ophthalmoscopic examinations when prolonged dilation is needed (tropicamide, homatropine)
   g. **"Colds" (over-the-counter remedies)**
      (1) Some symptomatic relief as the result of a drying effect
      (2) Useful as sleep aids
   h. **Parasympathomimetic toxicity: atropine**
      (1) Overdose of AChE inhibitors
      (2) Mushroom (*Amanita muscaria*) poisoning
3. Adverse effects
   a. Overdose
      (1) **Common signs:** dry mouth; dilated pupils; blurring of vision; hot, dry, flushed skin; tachycardia; fever; CNS changes
      (2) **Death** follows coma and respiratory depression.

Atropine toxicity: "mad as a hatter, dry as a bone, blind as a bat, red as a beet, hot as hell"

b. Treatment of overdose
  (1) Gastric lavage
  (2) Supportive therapy
  (3) Diazepam to control excitement and seizures
  (4) Effects of muscarinic receptor antagonists may be overcome by increasing levels of ACh in the synaptic cleft (usually by administration of AChE inhibitors such as physostigmine).

B. Nicotinic receptor antagonists

1. Ganglionic blockers
- Block nicotinic receptor at ganglion
- Primarily used in mechanistic studies

a. Hexamethonium: prototypic ganglionic blocking agent
b. Trimethaphan

2. Neuromuscular blockers

a. Mechanism of action: block nicotinic receptors at the neuromuscular junction (e.g., atracurium, d-tubocurarine) (see Chapter 6)
b. Use: relaxation of striated muscle
- Relaxation may be reversed by cholinesterase inhibitors.

5

Adrenergic Drugs

Target Topics

- Catecholamines
- α-Adrenergic agonists
- β-Adrenergic agonists
- Indirect-acting sympathomimetics
- α-Adrenoreceptor antagonists
- β-Adrenoreceptor antagonists

I. Adrenoreceptor Agonists

- Physiologic effects (Table 5-1)

A. Selected catecholamines (Box 5-1)

- Endogenous catecholamines (norepinephrine, epinephrine, and dopamine) are found in peripheral sympathetic nerve endings, the adrenal medulla, and the brain.
- Catecholamines affect blood pressure and heart rate (Figure 5-1).
- Monoamine oxidase (MAO) inhibitors, tricyclic antidepressants, and cocaine potentiate the effects of catecholamines.

1. Norepinephrine

- **Use: blood pressure elevation**, resulting from the ability of the drug to increase total peripheral resistance through arteriolar constriction

2. Epinephrine

a. Pharmacokinetics

(1) Usually injected **subcutaneously**

(2) Intracardiac or intravenous route used in cardiac arrest

b. Uses

(1) Treatment of **asthma**

(2) Treatment of **anaphylactic shock** or angioedema

Potency of α_1-adrenoreceptor agonists: epinephrine ≥ norepinephrine >> dopamine >>>>> isoproterenol

Potency of β_1-adrenoreceptor agonists: isoproterenol > epinephrine = norepinephrine = dopamine

TABLE 5-1 Pharmacologic Effects and Clinical Uses of Adrenoreceptor Agonists

Drug	Effect and Receptor Selectivity	Clinical Application
Direct-acting Adrenoreceptor Agonists		
Catecholamines		
Dobutamine	Cardiac stimulation (β_1) $\beta_1 > \beta_2$	Shock, heart failure
Dopamine	Renal vasodilation (D_1) Cardiac stimulation (β_1) Increased blood pressure (α_1) $D_1 = D_2 > \beta > \alpha$	Shock, heart failure
Epinephrine	Increased blood pressure (α_1) Cardiac stimulation (β_1) Bronchodilation (β_2) General agonist (α_1, α_2, β_1, β_2)	Anaphylaxis, open-angle glaucoma, asthma, hypotension, cardiac arrest, ventricular fibrillation, reduction in bleeding in surgery, prolongation of local anesthetic action
Isoproterenol	Cardiac stimulation (β_1) $\beta_1 = \beta_2$	Atrioventricular block, bradycardia
Norepinephrine	Increased blood pressure (α_1) α_1, α_2, β_1	Hypotension, shock
Noncatecholamines		
Albuterol	Bronchodilation (β_2) $\beta_2 > \beta_1$	Asthma
Clonidine	Decreased sympathetic outflow (α_2)	Chronic hypertension
Oxymetazoline	Vasoconstriction (α_1)	Decongestant
Phenylephrine	Vasoconstriction, increased blood pressure, and mydriasis (α_1) $\alpha_1 > \alpha_2$	Pupil dilation, decongestion, mydriasis, neurogenic shock, blood pressure maintenance during surgery
Ritodrine	Bronchodilation and uterine relaxation (β_2)	Asthma, premature labor
Terbutaline	Bronchodilation and uterine relaxation (β_2) $\beta_2 > \beta_1$	Asthma, premature labor
Indirect-acting Adrenoreceptor Agonists		
Amphetamine	Increased norepinephrine release General agonist (α_1, α_2, β_1, β_2)	Narcolepsy, obesity, attention deficit disorder
Cocaine	Inhibited norepinephrine release General agonist (α_1, α_2, β_1, β_2)	Local anesthesia
Mixed-acting Adrenoreceptor Agonists		
Ephedrine	Vasoconstriction (α_1) General agonist (α_1, α_2, β_1, β_2)	Decongestant, urine incontinence, hypotension
Phenylpropanolamine	Vasoconstriction (α_1)	Decongestant, no longer used because it may cause higher incidence of stroke
Pseudoephedrine	Vasoconstriction (α_1)	Decongestant

BOX 5-1 Adrenoreceptor Agonists

Direct-acting Agonists	
Catecholamines	
Dobutamine	β_1 (α_1)
Dopamine	D_1 (α_1 and β_1 at high doses)
Epinephrine	α_1, α_2, β_1, β_2
Isoproterenol	β_1, β_2
Norepinephrine	α_1, α_2, β_1
Noncatecholamines	
Albuterol	β_2
Clonidine	α_2
Methoxamine	α_1
Methyldopa	α_2
Oxymetazoline	α_1, α_2
Phenylephrine	α_1
Ritodrine	β_2
Salmeterol	β_2
Terbutaline	β_2
Indirect-acting Agonists	
Releasers	
Amphetamine	
Tyramine	
Monoamine Oxidase Inhibitors	
Phenelzine	
Selegiline	
Tranylcypromine	
Reuptake Inhibitors	
Cocaine	
Imipramine	
Mixed-acting Agonists	
Ephedrine	

(3) Prolongation of action of **local anesthetics**, due to the vasoconstrictive properties of epinephrine

(4) Treatment of **cardiac arrest**, bradycardia, and complete heart block in emergencies

3. **Dopamine**
   a. **Mechanism of action:** stimulates **specific dopamine receptors** on renal vasculature
      (1) High doses also stimulate α and β receptors.
      (2) Low doses stimulate renal dopamine receptors.
   b. **Use:** cardiogenic and noncardiogenic **shock** (dopamine increases blood flow through the kidneys)
   c. **Adverse effects**
      (1) Premature ventricular tachycardia, sinus tachycardia
      (2) Angina pectoris

Potency of β_2-adrenoreceptor agonists: isoproterenol > epinephrine >>>>> norepinephrine >> dopamine

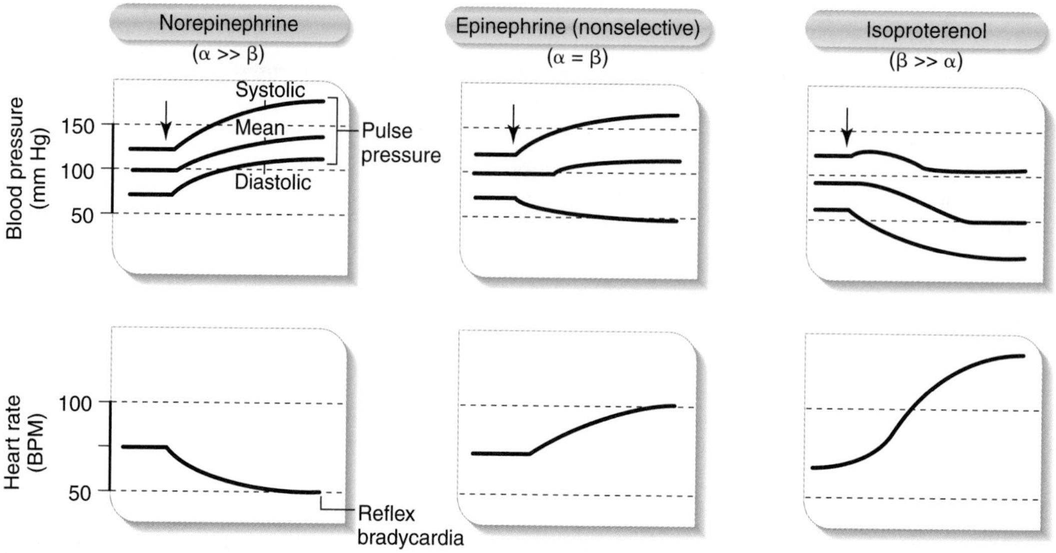

Figure 5-1 Graphic representations of the effects of catecholamines on blood pressure and heart rate. Note that the pulse pressure is greatly increased with epinephrine and isoproterenol. Norepinephrine causes reflex bradycardia.

B. α-Adrenergic receptor agonists (see Box 5-1)

1. α_1-Adrenergic receptor agonists

- **Examples: methoxamine, phenylephrine**

a. Mechanism of action: directly stimulate α_1-receptors

b. Uses (similar effects to those that occur after an injection of norepinephrine)

(1) **Blood pressure elevation**

(2) **Nasal decongestant**

(3) **Mydriasis induction**

2. α_2-Adrenergic receptor agonists

- **Examples: methyldopa, clonidine**
- Used to treat **hypertension** (see Chapter 13)

C. β-Adrenergic receptor agonists (see Box 5-1)

1. β_1-Adrenergic receptor agonists

a. Example: dobutamine

b. Use: selective inotropic agent in the management of advanced cardiovascular failure associated with low cardiac output

2. β_2-Adrenergic receptor agonists

a. Examples: terbutaline, albuterol, salmeterol

b. Uses

(1) **Asthma** and **chronic obstructive pulmonary disease (COPD)** (albuterol, salmeterol)

(2) **Hyperkalemia**

(3) **Delay of premature labor** (terbutaline)

c. Adverse effects

(1) Fine skeletal muscle tremor (most common)

(2) Minimal cardiac adverse effects (palpitations)

(3) Nervousness

D. Indirect stimulants (see Box 5-1)

1. Tyramine

- Releases norepinephrine from storage granules, thus producing both alpha and beta stimulation

a. Leads to **tachyphylaxis,** because of depletion of norepinephrine stores after repeated use

b. Results in **hypertensive crisis** in patients who are taking MAO inhibitors when tyramine is ingested (foods, wine)

Hypertensive crisis: MAO inhibitors and tyramine-rich foods ("cheese effect")

2. Amphetamine

- Indirect-acting amine that releases norepinephrine and epinephrine

a. Uses

(1) Central nervous system (CNS) stimulant: stimulates mood and alertness

(2) Appetite suppression

(3) Attention-deficit hyperactivity/attention deficit disorder in children (**methylphenidate** is preferable)

b. Adverse effects (due to sympathomimetic effects)

(1) Nervousness, insomnia, anorexia

(2) Growth inhibition (children)

3. Monoamine oxidase (MAO) inhibitors

a. Examples: phenelzine, tranylcypromine, selegiline

b. Use: occasional treatment of **depression** and **Parkinson's disease** (see Chapters 10 and 11)

4. Norepinephrine reuptake (uptake I) inhibitors

a. Examples: cocaine, imipramine

b. Potentiate effects of norepinephrine, epinephrine, and dopamine, but not isoproterenol (not taken up by uptake I; see Figure 3-2, *B*)

E. Direct and indirect stimulants (see Box 5-1)

1. Example: ephedrine

2. Mechanism of action

a. Releases norepinephrine (like tyramine)

b. Also has a direct effect on α-adrenergic receptors

3. Uses: mild asthma, nasal decongestion

II. Adrenoreceptor Antagonists

A. α-Adrenergic receptor antagonists

- **Mechanism of action:** block α-mediated effects of sympathomimetic drugs or sympathetic nerve stimulation

1. Nonselective α-adrenergic receptor antagonists (Box 5-2)

a. Phentolamine

(1) Pharmacokinetics: reversible, short-acting

(2) Uses

(a) Diagnosis and treatment of **pheochromocytoma**

(b) Reversal of effects resulting from accidental subcutaneous injection of epinephrine

b. Phenoxybenzamine

(1) Pharmacokinetics: irreversible, long-acting

(2) Use: preoperative management of **pheochromocytoma**

BOX 5-2 Adrenoreceptor Antagonists

Nonselective α-Receptor Antagonists
Phenoxybenzamine
Phentolamine

α_1-Receptor Antagonists
Doxazosin
Prazosin
Terazosin

α_2-Receptor Antagonists
Yohimbine

Nonselective β-Receptor Antagonists
Propranolol
Timolol

β_1-Receptor Antagonists
Atenolol
Esmolol
Metoprolol

Nonselective α- and β-Receptor Antagonists
Carvedilol
Labetalol

β-Receptor Antagonists with Intrinsic Sympathomimetic Activity (ISA)
Acebutolol
Pindolol

2. **Selective α_1-adrenergic receptor antagonists** (see Box 5-2)
   - **Examples: doxazosin, prazosin, terazosin**
   a. **Mechanism of action:** block α_1 receptors selectively on arterioles and venules, producing less reflex tachycardia than nonselective α-receptor antagonists
   b. **Uses**
      (1) **Hypertension**
      (2) **Benign prostatic hyperplasia (BPH)** (tamsulosin)
   c. **Adverse effects**
      (1) Orthostatic hypotension
      (2) Impaired ejaculation

Tamsulosin, which relaxes the bladder neck and the prostate, is used to treat BPH.

3. **Selective α_2-adrenergic receptor antagonist: yohimbine**
   - No clinical use (ingredient in herbal preparations)
   - May inhibit the hypotensive effect of clonidine or methyldopa

B. **β-Adrenergic receptor antagonists** (β-blockers)
   1. **Pharmacologic properties**
      a. **Mechanism of action**
         (1) Block β-receptor sympathomimetic effects
         (2) Exert cardiovascular effects: decreased cardiac output and renin secretion

(a) Decreased vasoconstriction
(b) Decreased salt and water retention
(c) Decreased heart and vascular remodeling

b. Uses
(1) **Cardiac problems: arrhythmias, "classical" angina** (angina of effort), **hypertension, moderate heart failure**
(2) **Thyrotoxicosis**
(3) **Performance anxiety**
(4) **Essential tremor**
(5) **Migraine** (prevention)

c. Adverse effects
(1) Bradycardia, heart block
(2) Bronchiolar constriction
(3) Increased triglycerides, decreased high-density lipoprotein (HDL) levels
(4) Mask symptoms of hypoglycemia (in diabetics)
(5) Depression

d. Precautions
(1) Abrupt withdrawal of β-adrenoreceptor antagonists can produce nervousness, increased heart rate, and increased blood pressure.
(2) These drugs should be used with caution in patients with **asthma, heart block, COPD,** and **diabetes.**

Use β-blockers with caution in the following conditions: heart block, asthma, COPD, diabetes

2. Nonselective β-adrenergic receptor antagonists (see Box 5-2)

a. Propranolol: β_1- and β_2-receptor antagonist
(1) **Mechanism of action**
(a) Decreases heart rate and contractility
(b) Decreases cardiac output, thus reducing blood pressure
(c) Decreases renin release
(2) **Use: pheochromocytoma**

b. Timolol
(1) **Mechanism of action:** lowers intraocular pressure, presumably by reducing production of aqueous humor
(2) **Use:** wide-angle **glaucoma** (topical preparation)

Contraindication to use of nonselective β-adrenergic receptor antagonists: asthma

3. Selective β_1-adrenergic receptor antagonists (see Box 5-2)

a. Metoprolol and atenolol: cardioselective β_1-adrenergic blockers
(1) Uses
(a) **Hypertension, angina, acute myocardial infarction (MI), heart failure, tachycardia**
(b) **MI (prevention)**
(2) These β_1-adrenergic blockers may be safer than propranolol for patients who experience bronchoconstriction because they produce less blockade of β_2-receptors.

Use selective β_1-adrenergic receptor antagonists with caution in the following conditions: asthma, COPD

b. Esmolol
(1) **Pharmacokinetics**
(a) Short half-life
(b) Given by intravenous infusion

(2) **Uses: hypertensive crisis, acute supraventricular tachycardia**

4. **Nonselective β- and α_1-adrenergic receptor antagonists** (see Box 5-2)
   a. **Labetalol**
      (1) **Mechanism of action:** α and β blockade (β blockade is predominant)
         - Reduces blood pressure without a substantial decrease in resting heart rate, cardiac output, or stroke volume

      (2) Uses
         (a) **Hypertension** and hypertensive emergencies
         (b) **Pheochromocytoma**

   b. Carvedilol
      (1) **Mechanism of action:** α and β blockade
      (2) **Uses: heart failure**

5. **β-Adrenoreceptor antagonists with intrinsic sympathomimetic activity (ISA)** (see Box 5-2)
   a. **Examples: acebutolol, pindolol**
      - These agents have partial agonist activity.

   b. Uses
      (1) Preferred in patients with **moderate heart block**
      (2) May be an advantage in the treatment of **patients with asthma**

6 Muscle Relaxants

Target Topics

- Spasmolytics
- Nondepolarizing neuromuscular blockers
- Depolarizing neuromuscular blockers

I. **Spasmolytics**
- Certain chronic diseases (e.g., cerebral palsy, multiple sclerosis) are associated with abnormally high reflex activity in neuronal pathways controlling skeletal muscles, resulting in painful spasms or spasticity.

A. Goals of spasmolytic therapy
1. Reduction of excessive muscle tone without reduction in strength
2. Reduction in spasm, which reduces pain and improves mobility

B. γ-Aminobutyric acid (GABA)–mimetics (Box 6-1)
1. Baclofen ($GABA_B$ agonist)
a. Mechanism of action: interferes with release of excitatory transmitters in the brain and spinal cord
b. Uses: spasticity in patients with **central nervous system (CNS) disorders**, such as multiple sclerosis, spinal cord injuries, and stroke
c. Adverse effects: sedation, hypotension, muscle weakness
2. Diazepam
a. Benzodiazepine, which acts on the $GABA_A$ receptor
b. Facilitates **GABA-mediated presynaptic inhibition** in the brain and spinal cord (see Chapter 7)
3. Tizanidine
a. Mechanism of action
(1) Stimulates presynaptic α_2 receptors

BOX 6-1 Spasmolytics

GABA-Mimetics
Baclofen
Diazepam

Other Relaxants
Botulinum toxin
Cyclobenzaprine
Dantrolene
Tizanidine

(2) Inhibits spinal interneuron firing
b. Use: spasticity associated with conditions such as cerebral palsy and spinal cord injury
c. Adverse effects: sedation, hypotension, muscle weakness (less than with baclofen)

C. Other relaxants (see Box 6-1)

1. Cyclobenzaprine
a. Relieves local skeletal muscle spasm through central-acting muscle relaxants
b. Ineffective in spasticity caused by CNS disorders

2. Dantrolene
a. Mechanism of action: decreases the release of intracellular calcium from the sarcoplasmic reticulum, "uncoupling" the excitation-contraction process
b. Uses
(1) **Spasticity** from CNS disorders such as cerebral palsy or spinal cord injury
(2) **Malignant hyperthermia** after halothane exposure
(3) **Neuroleptic malignant syndrome**
c. Adverse effects: hepatotoxicity, significant muscle weakness

II. Nicotinic Receptor Antagonists

- Nicotinic receptor antagonists include ganglionic blockers (see Chapter 4) and neuromuscular blockers (Box 6-2).
- Neuromuscular blockers may be classified as either depolarizing or nondepolarizing (Table 6-1).

A. Nondepolarizing neuromuscular blockers
- Also known as curariform drugs, of which **tubocurarine** is the prototype

1. Mechanism of action
- These drugs compete with acetylcholine (ACh) at nicotinic receptors at the neuromuscular junction, producing muscle relaxation and paralysis.

2. Uses
a. Induction of **muscle relaxation** during surgery
b. Facilitation of **intubation**
c. Adjunct to electroconvulsive therapy for prevention of injury

BOX 6-2 Neuromuscular Blockers

Nondepolarizing Drugs
Atracurium
Mivacurium
Pancuronium
Rocuronium
Tubocurarine
Vecuronium

Depolarizing Drugs
Succinylcholine

TABLE 6-1 Comparison of Nondepolarizing and Depolarizing Neuromuscular Blockers

Effect	Competitive	Depolarizing
Action at receptor	Antagonist	Agonist
Effect on motor end plate depolarization	None	Partial persistent depolarization
Initial effect on striated muscle	None	Fasciculation
Muscles affected first	Small muscles	Skeletal muscle
Muscles affected last	Respiratory	Respiratory
Effect of AChE inhibitors	Reversal	No effect or increased duration
Effect of ACh agonists	Reversal	No effect
Effect on previously administered D-tubocurarine	Additive	Antagonism
Effect on previously administered succinylcholine	No effect of antagonism	Tachyphylaxis or no effect
Effect of halothane	Increase potency	Decrease potency
Effect of antibiotics	Increase potency	Decrease potency
Effect of calcium channel blockers	Increase potency	Increase potency

ACh, Acetylcholine; *AChE,* acetylcholinesterase.

3. **Drug interactions**
   a. **Muscle relaxation is reversed** by acetylcholinesterase (AChE) inhibitors such as neostigmine.
   b. Use with **inhaled anesthetics** (isoflurane) or **aminoglycoside antibiotics** (gentamicin) **may potentiate or prolong blockade.**

Nondepolarizing neuromuscular blockers are reversed by AChE inhibitors.

B. **Depolarizing neuromuscular blockers** (succinylcholine)
   1. **Mechanism of action**
      a. These drugs **bind to nicotinic receptors** in skeletal muscle, causing persistent depolarization of the neuromuscular junction.
      b. This action initially produces an agonist-like stimulation of skeletal muscles (fasciculations) followed by sustained muscle paralysis.

Depolarizing neuromuscular blockers may be potentiated by AChE inhibitors.

Succinylcholine may cause malignant hyperthermia.

c. The response changes over time.

(1) Phase I: continuous depolarization at end plate

- Cholinesterase inhibitors prolong paralysis.

(2) Phase II: resistance to depolarization

- Cholinesterase inhibitors may reverse paralysis.

2. Use: production of **muscle relaxation** during surgery or electroconvulsive therapy

3. Adverse effects: hyperkalemia, muscle pain, malignant hyperthermia

4. Precaution

- Blockade may be prolonged if the patient has a genetic variant of plasma cholinesterase that metabolizes the drug very slowly.

SECTION III

Drugs That Affect the Central Nervous System

7

Sedative-Hypnotic and Anxiolytic Drugs

Target Topics

- Sedative-hypnotics
- Benzodiazepines
- Barbiturates
- Other sedative-hypnotics
- Alcohols

I. Basic Properties

- Sedative-hypnotics and anxiolytics are used to **reduce anxiety** or to **induce sleep** (Box 7-1).
- These agents, especially the barbiturates, produce central nervous system (CNS) depression at the level of the brain, spinal cord, and brain stem.
- These agents cause tolerance and physical dependence (**withdrawal**) if used for long periods.
- **Barbiturates** and other **older sedative-hypnotics cause complete CNS depression**, whereas benzodiazepines do not (Figure 7-1).

A. Pharmacokinetics

1. **Metabolism** primarily occurs by the microsomal system in the **liver.**
2. **Duration of action** is **variable.**
    - The half-life ($t_{1/2}$) of these drugs ranges from minutes to days.

BOX 7-1 Sedative-Hypnotics and Anxiolytics

Benzodiazepines
Alprazolam
Chlordiazepoxide
Clonazepam
Diazepam
Lorazepam
Midazolam
Oxazepam
Temazepam
Triazolam

Barbiturates
Pentobarbital
Phenobarbital
Secobarbital
Thiopental

Other Sedative-Hypnotics
Chloral hydrate
Diphenhydramine
Melatonin
Paraldehyde
Zolpidem

Nonsedating Anxiolytic
Buspirone

Benzodiazepine Antagonist
Flumazenil

- Many benzodiazepine metabolites are active, thus increasing the duration of action of the parent drug.

B. Mechanism of action
- Sedative-hypnotics facilitate chloride flux through the γ-aminobutyric acid (GABA) receptor chloride channel, which hyperpolarizes the neuron (Figure 7-2).

C. Uses: sedation, hypnosis, or anesthesia, depending on dose
1. **Sleep** induction (hypnosis)
2. **Anxiety** relief (anxiolytic)
3. **Sedation**
4. **Preanesthesia**
5. **Anticonvulsant** properties
   - **Phenobarbital** and **diazepam** are used clinically.
6. Central-acting **muscle relaxants**

D. Adverse effects
- **Chronic use may lead to toxicity.**

1. **General effects**
   a. Drowsiness
   b. Impaired performance and judgment
   c. "Hangover"
   d. Risk of drug abuse and addiction
   e. **Withdrawal syndrome** (most frequently seen with short-acting sedative-hypnotics that are used for long periods)
2. **Overdose** results in **severe CNS depression**, which may manifest as coma, hypotension, and respiratory cessation, especially when agents are given in combination.
3. **Treatment of overdose**
   a. **Observe continuously**
   b. **Prevent absorption of ingested drug** (charcoal, lavage)
   c. **Support respiration**
   d. Prevent or treat hypotension or shock
   e. Maintain renal function
   f. Increase rate of drug excretion

Sedative-hypnotic drugs should NOT be used in combination with alcohol.

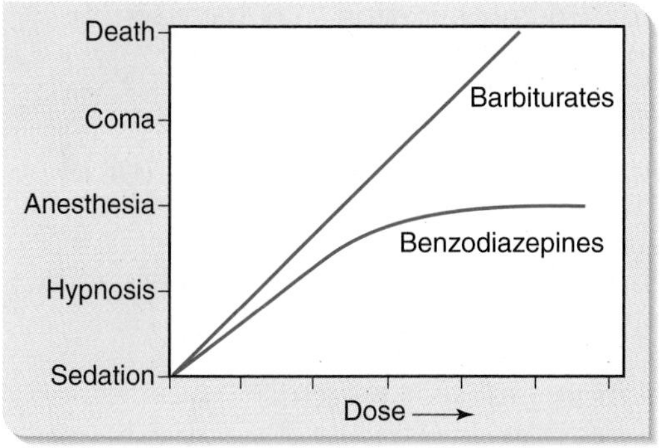

Figure 7-1 Dose-response curves for barbiturates and for benzodiazepines. Barbiturates produce complete central nervous system depression leading to anesthesia, coma, and death, even when given orally. Benzodiazepines may cause anesthesia and respiratory depression with intravenous, but not oral, administration.

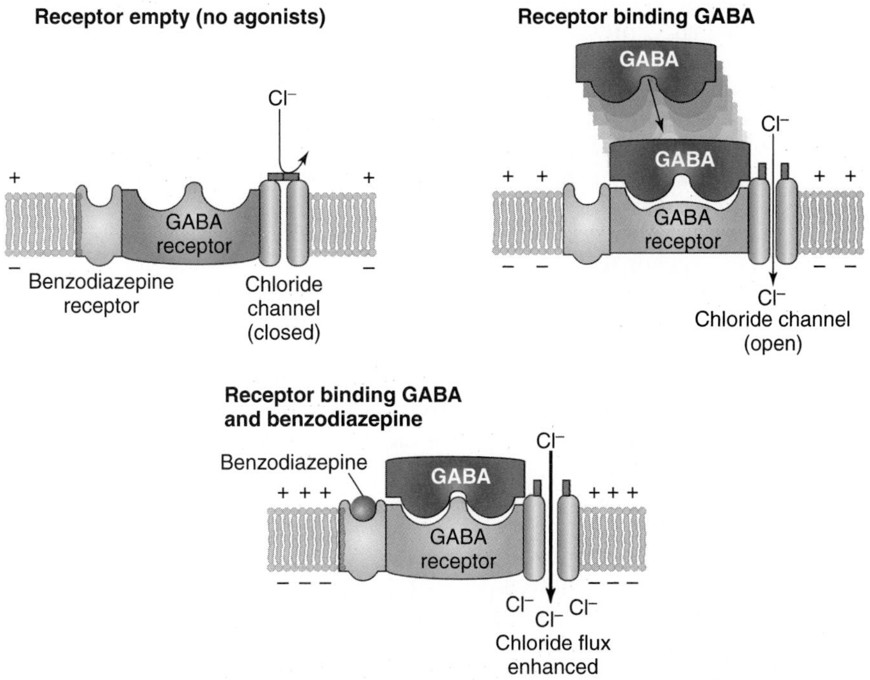

Figure 7-2 Benzodiazepine-GABA-chloride ionophore complex. Benzodiazepines increase the frequency of channel opening. Barbiturates increase the length of time that the channels remain open.

(1) Alkaline diuresis
- Useful for some barbiturates, such as phenobarbital

(2) Peritoneal dialysis
(3) Hemodialysis

E. Precautions

1. **Porphyria** or a family history of porphyria may be a problem.
   - **Barbiturates may increase porphyrin synthesis.**
2. **Hepatic or renal insufficiency** requires a reduced dose.

3. Additive effect of drugs in combination may have serious consequences.

II. Benzodiazepines (see Box 7-1)
- These **anxiolytic drugs** are associated with a reduced risk of respiratory depression and coma, which gives them a major advantage over the barbiturates (see Figure 7-1).
- The incidence of dependence is probably lower with benzodiazepines than with barbiturates.

A. Pharmacokinetics
1. Enterohepatic circulation with many agents
2. **Variable duration of action**
   - Most agents accumulate with multiple dosing due to long plasma half-lives.

   a. **Short-acting agents:** triazolam
   b. **Intermediate-acting agents:** lorazepam, oxazepam, temazepam, alprazolam
   c. **Long-acting agents:** chlordiazepoxide, clonazepam, diazepam

B. Mechanism of action (see Figure 7-1)
1. Benzodiazepines **bind to specific receptors on the $GABA_A$ receptor–ionophore complex.**
   - Alcohols, as well as barbiturates, interact at these receptors.
2. Benzodiazepines potentiate the activity of GABA on chloride ion influx by increasing the frequency of the openings of the chloride channels.

C. Uses
- **All of the general uses listed in section I C,** plus the following indications:

1. **Alcohol withdrawal**
2. **Status epilepticus**

D. Adverse effects
1. **Ataxia, retrograde amnesia**
2. Moderate addictive potential
   a. **Physical dependence** when used in high doses for several months
   b. **Withdrawal symptoms:** anxiety, agitation, depression, "rebound" insomnia

It is possible to reduce rebound effects by slowly reducing the dose of longer-acting benzodiazepines.

E. Benzodiazepine antagonist
- **Flumazenil,** a benzodiazepine antagonist, reverses toxicity.

III. Barbiturates

A. Pharmacokinetics
1. **Elimination** occurs by metabolism in the liver and excretion of the parent compound or its metabolites in the urine.
   a. **Phenobarbital** is a weak organic acid, whose excretion is enhanced by alkalinization of urine.
   b. The effects of **thiopental** are terminated by redistribution.
2. **Duration of action**

a. **Ultrashort-acting:** thiopental
b. **Intermediate-acting:** pentobarbital, secobarbital
c. **Long-acting:** phenobarbital

B. Mechanism of action

1. Barbiturates **facilitate the actions of GABA.**
   - Unlike benzodiazepines, these agents increase the **length of time** that the GABA-gated chloride channel remains open.
2. The multiplicity of barbiturate binding sites is the basis of the ability **to induce full surgical anesthesia** (see Figure 7-1).

C. Effects

1. **Low doses:** depression of sensory function, sedation without analgesia, drowsiness
2. **High doses:** depression of motor function, depression of medullary centers of brain (circulatory and respiratory depression), marked sedation, sleep, anesthesia

Adverse effects of barbiturates: ataxia, retrograde amnesia, impaired performance, dependence, withdrawal symptoms

IV. Other Sedative-Hypnotics

- Some of these agents are structurally related to the barbiturates and have similar properties.

A. Zolpidem: nonbenzodiazepine sedative-hypnotic for the short-term treatment of **insomnia**

B. Diphenhydramine: antihistamine found in over-the-counter (OTC) "sleep aids"

C. Buspirone

1. **Mechanism of action:** agonist at 5-HT_{1A} serotonin receptors in the brain
2. **Uses**
   a. **Antianxiety** (several days of use required for the drug to become effective)
   b. No hypnotic, anticonvulsant, or muscle relaxant properties
3. **Adverse effects**
   a. **Some sedation** but less than most benzodiazepines
   b. No evidence of tolerance, rebound anxiety on withdrawal of drug, cross-tolerance to benzodiazepines, drug abuse, or additive effects

D. Chloral hydrate

- Structurally related to alcohol, with trichloroethanol as active metabolite
- Paraldehyde is a short-acting congener.

1. **Use**
   a. **Very rapid-acting hypnotic**, which is often **used in children**
   b. Low incidence of abuse
2. **Adverse effect:** bad taste and smell

V. Alcohols

A. Ethanol

1. **Pharmacokinetics**

a. **Rapid, complete absorption**
   - Conversion to acetate by two enzymes: **alcohol dehydrogenase** and **acetaldehyde dehydrogenase**

b. **Zero-order kinetics**

2. **Mechanism of action:** potentiates actions at the GABA receptor
   a. **CNS depressant** with synergistic effects with many other CNS depressants
   b. **Cross-tolerant** with other sedative-hypnotic drugs
3. **Adverse effects**
   a. **Liver:** hepatic failure and cirrhosis
   b. **Gastrointestinal:** nutritional deficiencies (malabsorption) and bleeding
   c. **Nervous system**
      (1) **Peripheral neuropathy ("stocking glove" pattern)**
      (2) **Wernicke-Korsakoff syndrome: thiamine deficiency; ataxia, confusion, ophthalmoplegia**
   d. **Endocrine:** gynecomastia, testicular atrophy
   e. **Fetal alcohol syndrome:** teratogenic effects when used during pregnancy
      - Mental retardation, growth deficiency, microcephaly, wide-spaced eyes
   f. **Alcoholism**
      (1) **Withdrawal syndrome**
         (a) Insomnia
         (b) Tremor, anxiety, seizures, hallucinations **(delirium tremens)**
         (c) Diarrhea, nausea
      (2) **Management:** benzodiazepines (only in abstinent patients), antihypertensives
4. **Drug interactions:** drugs that **inhibit acetaldehyde dehydrogenase**
   a. **Disulfiram,** which is used in the treatment of alcoholism
   b. Metronidazole (has disulfiram-like effect)
   c. Oral hypoglycemic agents (chlorpropamide)

Disulfiram use leads to nausea, hypotension, headache, and flushing when patients drink alcohol; thus, it is used to help patients stop drinking.

B. Other alcohols
1. **Methanol**
   a. Conversion to **formic acid** can lead to **blindness** and **severe anion gap metabolic acidosis.**
   b. Intoxicated patients are treated with ethanol.
      - Ethanol competes with methanol for the dehydrogenase enzymes.
2. **Ethylene glycol**
   - **Antifreeze**
   - **Adverse effects:** severe **anion gap metabolic acidosis, hypocalcemia, renal damage**

8 Anesthetics

Target Topics

- Inhalation anesthetics
- Parenteral anesthetics
- Preanesthetic medications
- Local anesthetics

I. General Anesthetics

A. Goals of balanced anesthesia

1. **Analgesia:** elimination of perception and reaction to pain
2. **Amnesia:** loss of memory, which is not essential but desirable during most surgical procedures
3. **Loss of consciousness:** essential for many surgical procedures (e.g., cardiac, orthopedic)
4. **Muscle relaxation**
   a. Occurs in varying degrees
   b. Usually has to be further supplied by neuromuscular relaxants
5. **Suppression of autonomic and sensory reflexes:** requires use of additional medications to suppress the enhanced autonomic and sensory reactions that occur during surgical procedures

B. Inhalation anesthetics (Box 8-1; Table 8-1)

1. **General considerations**
   a. **Depth of anesthesia** directly relates to the partial pressure of the anesthetic in the brain.
   b. **Anesthetic potency** is expressed as the **minimum alveolar concentration (MAC).**
      - MAC is the concentration in inspired air at which 50% of patients have no response to a skin incision.
      - The higher the lipid solubility, the greater the potency.
   c. **Speed of induction** is influenced by several factors.

BOX 8-1 General Anesthetics

Inhalation Anesthetics	*Parenteral Anesthetics*
Desflurane	Alfentanil
Enflurane	Fentanyl
Halothane	Ketamine
Isoflurane	Lorazepam
Nitrous oxide	Midazolam
Sevoflurane	Propofol
	Sufentanil
	Thiopental

(1) **Higher inspired concentration** = more rapid induction
(2) **Lower solubility in blood** = more rapid induction
(3) **Higher ventilation rate** = more rapid induction
(4) **Lower pulmonary blood flow** = more rapid induction

The use of halothane may lead to hepatotoxicity and malignant hyperthermia.

2. Nitrous oxide (N_2O)
- Gaseous anesthetic

a. Characteristics
(1) Cannot produce surgical anesthesia by itself
- To produce unconsciousness, **N_2O must be used with other anesthetics.**

(2) Significantly reduces the MAC for halogenated anesthetics when used as an adjunct to anesthesia

b. Pharmacokinetics: extremely fast absorption and elimination, resulting in rapid induction and recovery from anesthesia

N_2O has excellent analgesic properties.

c. Uses: has good analgesic properties
- Analgesia in obstetrics and procedures that do not require unconsciousness, such as dental procedures

d. Contraindications: head injury, preexisting increased intracranial pressure, tumor
- N_2O can raise intracranial pressure.

3. Volatile halogenated hydrocarbons (see Box 8-1; see Table 8-1)
- These agents are of variable potency (MAC) and blood solubility; they may sensitize the heart to the arrhythmogenic effects of catecholamines.

C. Parenteral anesthetics (see Box 8-1)
- These anesthetics are useful for **procedures of short duration, induction of inhalation anesthesia** (wide use), and **supplementation of weak inhalation agents** such as N_2O.

1. Ultrashort-acting barbiturates (thiopental): poor analgesia

a. Pharmacokinetics
(1) Extremely rapid onset and action due to **high lipid solubility**
(2) **Brief duration of action** due to redistribution from brain to other tissues

TABLE 8-1 Properties of Inhalation Anesthetics

Agent	MAC (% vol/vol)	Blood:Gas Partition Coefficient	Rate of Induction and Emergence	Amount Metabolized	Skeletal Muscle Relaxation	Effect on Cardiovascular System	Effect on Liver and Kidney
Nonhalogenated (gaseous)							
Nitrous oxide	>100	0.47	Rapid	None	None	↓ Heart rate No arrhythmias	None
Halogenated (volatile)							
Desflurane	6.0	0.42	Rapid	< 2%	Medium	↑ Heart rate and blood pressure (transient)	None
Enflurane	1.7	1.9	Medium	5% (fluoride)	Medium	↓ Heart rate No arrhythmias; does not sensitize heart to catecholamines	Hepatotoxic
Halothane	0.75	2.3	Slow	20%	Low	None	Hepatotoxic
Isoflurane	1.3	1.4	Medium	< 2% (fluoride)	Medium	↓ Heart rate No arrhythmias; does not sensitize heart to catecholamines	None
Sevoflurane	1.9	0.65	Rapid	< 2%	Medium	None	Nephrotoxic (rare)

MAC, Minimum alveolar concentration.

b. Primary uses
   (1) Induction of anesthesia
   (2) Procedures of short duration
2. Propofol
   a. Preferred for **1-day surgical procedures** because patients can ambulate sooner and recover from the effects of anesthesia more rapidly
   b. May cause hypotension
3. Dissociative anesthetics
   - **Example: ketamine**
   - During induction, patients feel dissociated from the environment (i.e., in trancelike states).
   a. Mechanism of action: blocks the *N*-methyl-D-aspartate (NMDA) receptor
   b. Uses
      - **Allows patients**, particularly children, **to be awake and respond to commands** yet endure painful stimuli
      - **Example:** changing painful burn dressings
   c. Adverse effects
      (1) Increased heart rate, cardiac output, and arterial blood pressure
      (2) Postoperative psychotic phenomena **(hallucinations)**
         - **Rarely used in adults because of this effect**
4. High-dose opioid anesthetics
   - **Examples: fentanyl, alfentanil, sufentanil**
   - Used in cardiothoracic surgery to avoid the cardiac effects of many inhalation agents (see Chapter 19)
5. Neuroleptanalgesia
   - Droperidol plus fentanyl
   - Produces **quiescence, reduced responsiveness to painful stimuli**, and **decreased motor activity**
   a. Primary use: short procedures that require consciousness and cooperation such as **bronchoscopy** and **cystoscopy**
   b. Secondary uses
      (1) Premedication for anesthesia
      (2) Adjunct for induction and maintenance of anesthesia
6. Midazolam or lorazepam: used for procedures that require consciousness

D. Preanesthetic medications (Table 8-2)
   1. Increase analgesia, muscle relaxation
   2. Decrease vagal reflexes, postoperative nausea and vomiting

II. Local Anesthetics (Box 8-2)

- Local anesthetics reversibly abolish sensory perception, especially pain, in restricted areas of the body.

A. Pharmacokinetics
   - During administration, the **vasoconstrictors norepinephrine** and **epinephrine** are often added to **localize the anesthetic to the injection site, prolong the anesthetic effect**, and **slow absorption**, thus minimizing systemic toxicity.

Norepinephrine and epinephrine often localize anesthetics to the injection site, prolong the anesthetic effect, and slow absorption.

TABLE 8-2 Preanesthetic Drugs

Drug Class	Specific Agent	Effect(s)
Opioids	Morphine Meperidine Fentanyl	Sedation to decrease tension and anxiety Analgesia
Barbiturates	Pentobarbital Secobarbital Thiopental	Decreased apprehension Sedation Rapid induction
Benzodiazepines	Diazepam Lorazepam	Decreased apprehension Sedation Rapid induction
Phenothiazines	Promazine Promethazine	Sedation Antihistaminic effect Antiemetic Decreased motor activity
Anticholinergic drugs	Atropine Scopolamine Glycopyrrolate	Inhibition of secretions, vomiting, and laryngospasms
Antiemetics	Droperidol Hydroxyzine Benzquinamide	Prevention of postoperative vomiting

BOX 8-2 Local Anesthetics

Esters
Benzocaine
Cocaine
Procaine
Tetracaine

Amides
Bupivacaine
Lidocaine
Mepivacaine
Prilocaine

1. **Route of administration:** topical application or local injection
2. **Metabolism**
   a. **Esters** are metabolized by plasma pseudocholinesterases.
      - Therefore, many have a **shorter duration of action (minutes)**.

   b. **Amides** are metabolized by amidases in the **liver**.
      - Therefore, many have a **longer duration of action (hours)**.

The names of all amides contain two "**i**"s (e.g., l**i**doca**i**ne).

B. Mechanism of action
- Local anesthetics cause **reversible blockade of nerve conduction.**

1. Decrease the nerve membrane permeability to sodium by **binding to open or inactivated sodium channels**
2. Reduce the rate of membrane depolarization
3. Raise the threshold of electrical excitability

With local anesthetics, loss of sensation occurs in the following sequence: pain, temperature, touch, movement.

4. Affect pain fibers first because they are small and unmyelinated

C. Adverse effects

1. **Central nervous system (CNS):** seizures, lightheadedness, sedation
2. **Cardiovascular system:** myocardial depression, hypotension, cardiac arrest
    - Some agents, such as lidocaine, have antiarrhythmic effects.

D. Specific local anesthetics

1. **Esters**
    - **Examples: procaine, tetracaine, benzocaine, cocaine**

    a. **Uses:** topical, infiltration, nerve block, spinal anesthesia
    - Cocaine is also a vasoconstrictor because it blocks norepinephrine uptake.

    b. **Adverse effects:** CNS stimulation, higher incidence of seizures

Use of cocaine on the mucosa of the nose and paranasal sinuses causes shrinkage and minimizes bleeding.

2. **Amides**
    - **Examples: lidocaine, bupivacaine, mepivacaine, prilocaine**
    - These agents are preferred for all types of infiltration, nerve blocks, and spinal anesthesia because of their slower metabolism and longer half-life ($t_{1/2}$).

9 Anticonvulsant Drugs

Target Topics

- Treatment of generalized tonic-clonic seizures
- Treatment of partial seizures
- Treatment of absence seizures
- Treatment of status epilepticus

I. Anticonvulsant Therapy
- **Seizures** are **episodes of abnormal electrical activity in the brain** that may lead to involuntary movements and sensations, which are accompanied by characteristic changes on electroencephalography (EEG).

A. Classification of seizures (Table 9-1)
B. Drugs used in the treatment of seizures (Table 9-2)

Many patients receive two anticonvulsant drugs, because decreased doses of each individual drug can be given, minimizing adverse effects.

II. **Drugs Used in the Treatment of Partial Seizures and Generalized Tonic-Clonic Seizures** (Box 9-1; see Table 9-2)

A. Phenytoin and fosphenytoin
1. **Pharmacokinetics:** exhibit plasma protein-binding, which can affect drug levels and activity
   - **a.** Both zero-order (high blood levels) and first-order kinetics (low blood levels)
   - **b. Metabolism** in the **liver**
2. **Mechanism of action:** block voltage-sensitive sodium channels in the neuronal membrane
3. **Uses** (see Table 9-2)
4. **Adverse effects**
   - **a.** Sedation
   - **b.** Cerebellar ataxia, nystagmus, diplopia
   - **c.** Induction of liver enzymes, which leads to vitamin D deficiency
     - Affects the epiphyseal plate and results in osteomalacia

TABLE 9-1 International Classification of Partial and Generalized Seizures

Classification	Origin and Features
Partial (Focal) Seizures	Arising in one cerebral hemisphere
Simple partial seizure	No alteration of consciousness
Complex partial seizure	Altered consciousness, automatisms, and behavioral changes
Secondarily generalized seizure	Focal seizure becoming generalized and accompanied by loss of consciousness
Generalized Seizures	Arising in both cerebral hemispheres and accompanied by loss of consciousness
Tonic-clonic (grand mal) seizure	Increased muscle tone followed by spasms of muscle contraction and relaxation
Tonic seizure	Increased muscle tone
Clonic seizure	Spasms of muscle contraction and relaxation
Myoclonic seizure	Rhythmic, jerking spasms
Atonic seizure	Sudden loss of all muscle tone
Absence (petit mal) seizure	Brief loss of consciousness, with minor muscle twitches and eye blinking

TABLE 9-2 Choice of Antiepileptic Drugs for Seizure Disorders*

		Generalized Seizures				
Drug	**Partial Seizures**	**Tonic-Clonic**	**Absence**	**Myoclonic**	**Atonic**	**Status Epilepticus**
Carbamazepine	1	1	W	—	—	—
Phenytoin	1	1	W	—	—	2
Phenobarbital	2	2	—	—	—	3
Primidone	2	2	—	—	—	—
Gabapentin	A	—	—	—	—	—
Lamotrigine	A	A	A	—	A	—
Topiramate	A	—	—	—	—	—
Ethosuximide	—	—	1†	—	—	—
Valproate	2	1	2†	1	1	—
Clonazepam	—	W	3	2	1	—
Diazepam	—	—	—	—	—	1
Lorazepam	—	—	—	—	—	1

* *1,* Drugs of first choice; *2,* drug of second choice; *3,* drug of third choice; *A,* drug for adjunct use with other drugs; *W,* drug that may worsen seizure.

†For absence seizures in children, ethosuximide is the drug of first choice and valproate is the drug of second choice. For absence seizures in adults, valproate is probably the drug of first choice.

   - **d. Gingival hyperplasia**
   - **e.** Hirsutism
   - **f.** Folate deficiency, leading to megaloblastic anemia
   - **g.** Teratogenic ability (**fetal hydantoin syndrome**)

B. Phenobarbital (see Chapter 7)

1. **Mechanism of action:** enhances the inhibitory action of the γ-aminobutyric acid (GABA) receptor by increasing the time that the chloride channel remains open
2. **Adverse effects**
   - **a. Induction of liver enzymes**

BOX 9-1 Anticonvulsants

Drugs Used to Treat Partial and Generalized Tonic-Clonic Seizures
Carbamazepine
Phenobarbital
Phenytoin/fosphenytoin
Primidone
Valproate

Adjunct Drugs Used to Treat Partial Seizures
Clorazepate
Felbamate
Gabapentin
Lamotrigine
Topiramate

Drugs Used to Treat Absence, Myoclonic, or Atonic Seizures
Clonazepam
Ethosuximide
Lamotrigine
Valproate

Drugs Used to Treat Status Epilepticus
Diazepam
Lorazepam
Phenobarbital
Phenytoin

b. Sedation
c. Increase in irritability and hyperactivity in children (paradoxical effect)
d. Agitation and confusion in the elderly

C. Carbamazepine

- Structurally related to imipramine and other tricyclic antidepressants

1. Mechanism of action: blocks voltage-sensitive sodium channels, inhibiting sustained, repetitive firing

2. Uses

a. Drug of choice for partial seizures
- Often used first if the patient also has generalized tonic-clonic seizures

b. Trigeminal neuralgia and neuropathic pain
c. Bipolar affective disorder (alternative to lithium)

Many anticonvulsants are used to treat neuropathic pain.

3. Adverse effects

a. Diplopia and ataxia (most common)
b. Induction of liver microsomal enzymes
- Carbamazepine accelerates its own metabolism and the metabolism of other drugs.

c. Aplastic anemia and **agranulocytosis**
- Requires monitoring with complete blood counts (CBCs)

Carbamazepine interacts with phenobarbital, phenytoin, primidone, and valproic acid, reducing their therapeutic effect.

D. Valproate (valproic acid)

1. **Mechanism of action**
   a. **Increases concentrations of GABA** in the brain
   b. Suppresses repetitive neuronal firing through inhibition of voltage-sensitive sodium channels
2. **Uses**
   a. **Absence seizures**
      - Valproate is the preferred agent if the patient also has generalized tonic-clonic seizures.
   b. **Complex partial seizures** and myoclonic seizures
3. **Adverse effects**
   a. The most serious adverse reaction is **liver failure.**
   b. The incidence of central nervous system (CNS) and gastrointestinal (GI) effects is high.
   c. Valproate inhibits its own metabolism as well as the metabolism of other drugs.

Valproate inhibits the metabolism of phenytoin, phenobarbital, and carbamazepine, increasing the toxicity of these drugs.

E. Primidone

1. The action of primidone is due both to the parent compound and to its metabolites, phenobarbital and phenylethylmalonamide (PEMA).
2. This drug is **frequently added to the regimen when satisfactory seizure control is not achieved with phenytoin or carbamazepine.**

F. Vigabatrin

1. **Mechanism of action:** potentiates GABA by irreversibly inhibiting GABA-transaminase
2. **Use:** most effective in the treatment of **partial seizures**

G. Gabapentin

1. **Mechanism of action:** may alter GABA metabolism or its nonsynaptic release
2. **Uses**
   a. Adjunctive treatment of **partial seizures** with or without secondary generalized tonic-clonic seizures
   b. Neuropathic pain

H. Lamotrigine

1. **Mechanism of action:** acts at voltage-sensitive sodium channels to stabilize neuronal membranes
2. **Use:** adjunctive treatment for refractory partial seizures with or without secondary generalized tonic-clonic seizures

III. Absence (Petit Mal) Seizures and Drugs Used in Their Treatment (see Box 9-1 and Table 9-2)

- Absence seizures are primarily a **childhood disorder.**

A. Features

1. Brief lapses of consciousness
2. Characteristic **spike-and-wave pattern on EEG** (3/sec)

B. Therapeutic drugs

1. **Ethosuximide:** effective in a high percentage of cases
   a. **Mechanism of action:** reduces current in T-type calcium channel found on primary afferent neurons
   b. **Adverse effects:** GI upset, drowsiness
2. **Valproate** (used for both tonic-clonic and absence seizures)

3. Clonazepam
- Tolerance develops within a few months, making the drug **inappropriate for long-term therapy** (see Chapter 7).

IV. Status Epilepticus and Drugs Used in Its Treatment (see Box 9-1 and Table 9-2)

- Status epilepticus is a **life-threatening emergency** involving repeated seizures.

A. Treatment of choice

1. Diazepam (intravenous)
2. Lorazepam (intravenous)

B. Other therapeutic drugs

1. Phenytoin (intravenous) given by loading dose over 20–30 minutes
2. General anesthetics (intravenous thiopental)

10 Psychotherapeutic Drugs

Target Topics

- Antipsychotic drugs
- Antidepressants
- Mood stabilizers

I. **Antipsychotic Drugs** (Box 10-1)
- **Neuroleptics** are useful in the treatment of **schizophrenia.**
- These drugs **reduce positive symptoms** (e.g., paranoia, hallucinations, delusions) more than negative symptoms (e.g., emotional blunting, poor socialization, cognitive deficit) in patients with schizophrenia.

A. **Pharmacokinetics**
- Most antipsychotics are **metabolized to active and inactive metabolites.**

1. Immediate onset after intramuscular or intravenous injection
2. Slow and variable absorption after oral administration

B. **Mechanism of action** (Table 10-1)

Antipsychotic effects of neuroleptic agents are related to blockade of dopamine receptors.

1. **Blockade of dopamine D_2 receptor** correlates best with antipsychotic activity.
2. **Blockade of dopamine D_3 and D_4 receptors** may also contribute to therapeutic effects.
3. **Blockade of other receptors also occurs** (see Table 10-1).

C. Uses
1. **Schizophrenic reactions,** mania, psychosis
   - The actions of the neuroleptic agents in the mesolimbic and mesocortical pathways are most important for their antipsychotic effects.

BOX 10-1 Antipsychotic Drugs

Phenothiazines	***Azepines***
Chlorpromazine	Clozapine
Fluphenazine	Olanzapine
Thioridazine	Quetiapine
Trifluoperazine	***Other Drugs***
Thioxanthenes	Molindone
Thiothixene	Risperidone
Butyrophenones	
Droperidol	
Haloperidol	

TABLE 10-1 Mechanisms and Effects of Neuroleptic Agents

Mechanism	Action
Blockade of dopamine D_1 and D_2 receptors	Antipsychotic, extrapyramidal, and endocrine effects
Blockade of α-adrenergic receptors	Hypotension
Blockade of histamine H_1 receptors	Sedation
Blockade of muscarinic receptors	Anticholinergic effects (e.g., dry mouth, urinary retention)
Blockade of serotonin receptors	Antipsychotic effects

2. Nausea (**antiemetic**)
3. Intractable hiccoughs

D. Adverse effects
- Neuroleptics cause unpleasant effects.

1. **Behavioral effects**, such as "pseudodepression"
2. **Neurologic effects**
   a. Extrapyramidal effects and **iatrogenic parkinsonism**
   b. **Dystonic reactions** and **akathisia**
      - The **best treatment** is **diphenhydramine** or **benztropine** (antimuscarinic action).

      (1) **Acute dystonic reactions (1–5 days):** involvement of neck and head muscles
      (2) **Akathisia (5–60 days):** restlessness and agitation seen as continuous movement
      (3) **Parkinsonian syndrome (5–30 days):** extrapyramidal effects; tremors, rigidity, shuffling gait, postural abnormalities
      (4) **Neuroleptic malignant syndrome (weeks):** catatonia, stupor, fever, unstable blood pressure (autonomic instability); **may be fatal**
         - **Treatment** involves stopping the neuroleptic drug and using dantrolene or bromocriptine.

      (5) **Perioral tremor (months or years):** "rabbit syndrome" (involuntary movement of the lips)

Tardive dyskinesia: most important adverse effect of neuroleptics

TABLE 10-2 Effects of Antipsychotic Drugs

Drug	Relative Potency*	Extrapyramidal Effects	Sedative Action	Hypotensive Actions	Anticholinergic Effects
Phenothiazines					
Chlorpromazine (aliphatic)	Low	Medium	High	High	Medium
Fluphenazine (piperazine)	High	High	Low	Very low	Low
Thioridazine (piperadine)	Low	Low	High	High	Very high
Trifluoperazine (piperazine)	High	High	Low	Low	Medium
Thioxanthenes					
Thiothixene	High	Medium-high	Low	Medium	Very low
Butyrophenones					
Haloperidol	High	Very high	Low	Very low	Very low
Heterocyclics					
Clozapine	Medium	Very low	High	Medium	Very high
Olanzapine	High	Very low	Low	Low	Medium
Risperidone	High	Low	Low	Low	Very low

*Potency: low = 50–2000 mg/d; medium = 20–250 mg/d; high = 1–100 mg/d.

Use of neuroleptics leads to hyperprolactinemia, which results in amenorrhea-galactorrhea syndrome and infertility in women and loss of libido, impotence, and infertility in men.

- **Treatment** involves the use of anticholinergic agents.

(6) **Tardive dyskinesia (months or years):** stereotypical involuntary movements
   (a) **Frequently irreversible**
   (b) Results from effects on dopamine D_2 receptors

c. **Decrease in seizure threshold**
- Use **caution** when giving neuroleptics to individuals with **epilepsy.**
- **Avoid** giving to patients who are **undergoing withdrawal from central nervous system (CNS) depressants.**

E. **Specific drugs** (Table 10-2)
1. **Aliphatic phenothiazines:** chlorpromazine
   - **Least potent** phenothiazine
2. **Piperidine phenothiazines:** thioridazine
   a. Generally **low incidence of acute extrapyramidal effects**
   b. Requires regular eye examinations because of retinitis pigmentosa
3. **Piperazine phenothiazines:** fluphenazine
   - Generally **high incidence of acute extrapyramidal effects**
4. **Butyrophenones:** haloperidol, droperidol
   a. Additional uses for haloperidol: treatment of **Tourette's syndrome** and **acute psychosis**
   b. **Extremely high incidence of acute extrapyramidal effects**

BOX 10-2 Antidepressants

Tricyclic Antidepressants
Amitriptyline
Clomipramine
Desipramine
Imipramine
Nortriptyline

SSRIs
Citalopram
Fluoxetine
Fluvoxamine
Paroxetine
Sertraline

MAO Inhibitors
Phenelzine
Tranylcypromine

Other Antidepressants
Amoxapine
Bupropion
Maprotiline
Mirtazapine
Nefazodone
Trazodone
Venlafaxine

5. Azepines
- **a.** Clozapine
  - **(1)** **Mechanism of action: blocks serotonin and dopamine,** primarily the **dopamine D_1 and D_4 receptors,** with a greater effect on the serotonin receptors
    - **(a)** Has less effect on dopamine D_2 receptors than traditional antipsychotics
    - **(b)** Has a greater effect on negative symptoms of schizophrenia than other antipsychotics
  - **(2)** Adverse effects
    - **(a)** **Low incidence of extrapyramidal effects**
    - **(b)** **High incidence of agranulocytosis** (1–2%), which necessitates regular complete blood counts (CBCs)
- **b. Olanzapine:** newer clozapine-like agent with no notable incidence of agranulocytosis

6. Benzisoxazoles (risperidone): monoaminergic antagonist with a high affinity for both **serotonin 5-HT_2 and dopamine D_2 receptors**
- **a.** Widely used for long-term therapy
- **b.** Associated with fewer extrapyramidal symptoms

II. Antidepressants and Mood Stabilizers (Box 10-2)

- **Depression** can be classified as **reactive** (i.e., response to grief or illness); **endogenous** (i.e., genetically determined biochemical condition); or **bipolar affective** (i.e., manic-depressive disorder).
- **Antidepressant drugs** are used to treat **endogenous and bipolar affective forms** of depression.

A. Tricyclic antidepressants (TCAs) (see Box 10-2)

1. Pharmacokinetics
- Clinical improvement requires use for 2–3 weeks, thus reducing compliance.

TABLE 10-3 Pharmacologic Profile of Antidepressants*

Drug	Antimuscarinic Effects	Sedative Effects	Amine Pump Blockade: Serotonin	Amine Pump Blockade: Norepinephrine	Amine Pump Blockade: Dopamine
TCAs					
Amitriptyline	+++	+++	+++	++	0
Clomipramine	++	+++	+++	+++	0
Desipramine	+	+	0	+++	0
Imipramine	++	++	+++	++	0
Nortriptyline	++	++	+++	++	0
SSRIs					
Citalopram	0	0	+++	0	0
Fluoxetine	+	+	+++	0,+	0,+
Fluvoxamine	0	0	+++	0	0
Paroxetine	0	0	+++	0	0
Sertraline	+	0	+++	0	0
Other antidepressants					
Amoxapine	++	++	+	++	+
Bupropion	0	0	+,0	+,0	+
Maprotiline	++	++	0	+++	0
Mirtazapine†	0	+++	0	0	0
Nefazodone	+++	++	+,0	0	0
Trazodone	0	+++	++	0	0
Venlafaxine	0	0	+++	++	0,+

**0*, None; +, slight; ++, moderate; +++, extensive.
†Blocks α_2-adrenoreceptors and 5-HT_2 serotonin receptors.

TCAs produce conduction abnormalities: ECG needed prior to therapy to rule out AV block or other abnormalities

2. **Mechanism of action**
   - Most TCAs **block the reuptake of serotonin and norepinephrine,** causing accumulation of these monoamines in the synaptic cleft.
3. **Uses**
   a. **Depression,** chronic pain, and insomnia
   b. **Enuresis** (imipramine)
   c. **Obsessive-compulsive disorder** (clomipramine)
4. **Adverse effects**
   a. **Sedation,** which is due to blockade of histamine H_1 receptors
   b. Full range of anticholinergic effects, such as **dry mouth,** because agents are potent anticholinergics
   c. Full range of phenothiazine-like effects, especially **orthostatic hypotension,** resulting from α_1-receptor blockade
   d. Rare acute extrapyramidal signs, because the agents are not potent dopamine blockers

B. Selective serotonin reuptake inhibitors (SSRIs) (see Box 10-2; Table 10-3)

1. **Mechanism of action**
   a. Highly specific **serotonin reuptake blockade** at the neuronal membrane

b. Dramatically decreased binding to histamine, acetylcholine, and norepinephrine receptors, which leads to less sedative, anticholinergic, and cardiovascular effects when compared with TCAs

2. Uses: depression, obsessive-compulsive disorder, and bulimia nervosa

3. Adverse effects: nausea, nervousness, insomnia, headache, sexual dysfunction

C. Other antidepressants (see Box 10-2)

1. Mechanism of action: greater selectivity than TCAs for either norepinephrine or serotonin

2. Adverse effects: less cardiotoxicity and anticholinergic activity than TCAs

3. Selected antidepressants

a. Amoxapine
- **Use: depression in psychotic patients**
- Also has antipsychotic activity

b. Bupropion
- Structurally similar to amphetamine

(1) Uses: **depression, smoking cessation**

(2) Adverse effects: seizures, anorexia, aggravation of psychosis

c. Maprotiline: selective norepinephrine uptake inhibitor

d. Mirtazapine

(1) Mechanism of action: blockade of 5-HT_2 serotonin and α_2-adrenergic receptors

(2) Use: depression in patients who do not tolerate SSRIs

(3) Adverse effects (reputed): weight gain, sedation

e. Trazodone

(1) Mechanism of action

(a) Inhibits serotonin uptake into the presynaptic neurons

(b) Has no anticholinergic activity

(2) Uses

(a) Depression

(b) Insomnia (low doses), which causes sedation

Trazodone may cause priapism (prolonged, painful erection of the penis), which can lead to impotence.

f. Nefazodone: less sedating than trazodone

g. Venlafaxine: similar mechanism of action to the TCAs but a better side-effect profile, because it does not block α_1-adrenergic, histamine H_1, or muscarinic receptors

D. Monoamine oxidase (MAO) **inhibitors**

1. Pharmacokinetics

a. Long-lasting effects due to irreversible inhibition of the enzyme

b. Therapeutic effect develops after 2–4 weeks of treatment.

2. Mechanism of action: inhibition of MAO, thus increasing concentration of norepinephrine and serotonin in the brain

3. **Uses**
   a. **"Atypical" depression,** characterized by attendant anxiety and phobic features
   b. Depression in patients refractory to TCAs
4. **Adverse effects**
   a. **Postural hypotension**
   b. **CNS effects,** such as restlessness and insomnia
   c. **Hepatotoxicity**
   d. Possible hypertensive crisis

Ingestion of tyramine-containing foods (e.g., certain cheeses, wines, preserved meats) while taking MAO inhibitors may precipitate a hypertensive crisis.

5. **Drug interactions: meperidine, TCAs, SSRIs**
   - Due to "serotonin syndrome" (marked increase in synaptic serotonin)
   - **Possible severe reactions,** characterized by excitation, sweating, rigidity, hypertension, severe respiratory depression, coma, and vascular collapse, possibly resulting in death

Patients who are taking MAO inhibitors should not take meperidine, TCAs, or SSRIs.

E. **Mood stabilizers**
1. **Lithium:** used in the treatment of **bipolar disorders,** because it decreases the severity of the manic phase and lengthens the time between manic phases
   a. **Pharmacokinetics**
      (1) Narrow range of therapeutic serum levels
      (2) Delayed onset of action (6–10 days)
   b. **Mechanism of action:** unknown, but known to modify ion fluxes, neurotransmitter synthesis, turnover rates, and second messenger systems, particularly the inositol phosphate (IP_3) pathway
   c. Uses
      (1) **Bipolar disorders**
      (2) **Nonpsychiatric uses**
         (a) Neutropenia, thyrotoxic crisis, and migraine and cluster headaches
         (b) Considered a last choice for syndrome of inappropriate antidiuretic hormone (SIADH) secretion
   d. **Adverse effects:** evident at therapeutic serum concentrations
      (1) **Symptoms and signs**
         (a) **Fine hand tremor, dry mouth, weight gain**
         (b) Mild nausea and vomiting, diarrhea
         (c) Polydipsia, polyuria, impotence, decreased libido, nephrotic syndrome
      (2) **Electrocardiogram**
         - **Flattened or inverted T waves** produced by the inhibition of potassium cellular reuptake, leading to intracellular **hypokalemia**

Use of lithium causes nephrogenic diabetes insipidus and hypothyroidism.

2. **Alternatives to lithium use in bipolar disorders**
   - Carbamazepine, clonazepam, valproic acid

11

Drugs Used in the Treatment of Parkinson's Disease

Target Topics

- Pathogenesis of Parkinson's disease
- Levodopa-carbidopa
- Dopamine agonists
- Amantadine, tolcapone, and selegiline
- Anticholinergics

I. General Considerations

A. Parkinsonism is associated with **lesions** in the **basal ganglia,** especially the substantia nigra and the globus pallidus.

B. There is a reduction in the number of cells in the substantia nigra and a **decrease** in the **dopamine content.**

C. The lesions result in increased and **improper modulation** of motor activity by the **extrapyramidal system,** leading to a resting tremor, rigidity, and bradykinesia.

D. Therapy aims to **increase the dopamine** content through "replacement therapy" or **reducing acetylcholine (ACh) activity,** because proper function depends on the balance between the inhibitory neurotransmitter dopamine and the excitatory neurotransmitter ACh.

II. Drugs Used to Treat Parkinson's Disease (Box 11-1 and Figure 11-1)

A. Levodopa (L-dopa)

1. Pharmacokinetics

a. L-dopa has the ability to cross the blood-brain barrier.
  - Dopamine cannot be used to treat Parkinson's disease, because this agent does not readily enter the brain after systemic administration.

b. L-dopa is **rapidly metabolized**, predominantly by decarboxylation to dopamine, and excreted into the urine.

c. **L-dopa is usually given in combination with carbidopa**, a peripheral dopa decarboxylase inhibitor.

2. **Mechanism of action**
  - L-dopa enters the brain and is converted to dopamine, which reacts with dopamine receptors in the central nervous system (CNS).

Use of carbidopa with L-dopa allows more L-dopa to enter the brain.

BOX 11-1	**Drugs Used to Treat Parkinson's Disease**
Dopaminergic Drugs	*Dopamine Receptor Agonists*
Amantadine	Bromocriptine
Carbidopa	Pergolide
Levodopa	Pramipexole
Selegiline	Ropinirole
Tolcapone	
	Anticholinergics
	Benztropine
	Trihexyphenidyl

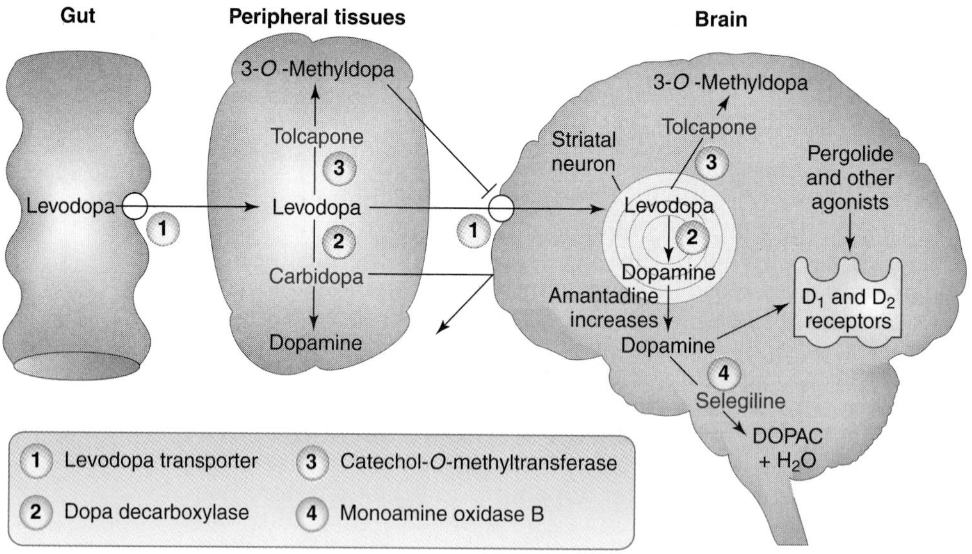

Figure 11-1 Mechanisms of dopaminergic drugs used in the treatment of Parkinson's disease. Dopa decarboxylase is inhibited by carbidopa in the peripheral tissues but not in the brain, because carbidopa does not cross the blood-brain barrier. Catechol-*O*-methyltransferase is inhibited by tolcapone in both the peripheral tissues and the brain. Monoamine oxidase B is inhibited by selegiline. *DOPAC,* Dihydroxyphenylacetic acid; *D_1* and *D_2*, dopamine receptor subtypes.

3. **Adverse effects**
   a. Severe **gastrointestinal problems:** nausea, vomiting, anorexia, peptic ulcer
   b. Postural hypotension
   c. **Dyskinesia:** development of abnormal involuntary movements
      - **Choreoathetosis,** the most common presentation, involves the face and limbs.
      - Effects resemble tardive dyskinesia induced by phenothiazines.
   d. Arrhythmias

B. Other Drugs Used to Treat Parkinson's Disease

1. **Bromocriptine**
   a. **Mechanism of action:** direct dopamine agonist that enters the CNS
   b. **Uses**
      - Lack of response to L-dopa or an unstable reaction to L-dopa
      - "On-off" symptoms, in which improved motility alternates with marked akinesia
2. **Pergolide**
   a. **Mechanism of action:** potent dopamine agonist that acts at the dopamine D_1 and D_2 receptors
   b. **Use:** "on-off" symptoms
3. **Pramipexole**
   a. **Mechanism of action:** dopamine agonist that binds to both the dopamine D_2 and D_3 receptors in the striatum and substantia nigra
   b. **Uses:** can delay the need for L-dopa and reduce the "off" symptoms

Pramipexole is now used as monotherapy for mild Parkinson's disease.

4. **Ropinirole**
   a. **Mechanism of action:** agonist that acts at both the dopamine D_2 and D_3 receptors
   b. **Uses:** can delay the need for L-dopa and reduce the "off" symptoms
5. **Amantadine**
   a. **Mechanism of action:** antiviral agent that releases dopamine and may block dopamine reuptake
   b. **Uses:** tremor, bradykinesia, rigidity
6. **Selegiline**
   a. **Mechanism of action:** indirect dopamine agonist that selectively inhibits monoamine oxidase B, an enzyme that inactivates dopamine
   b. **Use:** most commonly given in conjunction with L-dopa, but may be effective by itself as a "neuroprotectant" due to its antioxidant and antiapoptotic effects
7. **Tolcapone**
   a. **Mechanism of action:** catechol-*O*-methyltransferase (COMT) inhibitor that decreases the activation of dopamine
   b. **Use:** adjunct to L-dopa–carbidopa

8. Anticholinergic drugs

- **Examples: benztropine, trihexyphenidyl**

a. Only those agents with anticholinergic activity that enter the CNS are prescribed.

b. These drugs **decrease the tremor and symptoms produced by a dopamine D_2 receptor antagonist** such as haloperidol.

SECTION IV

Drugs That Affect the Cardiovascular, Renal, and Hematologic Systems

12

Antiarrhythmic Drugs

Target Topics

- Electrophysiology of the heart
- Class I antiarrhythmic drugs (sodium channel blockers)
- Class II antiarrhythmic drugs (β-blockers)
- Class III antiarrhythmic drugs (potassium channel blockers)
- Class IV antiarrhythmic drugs (calcium channel blockers)

I. General Considerations

A. Cardiac contraction (Figure 12-1): five-step process

1. Spontaneous development of the **action potential in the sinoatrial (SA) node**
2. Spread of the impulse **through the atrium**
3. Temporary delay of the impulse at the **atrioventricular (AV) node**
4. Rapid spread of the impulse along the **two branches of the bundle of His and the Purkinje fibers**
5. Spread of the impulse along the **cardiac muscle fibers of the ventricles**

B. Electrophysiology of the heart

1. **Action potential** (Figure 12-2)
   a. The action potential is the **resting membrane potential of the myocardium** (approximately **–90 mV**).
   b. It results from an unequal distribution of ions (high Na^+ outside, high K^+ inside).

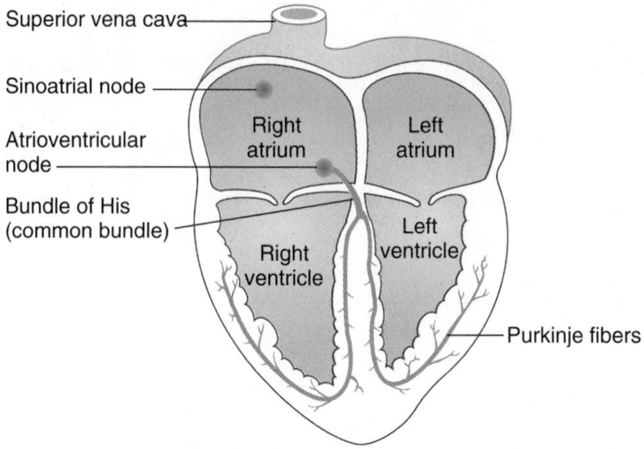

Figure 12-1 Schematic drawing of the heart.

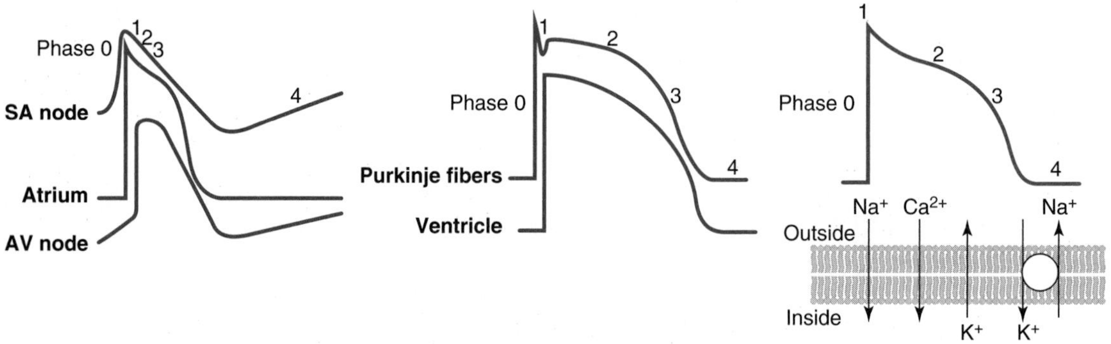

Figure 12-2 Schematic representation of cardiac electrical activity in the sinoatrial *(SA)* node and Purkinje fibers as well as ion permeability changes and transport processes that occur during an action potential. *AV,* Atrioventricular.

2. Five phases of the action potential

a. Rapid depolarization (phase 0)

(1) Rapid inward movement of Na^+ due to the opening of voltage-gated sodium channels

(2) Variation in resting membrane potential: –90 mV → +15 mV

b. Initial rapid repolarization (phase 1)

- Inactivation of sodium channels and influx of Cl^-

c. Plateau phase (phase 2)

- Slow but prolonged opening of voltage-gated calcium channels

d. Repolarization (phase 3)

(1) Closure of calcium channels and K^+ efflux through potassium channels

(2) Return of inactivated sodium channels to resting phase

e. Diastole (phase 4)

- Restoration of ionic concentrations by Na^+/K^+-activated ATPase and restoration of resting potential

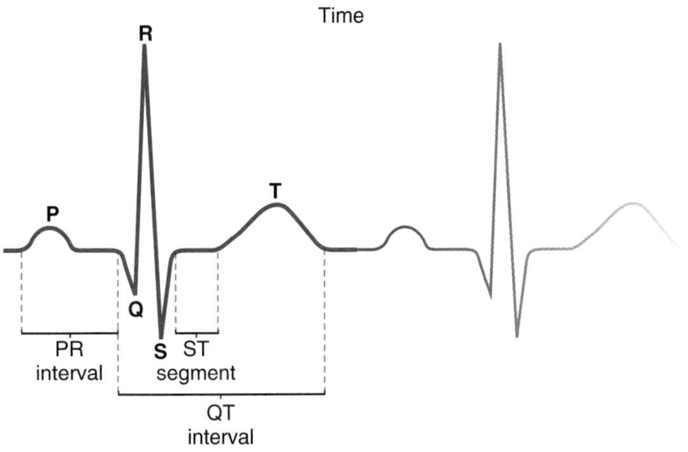

Figure 12-3 Schematic electrocardiogram (ECG) showing depolarization and repolarization of the heart. The P wave is produced by atrial depolarization, the QRS complex by ventricular polarization, and the T wave by ventricular repolarization. The PR interval measures the conduction time from atrium to ventricle, the ST segment represents the period when the ventricles are polarized, and the QT interval measures the duration of the ventricular action potential. The QRS complex measures the intraventricular conduction time.

3. **Important electrocardiographic (ECG) parameters** (Figure 12-3)
   a. **P wave** = atrial depolarization
   b. **PR interval** = delay of conduction through the AV node
   c. **QRS complex** = ventricular depolarization
   d. **T wave** = ventricular repolarization
   e. **QT interval** = duration of action potential in the ventricles

II. Arrhythmias and Their Treatment

- Arrhythmias are **irregularities in heart rhythm** that result from disturbances in pulse formation, impulse conduction, or both.

A. **Antiarrhythmic drugs produce effects** by altering one or more of the following factors:
   1. Automaticity
   2. Conduction velocity
   3. Refractory period
   4. Membrane responsiveness

B. These agents have varying effects on the electrophysiology of the heart (Table 12-1).

III. Antiarrhythmic Drugs (Box 12-1)

A. **Class I drugs: sodium channel blockers**
   - All class I agents, which are generally local anesthetics, bind to open and inactivated sodium channels, thus **inhibiting phase 0 depolarization of the action potential** (Figure 12-4).
   - **Lidocaine** is more effective in the treatment of **ventricular**

TABLE 12-1 Effects of Antiarrhythmic Drugs on the Electrophysiology of the Heart

Drug (Class)	SA Node Rate	AV Node Refractory Period	PR Interval	QRS Duration	QT Interval
Quinidine (IA)	↑↓	↑↓	↑↓	↑↑↑	↑↑
Lidocaine (IB)	N	N	N	N	N
Propranolol (II)	↓↓	↑↑	↑↑	N	N
Sotalol (III)	↓↓	↑↑	↑↑	N	↑↑↑
Verapamil (IV)	↓↓	↑↑	↑↑	N	N

AV, Atrioventricular; *N,* no major effect; *SA,* sinoatrial.

BOX 12-1 Antiarrhythmic Drugs

Sodium Channel Blockers

Class IA
Disopyramide
Procainamide
Quinidine

Class IB
Lidocaine
Mexiletine
Tocainide

Class IC
Flecainide
Propafenone

Other Antiarrhythmic Drugs

Class II
Esmolol
Metoprolol
Propranolol

Class III
Amiodarone
Bretylium
Ibutilide
Sotalol

Class IV
Diltiazem
Verapamil

Miscellaneous Antiarrhythmic Drugs
Adenosine
Magnesium

arrhythmias, whereas **quinidine** and **procainamide** are more effective in the treatment of **atrial arrhythmias.**

Quinidine and procainamide are particularly effective in the control of atrial arrhythmias.

Class I drugs and ERP: class IA, extend ERP; class IB, reduce ERP; class IC, no change

1. **Class IA drugs**
   - **Examples: quinidine, procainamide**

   a. **Quinidine**
      (1) **Mechanism of action**
         (a) **Inhibition of sodium channels,** extending the effective refractory period (ERP) of the myocardial cell membrane, thereby decreasing myocardial conduction velocity, excitability, and contractility
         (b) **Blockade of α-adrenergic receptors,** leading to a reflex increase in the SA node rate and producing vasodilation
      (2) Uses
         (a) **Conversion to or maintenance of sinus rhythm** in patients with atrial fibrillation, flutter, or ventricular tachycardia

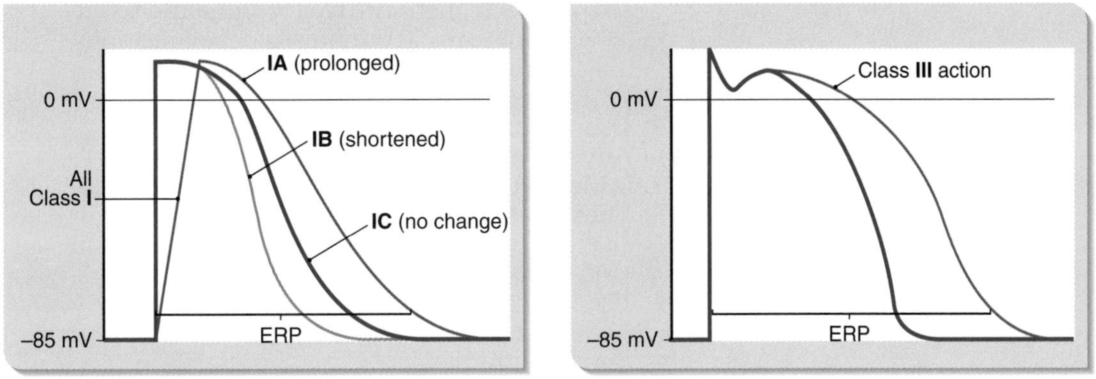

Figure 12-4 Effects of class I and class III antiarrhythmics on the action potential and the electrocardiogram (ECG). *ERP,* Effective refractory period.

- **(b) Treatment of paroxysmal supraventricular tachycardia (PSVT)**
- **(c) Prevention of PSVT** in patients with reentrant tachycardias, including Wolff-Parkinson-White syndrome

(3) Adverse effects
- **(a) Torsades de pointes**
- **(b) ECG changes:** prolonged QRS complex, giant U wave, ST-segment depression, flattened T wave
- **(c) Diarrhea**
- **(d) Cinchonism:** giddiness, light-headedness, ringing in the ears, impaired hearing, blurred vision

b. Procainamide
- This **local anesthetic** is equivalent to quinidine as an antiarrhythmic agent and has similar cardiac and toxic effects.
- Additional adverse effect: **induces systemic lupus erythematosus**

About one third of patients who receive long-term procainamide therapy develop reversible lupus-related symptoms.

2. Class IB drugs
- **Examples: lidocaine, tocainide, mexiletine**
- Class IB drugs **decrease the duration of the action potential.**

a. Lidocaine (see Chapter 8)

(1) Pharmacokinetics
- **(a)** Short-acting because of **rapid hepatic metabolism**
- **(b)** Loading dose should be followed by continuous intravenous infusion.

(2) Mechanism of action
- **(a) Acts primarily on the Purkinje fibers,** depressing automaticity and shortening the refractory period

Lidocaine is particularly useful in the control of ventricular arrhythmias.

- (b) Has a higher **affinity for ischemic tissue,** suppressing spontaneous depolarizations in the ventricles by inhibiting reentry mechanisms
- **(3) Use:** suppression of ventricular tachycardia
- **(4) Adverse effects: seizures** (in elderly patients)

b. Tocainide and mexiletine: congeners of lidocaine
- **(1) Pharmacokinetics**
  - **(a)** Resistant to first-pass hepatic metabolism
  - **(b)** Half-life ($t_{1/2}$): 8–20 hours
- **(2) Use** (oral administration): **ventricular arrhythmias**
- **(3) Adverse effects:** dizziness, vertigo, nausea, vomiting, arrhythmias

B. Class II drugs: β-adrenergic receptor antagonists (see Chapter 5)
- **Examples: propranolol, esmolol**
- Class II drugs **slow phase 4 depolarization in the SA node.**

1. Mechanism of action: blockade of β_1-receptors
- **a.** Reduce heart rate
- **b.** Reduce myocardial contraction
- **c.** Prolong AV conduction
- **d.** Prolong the AV refractory period

2. Propranolol
- **a. Uses**
  - **(1)** Treatment and prophylaxis of **PSVT** and **atrial fibrillation** (orally effective)
  - **(2)** Possible prevention of recurrent infarction in patients recovering from myocardial infarction (MI)
- **b. Adverse effects:** sedation, sleep disturbance, sexual dysfunction, cardiac disturbance, asthma

3. Esmolol
- **a. Pharmacokinetics**
  - **(1)** Short-acting
  - **(2)** Administered by intravenous infusion
- **b. Uses**
  - **(1)** Short-term control of **supraventricular tachyarrhythmias,** including sinus tachycardia and PSVT
  - **(2)** Control of ventricular rate in patients with atrial fibrillation or atrial flutter
- **c. Adverse effects:** AV block, cardiac arrest

C. Class III: potassium channel blockers
- **Examples: sotalol, bretylium, amiodarone**
- Class III drugs **increase the duration of the action potential** (see Figure 12-4).

1. Mechanism of action
- **a. Prolong repolarization**
- **b. Increase the ERP**

2. Amiodarone

Amiodarone, a class III drug, also has class I, II, and IV antiarrhythmic effects.

- **a. Pharmacokinetics**
  - **(1) Long $t_{1/2}$ (13–103 days)**
  - **(2)** Time required to achieve steady-state therapeutic levels: 15–30 days

b. Use: approved only for **ventricular arrhythmias**
- Amiodarone is very effective against both supraventricular and ventricular arrhythmias (atrial fibrillation or flutter, supraventricular tachycardia), but its **toxicity** is worthy of consideration.

c. Adverse effects
- **(1) Cardiovascular effects:** torsades de pointes, ECG changes (prolonged QT interval and QRS complex)
- **(2) Other effects**
  - **Pulmonary reactions** such as pneumonitis, **fibrosis (most severe)**
  - Photodermatitis, paresthesias, tremor, ataxia, thyroid dysfunction, constipation

3. Sotalol
- This drug is an oral, **nonselective β-adrenergic receptor antagonist.**

a. Uses: life-threatening sustained ventricular tachycardia, atrial fibrillation

b. Adverse effects: prolonged QT interval, torsades de pointes

4. Bretylium

a. Mechanism of action
- **(1)** The initial release of catecholamines produces an initial **positive inotropic effect.**
- **(2)** An **inhibition of catecholamine release** follows.
- **(3)** Antiarrhythmic properties may be due to prolongation of the refractory period unrelated to its catecholamine-related effects.

b. Uses
- **(1) Ventricular fibrillation** in combination with electrical defibrillation during cardiopulmonary resuscitation
- **(2) Unstable ventricular tachycardia and arrhythmias** other than ventricular fibrillation

c. Adverse effects
- **(1) Early:** precipitation of **ventricular arrhythmias** due to catecholamine release
- **(2) Late:** possible production of **orthostatic hypotension** due to blockade of catecholamine release

D. Class IV: **calcium channel blockers** (Figure 12-5)
- **Examples: verapamil, diltiazem**
- Class IV drugs **slow phase 4 depolarization in the SA node and decrease the heart rate.**

1. Mechanism of action: blockade of calcium uptake via a voltage-sensitive channel (L-type), thereby **reducing inward flow of calcium into myocardial cells**

2. Effects on the myocardium

a. Reduce the rate of SA node discharge

b. Slow conduction through the AV node

c. Prolong the AV node refractory period (prolong the PR interval)

d. Decrease myocardial contraction

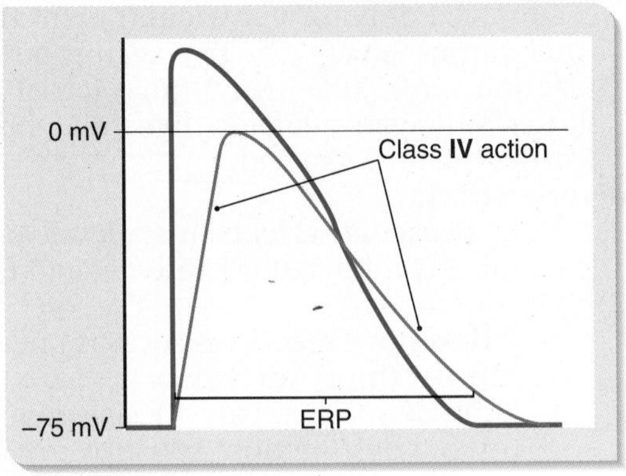

Figure 12-5 Effects of class II and class IV antiarrhythmics on the action potential. *ERP,* Effective refractory period.

3. **Other effects:** vasodilation, reflex tachycardia (greatest with dihydropyridines)
4. **Uses**
   a. **Treatment of PSVT**
   b. **Control of ventricular rate** in atrial flutter or atrial fibrillation
      - Verapamil is more effective than digoxin.
5. **Adverse effects:** hypotension, dizziness, constipation, edema, AV block

Verapamil is often used to control the ventricular rate of patients with atrial fibrillation.

E. Miscellaneous antiarrhythmic drugs

1. **Adenosine**
   a. **Pharmacokinetics**
      (1) $t_{1/2}$ (blood): about **10 seconds**
      (2) Route of administration: **intravenous**
   b. **Mechanism of action:** enhanced potassium conductance with inhibition of cyclic adenosine monophosphate (cAMP)–dependent calcium influx
2. **Digoxin** (see Chapter 14)
   - **Uses:** atrial fibrillation (decreases AV conduction), heart failure
3. **Magnesium (intravenous)**
   a. **Mechanism of action:** unknown
   b. **Uses:** digitalis-induced arrhythmias, torsades de pointes

Adenosine is the drug of choice for prompt conversion of PSVT to sinus rhythm.

13 Antihypertensive Drugs

Target Topics

- Approaches to the treatment of hypertension
- Diuretics
- Sympatholytic drugs
- Vasodilators
- Drugs that affect the renin-angiotensin system

I. General Considerations

- The diagnosis of **hypertension** in adults is confirmed when, on two subsequent visits, the **average diastolic blood pressure exceeds 90 mm Hg** or the **average systolic blood pressure exceeds 140 mm Hg.**

A. Treatment rationale

- **Sustained hypertension** leads to cardiovascular and renal damage, especially myocardial infarction (MI) and stroke.
- **Reducing blood pressure decreases morbidity and mortality.**

B. Treatment methods

1. **First-line treatment:** diet and lifestyle changes
2. **Second-line treatment:** pharmacologic intervention (Box 13-1)
   - Selection of pharmacologic treatment is based on concomitant conditions (Table 13-1).

II. Diuretics (see Chapter 15)

- **Thiazide diuretics** are most often used because they have antihypertensive properties in addition to diuretic effects.

A. Use: hypertension (first-line therapy)

- Thiazides are administered alone or in combination with other drugs.

BOX 13-1 Antihypertensive Drugs

Diuretics
Loop diuretics
Potassium-sparing diuretics
Thiazide diuretics

Sympatholytics
β-Receptor Antagonists
Atenolol
Labetalol
Metoprolol
Propranolol

α_1-Receptor Antagonists
Doxazosin
Prazosin
Terazosin

α_2-Receptor Agonists
Clonidine
Methyldopa

Vasodilators
Calcium channel blockers
Hydralazine
Minoxidil
Sodium nitroprusside

Angiotensin Inhibitors
Angiotensin-Converting Enzyme (ACE) Inhibitors
Captopril
Enalapril
Lisinopril

Angiotensin Receptor Blockers
Losartan
Valsartan

B. Adverse effects: hypokalemia (except with potassium-sparing diuretics), hyperuricemia, sexual dysfunction, hyperglycemia, hyperlipidemia

III. Sympatholytic Drugs

A. β-Adrenergic receptor antagonists (see Chapter 5)

1. Pharmacologic properties

a. Mechanism of action: blockade of β receptors
- **(1)** Decrease heart rate and contractility
- **(2)** Decrease blood pressure
- **(3)** Decrease renin release

b. Use: first-line therapy for hypertension, especially in patients with heart failure and previous MI

c. Adverse effects: central nervous system (CNS) depression, increased serum lipids, asthma, cardiac disturbances, sexual dysfunction

2. Selected drugs

a. Propranolol (nonselective): inhibitor of both β_1 and β_2 receptors

b. Atenolol (selective): β_1-selective, with a longer half-life ($t_{1/2}$) (6–9 h)
- **(1)** Better tolerated than propranolol in patients with **asthma**
- **(2)** Fewer CNS-related adverse effects than other β-adrenergic receptor antagonists (less lipid-soluble)

B. α_2-Adrenergic receptor agonists

1. Methyldopa

a. Mechanism of action
- This **centrally acting** agent is converted to α-methylnorepinephrine, which stimulates

TABLE 13-1 Selection of Antihypertensive Drugs

Patient Characteristic	Most Preferred Drugs	Least Preferred Drugs
Demographic Traits		
African heritage	Calcium channel blocker, thiazide diuretic	
Pregnancy	Methyldopa, hydralazine	ACE inhibitor, angiotensin receptor antagonist
Lifestyle Traits		
Physically active	ACE inhibitor, calcium channel blocker, α-blocker	β-Blocker
Noncompliance	Drug with once-daily dosage regimen	Centrally acting α-adrenoceptor agonist
Concomitant Conditions		
Angina pectoris	β-Blocker, diltiazem, verapamil	Hydralazine, minoxidil
Asthma, COPD	Calcium channel blocker, ACE inhibitor	β-Blocker
Benign prostatic hyperplasia	α-Blocker	—
Collagen disease	ACE inhibitor (but not captopril), calcium channel blocker	Hydralazine, methyldopa
Depression	ACE inhibitor, calcium channel blocker	Centrally acting α-adrenoceptor agonist, β-blocker, reserpine
Diabetes mellitus	ACE inhibitor, calcium channel blocker, angiotensin receptor antagonist	β-Blocker, diuretic
Gout	—	Diuretic
Heart failure	ACE inhibitor, diuretic, hydralazine	Calcium channel blocker
Hypercholesterolemia	α-Blocker, ACE inhibitor, calcium channel blocker	β-Blocker, thiazide
Migraine	β-Blocker, calcium channel blocker	—
Myocardial infarction	β-Blocker, ACE inhibitor	—
Osteoporosis	Thiazide	—
Peripheral vascular disease	ACE inhibitor, calcium channel blocker, α-blocker	β-Blocker

ACE, Angiotensin-converting enzyme; *COPD,* chronic obstructive pulmonary disease.

α_2-adrenergic receptors in the CNS to decrease sympathetic outflow.

b. Adverse effects: sedation, dry mouth, postural hypotension, failure of ejaculation, anemia
- Methyldopa, which triggers antibody production (positive Coombs' test), causes **autoimmune hemolytic anemia.**

Patients receiving methyldopa may have a positive Coombs' test.

2. Clonidine

a. Mechanism of action: direct stimulation of **central α_2-receptors,** decreasing sympathetic and increasing parasympathetic tone to reduce both blood pressure and heart rate

Withdrawal from clonidine should occur slowly (over 1 week) to avoid a hypertensive crisis.

b. Adverse effects: dry mouth, sedation, postural hypotension
- **Withdrawal from high-dose therapy may result in life-threatening hypertensive crises due to increased sympathetic activity.**

C. α_1-Adrenergic receptor antagonists
- **Examples: prazosin, doxazosin, terazosin** (see Chapter 5)

1. Mechanism of action
- α_1-Adrenergic receptor antagonists **block α_1-receptors** selectively on arterioles and venules, thus decreasing peripheral vascular resistance.
- These drugs **relax the bladder neck** and the **prostate** by blocking the α_1-adrenergic receptors located in smooth muscle.

Terazosin is recommended for the treatment of BPH.

2. Uses: hypertension, benign prostatic hyperplasia (BPH)

3. Adverse effects: postural hypotension, dizziness

IV. Vasodilators
- Directly relax vascular smooth muscles (Figure 13-1)

A. Hydralazine

1. Pharmacokinetics
- **Oral bioavailability** is dependent on the acetylation phenotype (*N*-acetyltransferase) of patients.
- About 50% of patients are "slow" acetylators and 50% are "fast" acetylators.

2. Mechanism of action
- **Relaxation of the vascular smooth muscle of the arterioles** causes reflex tachycardia and increased renin secretion, which may be blocked by propranolol (or by centrally acting agents).

3. Uses: heart failure (with nitrates), **hypertension** (safe in pregnancy)

4. Adverse effects

a. Drug-induced systemic lupus erythematosus–like syndrome, which is reversible on drug withdrawal (10–20%)

b. Peripheral neuritis with paresthesias (numbness, pain, and tingling in the hands and feet)
- This effect can be prevented by the administration of **pyridoxine.**

B. Minoxidil: potent arteriolar dilator

1. Mechanism of action
- Induction of delay in the hydrolysis of cyclic adenosine monophosphate (cAMP) via inhibition of phosphodiesterase may contribute to vasodilatory action.

2. Uses: hypertension, facilitation of hair growth

3. Adverse effects: tachyphylaxis, palpitations

C. Sodium nitroprusside

1. Pharmacokinetics
- **Metabolic conversion to cyanide and thiocyanate** may cause severe toxic reactions if the infusion of sodium nitroprusside is continued for several days.

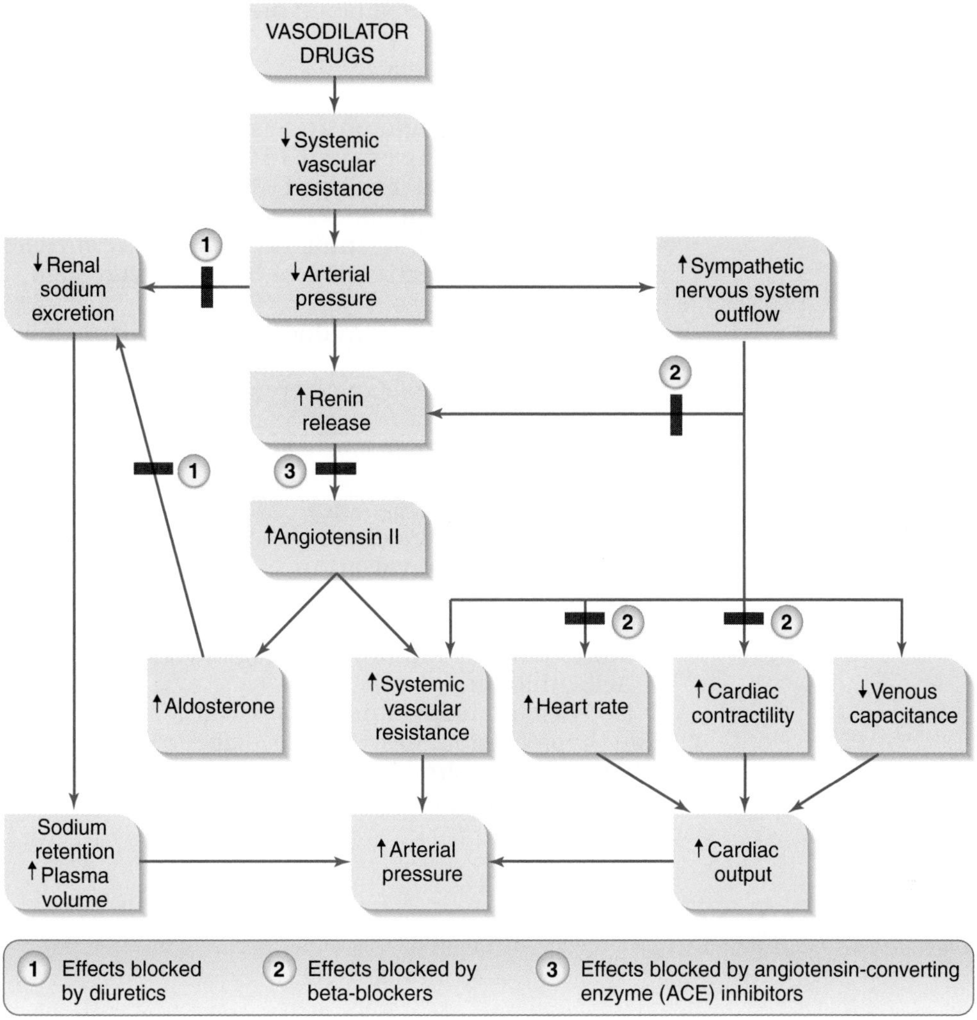

Figure 13-1 Compensatory response to vasodilators when used to treat hypertension.

- Arterial pressure may be titrated by intravenous administration because of its **rapid action** and **short $t_{1/2}$** (minutes).

2. **Mechanism of action**
   a. Occurs via the **release of nitric oxide**
   b. Involves relaxation of smooth muscle in arterioles and venules
   c. Decreases both preload and afterload
3. **Uses: hypertensive emergencies,** acute MI, aortic dissection
4. **Adverse effects:** hypertension, tachycardia, cyanide toxicity

D. Calcium channel blockers (see Chapter 12)
- **Examples: nifedipine, diltiazem, verapamil** (slow-release or long-acting preparations)

Relative efficacy of calcium channel blockers as vasodilators: nifedipine > diltiazem > verapamil

Relative efficacy of calcium channel blockers in control of heart rate: verapamil > diltiazem > nifedipine

Hyperkalemia, dry cough, and angioedema often occur in patients taking ACE inhibitors.

1. **Uses:** control of elevated blood pressure by relaxation of smooth muscles
2. **Adverse effects:** edema

V. Drugs That Affect the Angiotensin System

A. Angiotensin-converting enzyme (ACE) inhibitors

- **Examples: captopril, enalapril**

1. **Mechanism of action:** blockade of conversion of angiotensin I to angiotensin II by inhibiting converting enzyme
   a. **Inhibition of inactivation of bradykinin** (cough, angioedema)
   b. **Increased plasma renin** due to decrease in angiotensin II and aldosterone
2. **Uses:** hypertension, diabetic nephropathy, heart failure, post-MI
3. **Adverse effects:** proteinuria, acute renal failure in patients with renal artery stenosis
4. **Contraindication:** pregnancy

B. Angiotensin receptor blockers

- **Examples: losartan, valsartan**

1. **Mechanism of action:** blockade of angiotensin II type 1 (AT_1) receptors
   - More complete inhibition of angiotensin effects than ACE inhibitors
   - No effect on bradykinin metabolism
2. **Uses:** hypertension, heart failure, diabetic nephropathy
3. **Adverse effects:** similar to those of the ACE inhibitors, but no cough and angioedema

14

Other Cardiovascular Drugs

Target Topics

- Drugs used to treat angina
- Drugs used to lower lipid levels
- Drugs used to treat heart failure

I. General Considerations

A. The goal of antianginal therapy is to **decrease oxygen demand** on myocardial tissue or **increase oxygen supply** (Figure 14-1).

B. Antianginal drugs are used to treat **angina pectoris** caused by myocardial ischemia (Box 14-1).

C. Coronary blood flow depends on aortic diastolic pressure, duration of diastole, and resistance of the coronary vascular bed.

D. Antianginal drugs have vasodilator action on the coronary, cerebral, and peripheral vascular beds.

Objective of antianginal therapy: to balance O_2 demand with O_2 supply in myocardial tissue

II. Antianginal Drugs

A. Nitrites and nitrates

1. Pharmacokinetics

- Classification is primarily based on **duration of action.**

a. Rapid-acting agents: amyl nitrite (inhalation); nitroglycerin (intravenous, sublingual)

b. Long-acting agents: isosorbide dinitrate (oral, sublingual); nitroglycerin (transdermal, ointment)

2. Mechanism of action

- **Release of the nitrite ion,** which is metabolized to nitric oxide, activates guanylyl cyclase, increasing cGMP levels, which in turn relaxes vascular smooth muscle.

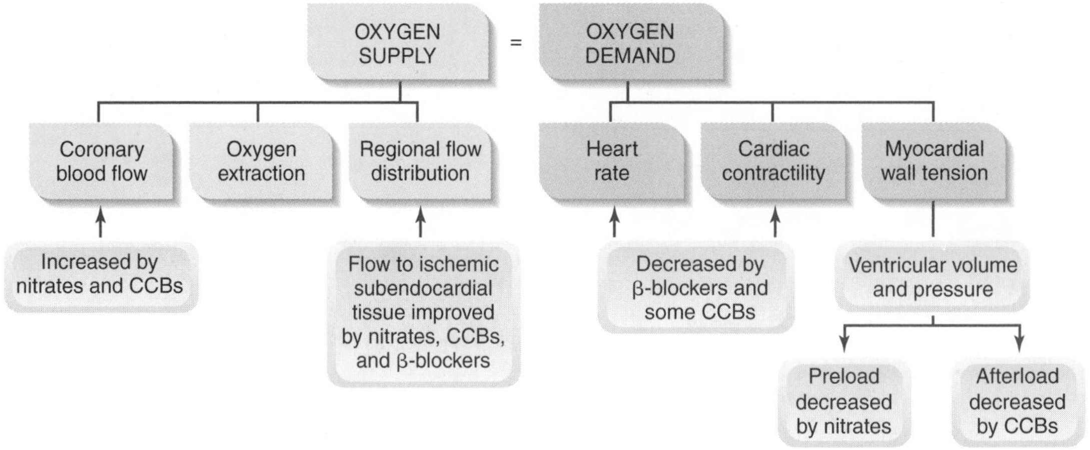

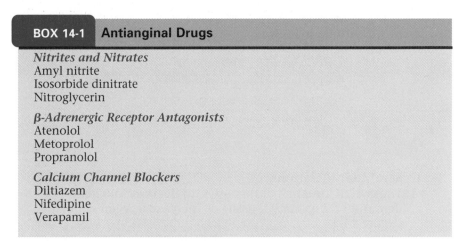

Figure 14-1 Effects of nitrates, calcium channel blockers *(CCBs),* and β-blockers on myocardial oxygen supply and demand.

BOX 14-1 Antianginal Drugs

Nitrites and Nitrates
Amyl nitrite
Isosorbide dinitrate
Nitroglycerin

β-Adrenergic Receptor Antagonists
Atenolol
Metoprolol
Propranolol

Calcium Channel Blockers
Diltiazem
Nifedipine
Verapamil

Nitrate-induced vasodilation results in lower cardiac oxygen demand.

a. **Nitrates** do *not* increase total coronary blood flow in patients with ischemia, but they **redistribute blood to ischemic areas**, thus correcting the myocardial oxygen imbalance (see Figure 14-1).
b. Nitrate-induced **vasodilation increases venous capacitance and decreases arteriole resistance**, thereby reducing preload and afterload and lowering oxygen demand.

3. **Uses**
   a. Treatment of acute **angina pectoris**, prophylaxis of angina attacks
   b. Treatment of **heart failure** (with hydralazine)
   c. Treatment of **hypertensive emergencies**, control of perioperative hypertension
4. **Adverse effects**
   a. **Headaches** (usually transient), dizziness, hypotension, flushing

b. Reflex tachycardia
c. Methemoglobinemia (nitrites)
5. Tolerance
a. Develops and disappears rapidly (2–3 days)
- **Headaches disappear as tolerance develops.**

b. Limits the usefulness of nitrates in continuous prophylaxis
- To counter tolerance, patches are usually removed between 12:00 AM and 6 AM.

B. β-Adrenergic receptor antagonists (see Chapter 5)
1. Mechanism of action
- β-Adrenergic receptor antagonists **inhibit the reflex tachycardia** produced by nitrates.
- Subsequent reductions in heart rate and blood pressure decrease myocardial oxygen requirements.

2. Use: angina (in combination with other drugs, such as nitrates)

β Blockers reduce heart rate and blood pressure, leading to relief of angina and improved exercise tolerance.

C. Calcium channel blockers (see Chapter 12)
1. Mechanism of action
a. Block calcium movement into cells, inhibiting excitation-contraction coupling in myocardial and smooth muscle cells
b. Reduce heart rate, blood pressure, and contractility
2. Uses: coronary artery disease and Prinzmetal's or variant angina
3. Adverse effects: flushing, edema, dizziness

Calcium channel blockers are effective in the treatment of Prinzmetal's angina.

III. Drugs That Affect Cholesterol and Lipid Metabolism

A. General considerations
1. Hyperlipidemia is defined as **high levels of serum lipids.**
a. Primary hyperlipidemia is caused by **genetic predisposition.**
b. Secondary hyperlipidemia arises as a **complication of disease states,** such as diabetes, hypothyroidism, Cushing's disease, and acromegaly.
2. Atherosclerosis may result from high levels of plasma lipids, although the exact pathogenesis remains unknown.
3. Therapy
a. First-line treatment: control by diet and lifestyle modifications
b. Second-line treatment: pharmacologic intervention (Table 14-1)
- The metabolism of lipoproteins and the mechanism of action of some antihyperlipidemic drugs are summarized in Figure 14-2.

B. Bile acid–binding resins (Box 14-2)
- **Examples:** cholestyramine, colestipol

1. Mechanism of action
a. Resins **bind bile acids** in the intestine to form an insoluble, nonabsorbable complex that is excreted in the feces along with the unchanged resin.
b. This action causes an increase in the conversion of

plasma cholesterol to bile acids, thus **decreasing plasma cholesterol levels.**

2. Uses
   a. Elevated **low-density lipoprotein (LDL)** level (in combination with other drugs); heterozygous familial hypercholesterolemia
   b. Reduction of itching in cholestasis
3. **Adverse effects**
   a. **Nausea, malabsorption of fat-soluble vitamins** and other drugs such as digoxin, iron salts, tetracycline, and warfarin in the intestine due to the binding of these drugs to the resin
   b. **Constipation**

TABLE 14-1 Effects of Drug Therapy on Serum Lipid Concentrations

Drug or Class	LDL Concentration	HDL Concentration	Total Decrease in Triglyceride Concentration	Other Effects
HMG-CoA reductase inhibitors	↓ 10–15%	↑ 10%	↓ 10–20%	Increase in hepatic LDL receptors
Bile acid-binding resins	↓ 20–40%	↑ 0–2%	↑ 0–5%	Increase in hepatic LDL receptors
Gemfibrozil	↓ 10%	↑ 10–25%	↓ 40–50%	Activation of lipoprotein lipase
Niacin	↓ 10–15%	↑ 10%	↓ 20–80%	Decrease in lipolysis and lipoprotein levels

HDL, High-density lipoprotein; *LDL,* low-density lipoprotein.

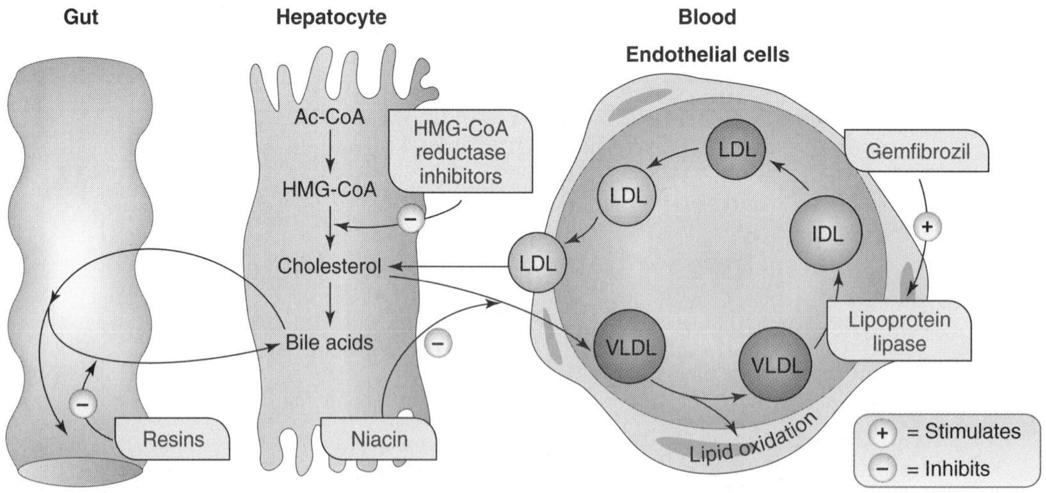

Figure 14-2 Sites of action and mechanisms of drugs used in the treatment of hyperlipidemia. The bile acid resins decrease the reabsorption of bile acids from the gut. The HMG-CoA reductase inhibitors block the rate-limiting step of cholesterol synthesis. Niacin affects lipid metabolism, transport, and clearance. Gemfibrozil stimulates lipoprotein lipase. *IDL,* Intermediate-density lipoproteins; *LDL,* low-density lipoproteins; *VLDL,* very low–density lipoproteins.

C. HMG-CoA reductase inhibitors
- **Examples: atorvastatin, lovastatin, pravastatin** ("statins")

1. **Mechanism of action**
   a. The "**statins**" **inhibit action of HMG-CoA reductase** (the rate-limiting step in cholesterol synthesis), thereby decreasing cholesterol levels.
   b. The resulting increase in synthesis of LDL cholesterol receptors in cell walls decreases plasma cholesterol.
2. **Use: elevated LDL plasma levels**
3. **Adverse effects**
   a. **Elevated hepatic enzymes**
   b. **Skeletal muscle toxicity** (elevated creatine kinase), myositis

D. Lipoprotein lipase stimulators

1. **Gemfibrozil**
   a. **Mechanism of action**
      (1) Activates **lipoprotein lipase,** promoting delivery of triglycerides to adipose tissue
      (2) Decreases hepatic triglyceride production
      (3) Interferes with the formation of very low density lipoprotein (VLDL) in the liver
   b. **Uses:** hypertriglyceridemia, hyperlipoproteinemia
   c. **Adverse effects:** myalgias, cholelithiasis
2. **Niacin (nicotinic acid)**
   a. **Mechanism of action**
      (1) **Reduces hepatic VLDL secretion** (like gemfibrozil)
      (2) **Enhances VLDL clearance** by activating lipoprotein lipase (like gemfibrozil)
      (3) **Decreases LDL and triglycerides** and **increases** high-density lipoproteins (**HDLs**)
   b. **Uses:** almost **all types of hyperlipidemia,** especially those that are genetically induced
      - Used in combination with bile acid resins

Peripheral vasodilation occurs frequently with niacin; pretreatment with aspirin prevents this development.

BOX 14-2 Drugs Used in the Treatment of Hypercholesterolemia

Bile Acid–Binding Resins
Cholestyramine
Colestipol

HMG-CoA Reductase Inhibitors
Atorvastatin
Fluvastatin
Lovastatin
Pravastatin
Simvastatin

Lipoprotein Lipase Stimulators
Gemfibrozil
Niacin

BOX 14-3 Drugs Used in the Treatment of Heart Failure

Digitalis Glycosides
Digitoxin
Digoxin

Vasodilators
Hydralazine
Nitrates
Sodium nitroprusside

Diuretics
Loop
Furosemide

Potassium-sparing
Spironolactone

Thiazide
Hydrochlorothiazide

ACE Inhibitors
Captopril
Enalapril
Lisinopril

Angiotensin Receptor Antagonists
Losartan
Valsartan

β-Receptor Antagonists
Atenolol
Carvedilol
Metoprolol

c. Adverse effects
- **(1)** Generalized **pruritus** as a result of peripheral vasodilation, characterized by flushing, warmth, and burning or tingling of the skin, especially of the face or neck
- **(2)** Increased hepatic enzymes

IV. Inotropic Agents and Treatment of Heart Failure (Box 14-3)

- Drugs that should be considered in the treatment of heart failure include digitalis, β-adrenergic receptor antagonists, vasodilators (nitrates and hydralazine), diuretics, angiotensin receptor antagonists, and ACE inhibitors.

A. Digitalis glycosides (see Chapter 12)
- Digitalis glycosides have positive inotropic and electrophysiologic effects on the heart (Figure 14-3).
- These agents are derived from the leaves of the plant *Digitalis purpurea* (foxglove) or *D. lanata.*

1. Pharmacokinetics (Table 14-2)

2. Mechanism of action: inhibition of Na^+/K^+-activated ATPase, thus increasing the force of myocardial contraction by increasing available intracellular calcium

Digoxin has a low therapeutic index.

- **a.** Increase **vagal stimulation,** leading to decreased heart rate
- **b. Slow conduction** through the atrioventricular **(AV) node**

3. Uses: treatment of heart failure and control of ventricular rate in the management of atrial fibrillation

4. Adverse effects

a. Toxicity
- **(1) Nausea and vomiting**
- **(2) Mental status changes**

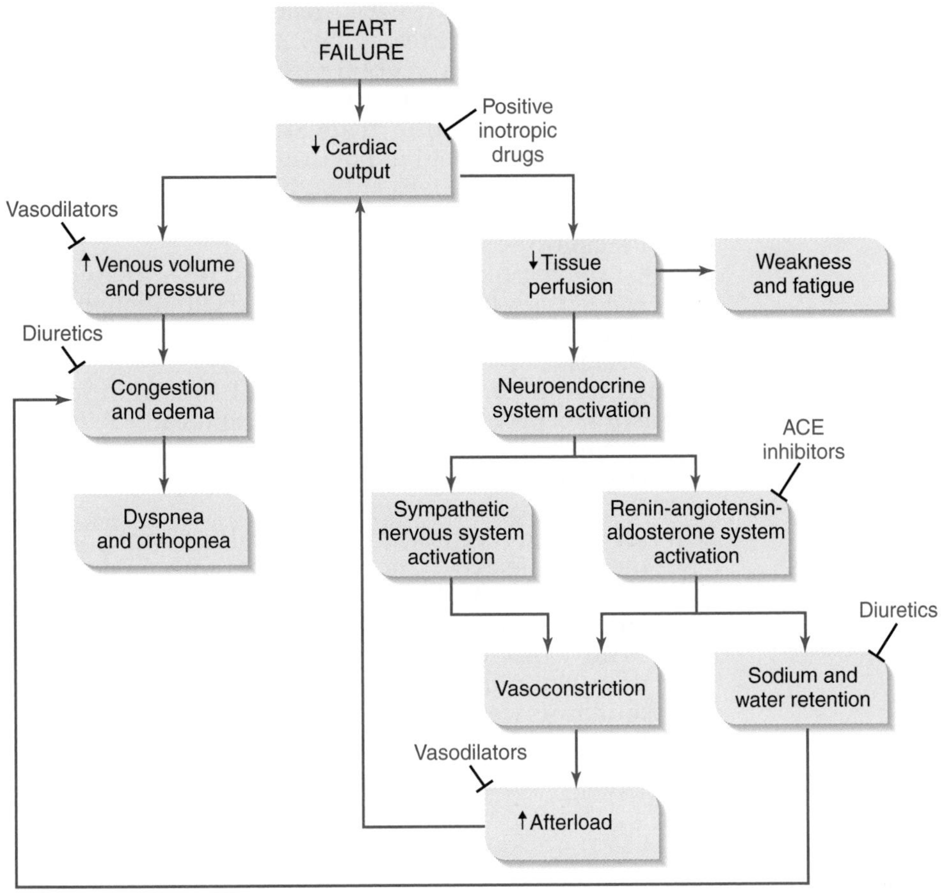

Figure 14-3 Algorithm of the pathogenesis and treatment of heart failure, indicating the sites where certain drugs may interfere with the development of heart failure. *ACE,* Angiotensin-converting enzyme.

TABLE 14-2 Pharmacokinetic Parameters of Digitalis Glycosides

Parameter	Digitoxin	Digoxin
Route of administration	Oral, intravenous	Oral, intravenous
Oral bioavailability (%)	> 90	75
Time to peak effect (hours)	6–12	3–6
Volume of distribution (L/kg)	0.6	6.3*
Plasma protein binding (%)	> 90	20–40
Half-life (hours)	168	40
Elimination	Hepatic and renal	Renal

*The large volume of distribution of digoxin is due to tissue protein binding; it is displaced by quinidine.

(3) **Changes on electrocardiogram:** decreased QT interval, increased PR interval, ST-segment depression

(4) **Changes in color vision** (green or yellow halos)

b. **Treatment of toxicity**

(1) **Discontinue medication**

(2) Correct either potassium or magnesium deficiency

(3) Give digitalis antibody (digoxin immune Fab, or Digibind) for severe toxicity

5. **Precautions**

- The **hypokalemia** that often occurs with diuretic therapy increases the toxicity associated with digitalis therapy.

B. Diuretics (see Chapter 15)

- Decrease edema

C. Angiotensin-converting enzyme (ACE) inhibitors and **angiotensin receptor antagonists** (see Chapter 13)

1. Decrease peripheral resistance
2. Decrease salt and water retention
3. Decrease tissue remodeling

D. β-Adrenergic receptor antagonists (see Chapter 5)

- Increase life expectancy in patients with mild and moderate congestive heart failure

E. Agonists in severe heart failure (dobutamine and dopamine)

- Positive inotropic agents that should be used for acute treatment only

F. Vasodilators (see Chapter 13)

- Decrease preload and afterload

15

Diuretics

Target Topics

- Carbonic anhydrase inhibitors
- Loop diuretics
- Thiazide diuretics
- Potassium-sparing diuretics
- Osmotic diuretics
- Drugs that affect water excretion

I. General Considerations

A. Role of the kidney

1. The kidney is the most important organ in **maintaining body fluid composition.**
2. It is the chief means of **excreting most drugs** and nonvolatile **metabolic waste products**.
3. It plays a fundamental role in **maintaining pH**, controlling levels of electrolytes and water, and conserving substances such as glucose and amino acids.

B. Functions of the renal nephrons

1. **Glomerular filtration**
   - **a.** Blood is forced into the glomerulus and filtered through capillaries into the glomerular capsule.
     - The **glomerular filtration rate** (GFR) is **120 mL/min.** GFR = 120 mL/min
   - **b. Plasma filtrate** is composed of fluids and soluble constituents.
   - **c.** Substances normally *not* filtered include cells, plasma proteins or substances bound to them, lipids, and other macromolecules.
     - Approximately 99% of the filtrate is **reabsorbed.**
2. **Tubular secretion**

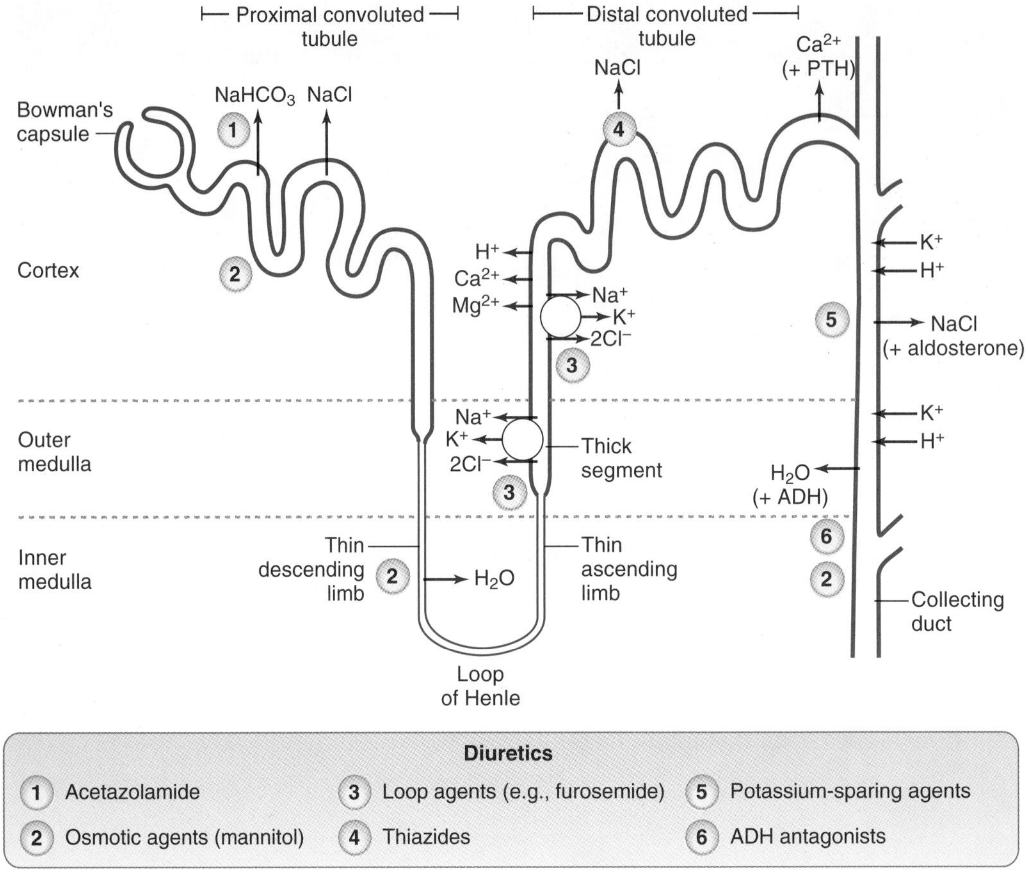

Figure 15-1 Tubule transport systems and sites of action of diuretics. *ADH,* Antidiuretic hormone; *PTH,* parathyroid hormone.

a. This process involves the movement of substances from the blood into the renal tubular lumen.

b. **Many drugs** (e.g., penicillins, glucuronide conjugates of drugs) are **actively secreted** by anion or cation transport systems.

II. Diuretics

- **Classification** is based on **sites** (Figure 15-1) and **mechanisms of action** (Table 15-1).

A. Carbonic anhydrase inhibitors (Box 15-1)

- **Examples: acetazolamide, dorzolamide**

1. Carbonic anhydrase inhibitors act in the proximal renal tubules, changing the composition of urine by increasing bicarbonate, sodium, and potassium excretion.

2. This effect lasts only 3–4 days.

B. Loop (high-ceiling) diuretics

- **Examples: ethacrynic acid, furosemide**

TABLE 15-1 Mechanisms, Uses, and Adverse Effects of Different Diuretics

Drug Class (Agent)	Mechanism	Uses	Adverse Effects
Carbonic anhydrase inhibitors (acetazolamide)	Inhibit carbonic anhydrase in proximal tubule, changing composition of urine	Glaucoma Urinary alkalinization Acute mountain sickness Pseudotumor cerebri	Hyperchloremic anion gap metabolic acidosis
Loop diuretics (furosemide)	Inhibit $Na^+/K^+/2Cl^-$ symport along thick ascending limb of loop of Henle	Acute pulmonary edema Refractory edema Hypertension Hyperkalemia Ascites	Hyperglycemia Hyperuricemia Hypocalcemia Dehydration Hypokalemia Metabolic alkalosis
Loop diuretics (ethacrynic acid)	Inhibit sulfhydryl-catalyzed enzyme systems responsible for reabsorption of sodium and chloride in proximal and distal tubules	Edema Sulfonamide sensitivity	Ototoxicity
Thiazide diuretics (hydrochlorothiazide)	Inhibit Na^+/Cl^- symport in distal convoluted tubule	Hypertension Heart failure Nephrolithiasis Nephrogenic diabetes insipidus	Hypokalemic metabolic alkalosis Hypomagnesemia Hypercalcemia Hyperlipidemia Hyperglycemia Hyperuricemia
Potassium-sparing diuretics (triamterene)	Inhibit Na^+/K^+ ion exchange in distal tubule and collecting duct	Adjunctive treatment of edema hypertension in combination with thiazides or loop diuretics Antagonize potassium loss associated with other diuretics	Cardiac arrhythmias from hyperkalemia
Potassium-sparing diuretics (spironolactone)	Block binding of aldosterone to receptors in cells of distal renal tubules	Diagnose primary hyperaldosteronism Treat polycystic ovary syndrome, hirsutism, ascites, and heart failure	Gynecomastia
Osmotic diuretics (mannitol)	Increase osmotic gradient between blood and tissues and remove water because diuretic is filtered and not reabsorbed	Maintain urine flow in acute renal failure Treat acute oliguria Reduce intracranial pressure and cerebral edema Treat acute glaucoma	Electrolyte imbalances Expansion of extracellular fluid

BOX 15-1 Diuretics

Carbonic Anhydrase Inhibitors
Acetazolamide
Dorzolamide

Loop Diuretics
Bumetanide
Ethacrynic acid
Furosemide
Torsemide

Thiazide and Thiazide-like Diuretics
Hydrochlorothiazide
Indapamide
Metolazone

Potassium-sparing Diuretics
Aldosterone Antagonists
Spironolactone

Sodium Channel Blockers
Amiloride
Triamterene

Osmotic Diuretics
Glycerol
Mannitol

- Loop diuretics cause a **profound diuresis** (much greater than that produced by thiazides) and a **decreased preload** to the heart.
- These drugs are useful in patients with renal impairment because they retain their effectiveness when creatinine clearance is less than 30 mL/min (normal = 120 mL/min).

1. **Ethacrynic acid**
   a. **Mechanism of action:** inhibition of sulfhydryl-catalyzed enzyme systems, which is responsible for reabsorption of sodium and chloride in the proximal and distal tubules
   b. **Uses**
      (1) **Hypersensitivity to sulfonamide diuretics** such as thiazides, furosemide (major use)
      (2) **Edema** related to heart failure or cirrhosis
   c. **Adverse effects:** ototoxicity, leading to hearing loss and tinnitus
2. **Furosemide**
   - This drug is structurally related to thiazides and has many of the properties of those diuretics.

   a. **Mechanism of action:** inhibition of reabsorption of sodium and chloride by **blocking $Na^+/K^+/2Cl^-$ symport in the ascending limb of the loop of Henle**
   b. **Uses:** hypertension, heart failure, ascites, hypercalcemia, pulmonary edema
   c. **Adverse effects:** dehydration, hyperglycemia, hypokalemia, hyperuricemia, metabolic alkalosis

Loop diuretics and thiazides cause hypokalemia; administer them in combination with a potassium-sparing diuretic.

C. Thiazide diuretics

- These diuretics differ from each other only in potency and duration of action.
- The most commonly used thiazide diuretic is **hydrochlorothiazide.**

1. **Mechanism of action:** reduction in plasma volume, which increases plasma renin activity and aldosterone excretion, resulting in a decrease in renal blood flow and GFR

Use thiazide diuretics in patients who form calcium calculi because these drugs decrease calcium excretion, thus preventing calculi formation.

2. **Uses:** hypertension, heart failure, edema, renal calculi
3. **Adverse effects:** hyperkalemia, metabolic alkalosis, hyperlipidemia, hyperuricemia, hypomagnesemia

D. Potassium-sparing diuretics

- These drugs are used in combination with other diuretics to protect against hypokalemia.

1. **Aldosterone antagonists**
   - **Example: spironolactone**

   a. **Mechanism of action:** competitive inhibition of the aldosterone receptor

   b. **Uses**
      (1) Diagnosis of **primary hyperaldosteronism**
      (2) Treatment of **heart failure**
      (3) **Adjunct with thiazides or loop diuretics to prevent hypokalemia**

   c. **Adverse effects: antiandrogenic effects,** such as impotence, gynecomastia, and hyperkalemia
2. **Sodium channel blockers**
   - **Examples: triamterene, amiloride**

   a. When potassium loss is minimal, sodium channel blockers cause only a slight reduction in potassium excretion.

   b. When potassium renal clearance is increased by loop diuretics or mineralocorticoids, these drugs cause a significant decrease in potassium excretion.

Use thiazide diuretics cautiously in patients with diabetes mellitus, gout, and hyperlipidemia, as well as those who are receiving digitalis glycosides.

E. Osmotic diuretics

- **Examples: mannitol, glycerol**
- Any agent that is filtered and not completely reabsorbed

1. **Mechanism of action:** rise in blood osmolality
   - This action **increases the osmotic gradient** between blood and tissues.
   - It **facilitates the flow of fluid** out of the tissues (including the brain and the eye) and into the interstitial fluid.
2. **Uses: increased intracranial pressure, glaucoma**
3. **Adverse effects:** circulatory overload, pulmonary edema

III. Agents That Affect Water Excretion

A. Vasopressin (antidiuretic hormone, or ADH)

- ADH is a **peptide hormone** synthesized in and secreted by the hypothalamus and stored in and released from the posterior pituitary.
- Its antidiuretic effects are due to **increased reabsorption of water** at the renal collecting ducts.

1. **Mechanism of action:** stimulation of adenylyl cyclase activity, which leads to:

   a. **Increased cyclic adenosine monophosphate** (cAMP) in the distal convoluted tubule and collecting duct

   b. **Increased reabsorption of water** and **decreased urine flow**

   c. **Increased urine osmolality,** with maintenance of serum osmolality within an acceptable physiologic range (280–307 mOsm/kg)

2. **Uses**
   a. **Central** (neurogenic) **diabetes insipidus** caused by a deficiency of pituitary vasopressin secretion
   b. Adjunct in treatment of esophageal varices, hemorrhage, upper gastrointestinal bleeding, variceal bleeding
3. **Adverse effect:** water intoxication (overhydration)

B. Desmopressin
- Administered orally and intranasally
- More potent and much longer acting than vasopressin

1. **Mechanism of action:** structural analogue of vasopressin
   - 4000:1 antidiuretic-to-vasopressor activity
2. **Uses**
   a. Usual agent for **central** (neurogenic) **diabetes insipidus**
   b. Nocturnal enuresis, hemophilia A, von Willebrand's disease
3. **Adverse effects:** water intoxication (overhydration)

C. ADH antagonists
- ADH antagonists inhibit effects of ADH at the collecting tubule.

1. **Lithium salts**
   a. **Mechanism of action: reduction in vasopressin (V_2) receptor–mediated stimulation** of adenylyl cyclase in the medullary collecting tubule of the nephron, thus increasing renal sodium and potassium clearance
   b. **Use:** syndrome of inappropriate ADH (**SIADH**)
      - **Last choice for treatment**
   c. **Adverse effects:** polyuria that is usually, but not always, reversible
2. **Demeclocycline**
   - Attenuates antidiuretic effects of vasopressin

   a. **Mechanism of action:** reduced formation of cAMP, limiting the action of demeclocycline in the distal portion of the convoluted tubules and collecting ducts of the kidneys
   b. **Use:** SIADH
   c. **Adverse effects: nephrogenic diabetes insipidus** (treated with thiazide diuretics or amiloride), renal failure

16

Drugs Used in the Treatment of Coagulation Disorders

Target Topics

- Antithrombotic drugs
- Heparins
- Oral anticoagulants
- Fibrinolytic drugs
- Hemostatic drugs

I. General Considerations

A. Clot formation at the tissue level results from complex interactions (Figure 16-1).

- **Enzymatic pathway for clot formation** (Figure 16-2)

B. Hematologic drugs

- These agents have various clinical indications (Table 16-1).

1. Drugs used to break up thrombi

a. Antithrombotic drugs

b. Anticoagulant drugs

c. Fibrinolytic drugs

2. Hemostatic drugs, which prevent bleeding

II. Antithrombotic Drugs (antiplatelet drugs)

- Antithrombotic drugs interfere with platelet adhesion and aggregation (Box 16-1; see Figure 16-2).

A. Aspirin

- This **nonsteroidal anti-inflammatory drug (NSAID)** is also used as an analgesic and as an antipyretic (see Chapter 18).

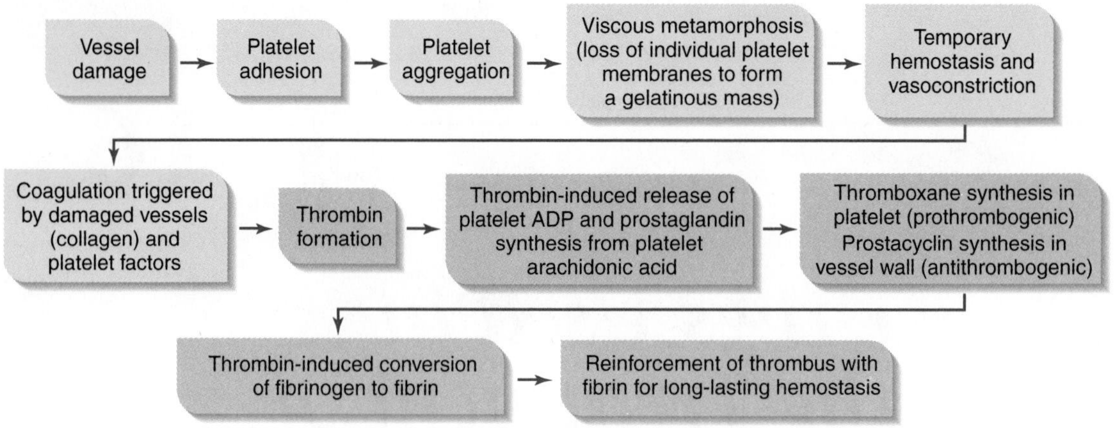

Figure 16-1 Events occurring after vessel damage that lead to the formation of fibrin clots. Note the involvement of both platelets and the coagulation pathway. *ADP,* Adenosine diphosphate.

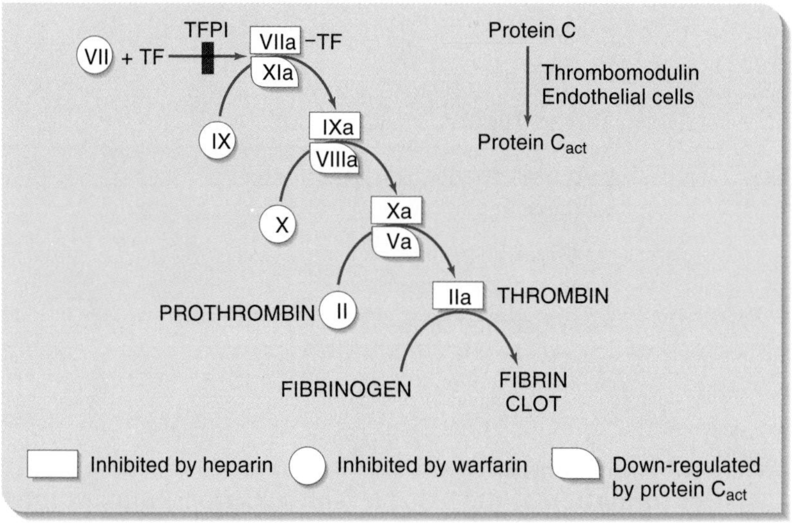

Figure 16-2 Intrinsic and extrinsic pathways of coagulation. Tissue factor is generated by the extrinsic pathway and is important in maintaining the velocity of the intrinsic pathway. Warfarin inhibits the hepatic synthesis of factors VII, IX, X, and II. Heparins accelerate the destruction of activated factors by antithrombin III. Unfractionated heparins have their greatest effect on factor IIa, whereas low molecular weight heparins have their greatest effect on factor Xa. *Protein C_{act},* Activated protein C; *TF,* tissue factor; *TFPI,* tissue factor pathway inhibitor.

1. **Mechanism of action**
   a. Aspirin inhibits synthesis of **thromboxane A_2 (TXA_2)**, a potent platelet aggregator, by **irreversible** acetylation of cyclooxygenase.
   b. TXA_2 increases cAMP in platelets, causing aggregation.
   c. Low-dose aspirin therapy **inhibits cyclooxygenase** to prevent synthesis of TXA_2 without decreasing the synthesis of prostacyclin (PGI_2), which inhibits platelet aggregation

TABLE 16-1 Clinical Uses of Anticoagulant, Antiplatelet, and Fibrinolytic Drugs

Clinical Use	Primary Drug*	Secondary Drug*
Acute thrombotic stroke	Fibrinolytic drug	—
Artificial heart valve	Warfarin or aspirin	Dipyridamole
Atrial fibrillation	Heparin, warfarin, or LMWH	Aspirin
Deep vein thrombosis		
Treatment	Heparin, warfarin, or LMWH	—
Surgical prophylaxis	LMWH	Heparin
Myocardial infarction		
Treatment	Fibrinolytic drug, heparin, aspirin, or abciximab	—
Prevention	Aspirin	—
Percutaneous transluminal coronary angioplasty	Abciximab, heparin, aspirin, or clopidogrel	—
Pulmonary embolism	Fibrinolytic drug, heparin, warfarin, or LMWH	—
Stroke	Aspirin, clopidogrel, or warfarin	—
Transient ischemic attacks	Aspirin	Warfarin
Unstable angina	Aspirin, abciximab, heparin, or LMWH	—

LMWH, Low molecular weight heparin.
*If aspirin is contraindicated or not tolerated, ticlopidine may be used. If warfarin is contraindicated or not tolerated, another oral anticoagulant may be used.

BOX 16-1 Antithrombotic Drugs

Platelet Aggregation Inhibitors
Aspirin
Anagrelide
Clopidogrel
Dipyridamole
Ticlopidine

Platelet-receptor Glycoprotein Inhibitors
Abciximab
Eptifibatide
Tirofiban

- Higher doses of aspirin inhibit synthesis of both TXA_2 and PGI_2.

2. **Uses** (see Table 16-1)
3. **Adverse effects**
   a. **Gastrointestinal (GI) irritation and bleeding**
   b. **Tinnitus,** respiratory alkalosis followed by metabolic acidosis (high doses)

Use low-dose aspirin to prevent thrombus formation.

B. Platelet aggregation inhibitors

1. **Ticlopidine and clopidogrel**
   a. **Mechanism of action**
      (1) Interferes with **adenosine diphosphate** (ADP)–induced binding of fibrinogen to platelet membrane at specific receptor sites

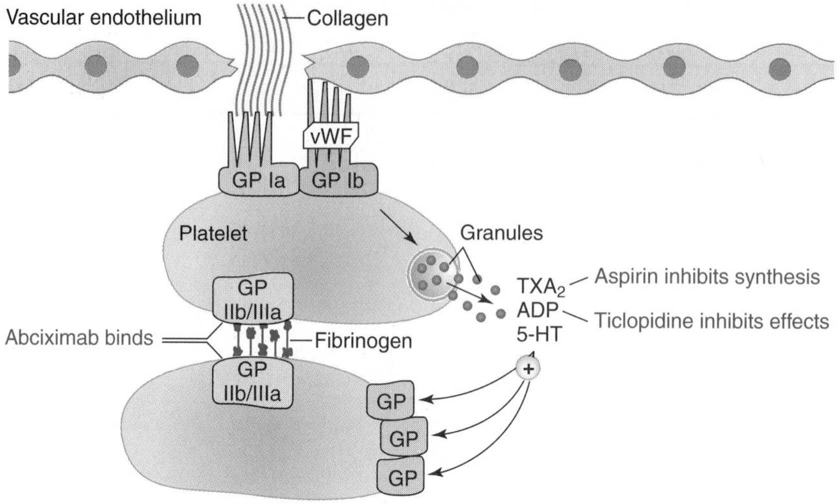

Figure 16-3 Platelet aggregation and sites of drug action. *ADP,* Adenosine diphosphate; *GP,* glycoprotein; *5-HT,* 5-hydroxytryptamine; *TXA_2,* thromboxane A_2; *vWF,* von Willebrand's factor.

(2) Inhibits **platelet aggregation** and platelet-platelet interactions

b. Uses

(1) Prevents **thrombotic stroke** (initial or recurrent) in patients who are intolerant or unresponsive to aspirin

(2) Prevents **thrombus formation** in patients with cardiac stents and in treatment of acute coronary syndromes (in combination with aspirin)

c. Adverse effects

- **Clopidogrel is associated with a lower incidence** of adverse cutaneous, GI, and hematologic reactions than ticlopidine.

(1) **Severe bone marrow toxicity,** including agranulocytosis, aplastic anemia, pancytopenia (rare)

(2) **Thrombotic thrombocytopenic purpura**

Because of the risk of bone marrow toxicity, patients who are receiving ticlopidine must have frequent CBCs with white cell differential.

2. Dipyridamole (vasodilator)

a. Mechanism of action

(1) Decreases platelet adhesion

(2) Potentiates action of prostacyclin, which is coupled to a cyclic adenosine monophosphate (cAMP)–generating system in platelets, causing vasodilation

b. Uses

(1) Prevention of **thrombotic stroke** (in combination with aspirin)

(2) As vasodilator during myocardial perfusion scans **(cardiac stress test)**

C. Abciximab (Figure 16-3): platelet-receptor glycoprotein inhibitor

- **Newer glycoprotein IIb and IIIa inhibitors** include eptifibatide and tirofiban.

BOX 16-2 Anticoagulants

Parenteral Anticoagulants
Heparin

Subcutaneous Anticoagulants
Low molecular weight heparins: enoxaparin, dalteparin

Oral Anticoagulants
Warfarin

TABLE 16-2 Comparison of the Properties of Heparin and Warfarin

Property	Heparin	Warfarin
Route of administration	Parenteral/subcutaneous	Oral
Site of action	Blood (in vivo and in vitro)	Liver
Onset of action	Immediate	Delayed; depends on half-lives of factors being replaced
Duration of action	4 hours	2–5 days
Mechanism of action	Accelerates action of antithrombin III to neutralize thrombin	Interferes with hepatic synthesis of vitamin K–dependent clotting factors
Laboratory control of dose	PTT	PT, INR
Antidote	Protamine sulfate	Vitamin K (phytonadione), fresh frozen plasma
Safety in pregnancy	Yes	No (fetal warfarin syndrome)

INR, International normalized ratio; *PT,* prothrombin time; *PTT,* partial thromboplastin time.

1. **Mechanism of action:** binds to the glycoprotein receptors IIb and IIIa on activated platelets
   - Abciximab **prevents binding of fibrinogen,** von Willebrand factor, and other adhesive molecules to the glycoprotein receptor.
   - When given intravenously, the drug produces rapid inhibition of platelet aggregation.
2. **Uses:** acute coronary syndromes, percutaneous transluminal coronary angioplasty
3. **Adverse effects:** bleeding, thrombocytopenia

III. **Anticoagulants** (Box 16-2)
- Anticoagulants may be differentiated on the basis of route of administration.
- These drugs have different pharmacologic properties (Tables 16-2 and 16-3).
-

A. **Parenteral anticoagulants (heparin)**
1. **Mechanism of action**
   - Heparin **accelerates** the **action of antithrombin III** to neutralize thrombin (factor IIa).
2. **Uses** (see Table 16-1)

Activated PTT (1.5–2× control): basis for calculation of the heparin dose

TABLE 16-3 Comparison Between Unfractionated Heparin and Low Molecular Weight Heparins

Property	Heparin	LMWH
Anti-Xa versus anti-IIa activity	1:1	2:1–4:1
PTT monitoring	Required	Not required
Inhibition of platelet function	++++	++
Endothelial cell-protein binding	Extensive	Minimal
Dose-dependent clearance	Yes	No
Elimination half-life	Short (50–90 min)	Long (2–5 times longer)

LMWH, Low molecular weight heparin; *PTT,* partial thromboplastin time.

PT (1.5× control) and INR (2–3): basis for calculation of the warfarin dose

Warfarin can cause fetal hemorrhage and skeletal malformations (fetal warfarin syndrome).

3. **Adverse effect:** bleeding, hyperkalemia, thrombocytopenia

B. Subcutaneous anticoagulants (low molecular weight heparins, or LMWHs)

- **Examples: enoxaparin, dalteparin**

1. **Mechanism of action:** antifactor Xa and antifactor IIa activity
2. **Uses**
   - **a.** Primary prevention of **deep vein thrombosis after hip replacement** (use is approved)
   - **b.** Other thrombolytic diseases (see Table 16-1)
3. **Adverse effects:** bleeding, allergic reactions

C. Oral anticoagulants (coumarin derivatives, including warfarin)

- Structurally related to vitamin K

1. **Mechanism of action:** inhibits γ-carboxylation of functional vitamin K–dependent clotting factors in the liver
2. **Uses** (see Table 16-1)
3. **Adverse effects:** bleeding
4. **Contraindications:** pregnancy, bleeding disorders
5. **Drug interactions**
   - Most relate to the cytochrome P450 system (Table 16-4).

IV. Fibrinolytic (Thrombolytic) Drugs (Box 16-3)

A. Basis of therapy

- When coagulation begins, plasminogen is converted to plasmin, a protease that limits the spread of new clots and dissolves the fibrin in established clots (Figure 16-4).

1. **Mechanism of action:** dissolution of clots by catalyzing formation of plasmin from its precursor, plasminogen
2. **Use** (see Table 16-1)
   - Thrombolytic drugs **must be given within 6 to 12 hours of a myocardial infarction** (MI) to limit cardiac damage and within 3 hours of a stroke.

B. Drugs used in thrombolytic therapy

1. **Alteplase and reteplase:** recombinant forms of human tissue plasminogen activator (t-PA)
   - **a. Mechanism of action:** direct cleavage of the bond in plasminogen

TABLE 16-4 Drugs That Interact With Warfarin

Drug	Mechanism of Interaction
Enhanced Response	
Allopurinol	Inhibits metabolism
Cimetidine	Inhibits metabolism
Ciprofloxacin	Inhibits metabolism
Co-trimoxazole	Inhibits metabolism
Erythromycin	Inhibits metabolism
Fluconazole	Inhibits metabolism
Metronidazole	Inhibits metabolism
Broad-spectrum antibiotics	Reduce availability of vitamin K
Sulfonamides	Displace from plasma albumin
Diminished Response	
Barbiturates	Induces hepatic microsomal enzymes
Carbamazepine	Induces hepatic microsomal enzymes
Primidone	Induces hepatic microsomal enzymes
Rifampin	Induces hepatic microsomal enzymes
Cholestyramine	Inhibits absorption
Estrogens	Stimulates synthesis of clotting factors
Vitamin K	Stimulates synthesis of clotting factors

BOX 16-3 Fibrinolytic Drugs

Forms of Recombinant Tissue Plasminogen Activator (t-PA)
Alteplase
Reteplase

Other Fibrinolytic Agents
Anistreplase
Streptokinase
Urokinase

- These thrombolytic drugs selectively work within the thrombi.

b. Uses
- In the United States, these agents are the most commonly used drugs for thrombolysis in **acute MI, pulmonary embolism**, and **acute stroke.**

Administer alteplase within 3 h of symptoms of ischemic stroke.

2. **Streptokinase:** nonenzymatic protein isolated from streptococci

a. Mechanism of action
- Streptokinase acts indirectly by **forming an activator complex** with plasminogen to **form plasmin.**
- Action occurs both within thrombi and in circulating blood, leading to lysis of both normal and pathologic thrombi.

b. Antidote: aminocaproic acid or tranexamic acid

3. **Urokinase:** enzyme derived from cultured human kidney cells

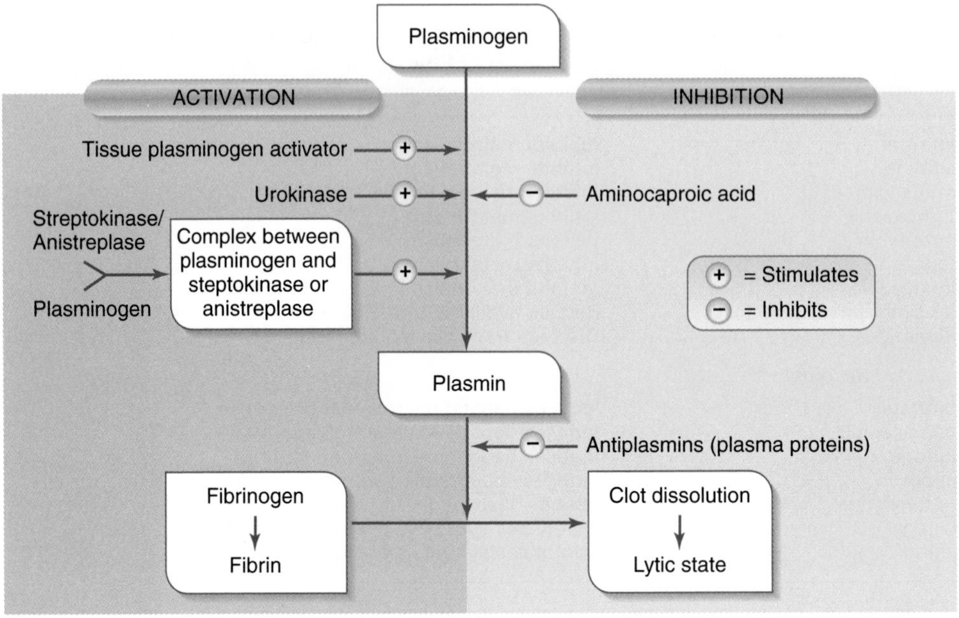

Figure 16-4 Site of action of drugs acting on the fibrinolytic system. Fibrinolytic drugs accelerate the conversion of plasminogen to plasmin, which is a protease that breaks down fibrinogen and fibrin to degradation products.

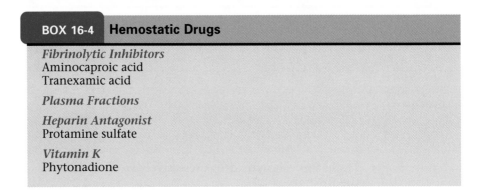

BOX 16-4 Hemostatic Drugs

Fibrinolytic Inhibitors
Aminocaproic acid
Tranexamic acid

Plasma Fractions

Heparin Antagonist
Protamine sulfate

Vitamin K
Phytonadione

4. Anistreplase
- Acetylated complex containing a combination of **streptokinase** and **human plasminogen**
- Preferentially works within the thrombi rather than converting free plasminogen to plasmin

V. Hemostatic Drugs (Box 16-4)

A. Vitamin K
- This **fat-soluble vitamin** is found in **leafy green vegetables.**
- It is produced by bacteria that colonize the human intestine and needs bile salts for absorption.
- It is required for γ-carboxylation of glutamate residues in prothrombin (factor II) and factors XII, IX, and X.

1. Uses
   a. **Prevention of hemorrhagic disease of the newborn** (intramuscular or subcutaneous)
   b. Treatment of dietary vitamin K deficiencies and **reversal of the effect of warfarin** (oral or parenteral)
2. **Adverse effects**
   - Hemolysis, jaundice, and hyperbilirubinemia occasionally occur in newborns.

B. Plasma fractions

- Available as factor VIII concentrate and factor IX concentrate, either from pooled human plasma or as recombinant antihemophilic factor

1. **Uses:** hemophilias A and B marked by deficiencies of factor VIII and factor IX
2. **Adverse effects:** risk of AIDS and hepatitis transmission from concentrated plasma fractions

C. Fibrinolytic inhibitor (aminocaproic acid)

- **Use:** systemic or urinary **hyperfibrinolysis** (as in aplastic anemia, abruptio placentae, hepatic cirrhosis)

D. Protamine sulfate

1. **Mechanism of action:** chemical antagonist of **heparin**
2. **Use:** hemorrhage associated with heparin overdose

17 Hematopoietic Drugs

Target Topics

- Treatment of iron deficiency anemia
- Treatment of folate and vitamin B_{12} deficiency anemia
- Treatment of deficiencies in hematopoietic factors

I. General Considerations

A. Causes of anemia

1. **Failure to produce sufficient red blood cells (RBCs)**
2. **Inadequate synthesis of hemoglobin**
3. **Destruction of RBCs**

B. Classification of types of anemia by mean corpuscular volume (MCV)

- Different conditions may lead to the development of the various types of anemia (Table 17-1).

1. **Microcytic:** smaller-than-normal RBCs and decreased MCV ($< 80\ \mu m^3$)
   - Iron deficiency results in small RBCs with insufficient hemoglobin (microcytic hypochromic anemia).
2. **Macrocytic:** larger-than-normal RBCs and increased MCV ($> 100\ \mu m^3$)
   - Both **folic acid deficiency** and **vitamin B_{12} deficiency** cause impaired production and maturation of erythroid precursors (macrocytic hyperchromic or megaloblastic anemia).
3. **Normocytic:** normal-sized RBCs and normal MCV (80–$100\ \mu m^3$)

C. Agents used to treat anemia (Box 17-1)

TABLE 17-1 Etiology of Anemia

Types of Anemia	Specific Cause/Pathophysiology
Microcytic Anemia	
Iron deficiency anemia	Increased need (e.g., growth, pregnancy, menstruation) Blood loss (e.g., gastrointestinal bleeding) Inadequate dietary intake Malabsorption
Anemia of chronic disease	Chronic infection, cancer, or liver disease Failure of increase in red blood cell production due to sequestration of iron in reticuloendothelial system
Thalassemia	Hereditary disorder characterized by decreased globulin chain production
Megaloblastic Anemia	
Folic acid deficiency anemia	Inadequate dietary intake Increased need during **pregnancy** Interference with utilization by other drugs (phenytoin, primidone, and phenobarbital; oral contraceptives; isoniazid) **Malabsorption syndromes** (e.g., high rates of cell turnover as in hemolytic anemia or alcoholism, or poor liver function)
Vitamin B_{12} deficiency anemia	**Pernicious anemia** (lack of intrinsic factor [IF]), which may occur following gastrectomy Lack of receptors for IF-vitamin B_{12} complex in ileum Fish tapeworm infestations Crohn's disease/ileotomy
Anemia due to bone marrow failure	Myelofibrosis and multiple myeloma: **direct effects** Myelosuppressive chemotherapy Deficiency of hematopoietic growth factors and hormones (as in chronic renal failure)

BOX 17-1 Hematopoietic Drugs

Minerals
Ferrous sulfate
Iron dextran

Vitamins
Folic acid
Vitamin B_{12}

Hematopoietic Growth Factors
Epoetin alfa
Filgrastim
Sargramostim

II. Minerals: Iron

A. Role of iron

1. Requirement for the **synthesis** of **hemoglobin** and **myoglobin**
2. **Cofactor** in enzymes (cytochromes)

B. Causes of iron deficiency (see Table 17-1)

C. Clinical use: iron deficiency anemia

- **Drug of choice: ferrous sulfate**

D. Adverse effects

Acute iron toxicity requires treatment with deferoxamine, an iron chelating drug.

1. **Acute toxicity** (when given orally): gastrointestinal (GI) irritation; necrosis; nausea; hematemesis; green, tarry stools
   - In children, acute iron toxicity is seen as **acute poisoning.**
2. **Chronic toxicity:** hemochromatosis

III. **Vitamins**

- Both **folic acid deficiency and vitamin B_{12} deficiency** can lead to **hematologic impairment** and show **hypersegmented polymorphonuclear neutrophils** as well as **anemia** on blood smear.

A. Folic acid

1. **Role of folic acid**
   - **a.** Folic acid is **essential for normal DNA synthesis** and **normal mitosis of proliferating cells.**
   - **b.** It is readily and completely **absorbed from the small intestine** by active transport.
2. **Causes of folic acid deficiency** (see Table 17-1)
3. **Clinical use**
   - **a. Treatment of folate deficiency**
   - **b. Prophylaxis of neural tube defects** (spina bifida) in pregnancy

B. Vitamin B_{12}

Neurologic changes may result from vitamin B_{12} deficiency.

1. **Role of vitamin B_{12}**
   - **a.** Vitamin B_{12} is essential for **normal DNA synthesis** (hematopoiesis).
   - **b.** It is essential for maintenance of myelin throughout the nervous system.
2. **Causes of vitamin B_{12} deficiency** (see Table 17-1)
3. **Tests for vitamin B_{12} deficiency**
   - **a.** The **Schilling test,** which uses radioactive cobalt to test the body's ability to take up vitamin B_{12} from the GI tract
   - **b.** The **gastric acidity test** and measurement of urinary methylmalonate levels
     - **Achlorhydria** (lack of gastric acidity) is associated with **lack of intrinsic factor.**
4. **Pharmacokinetics of vitamin B_{12}**
   - **a. Absorption** requires intrinsic factor, a glycoprotein synthesized by the parietal cells of the stomach.
     - Intrinsic factor binds vitamin B_{12}, and the intrinsic factor–vitamin B_{12} complex is absorbed in the ileum.
   - **b. Metabolism** involves enterohepatic circulation, and vitamin B_{12} is normally reabsorbed from the small intestine.
     - Depletion of the body's stores of vitamin B_{12} takes 3–6 years.
   - **c. Excretion** occurs mainly in **bile.**

5. Use: vitamin B_{12} deficiency
   a. Vitamin B_{12} is given intramuscularly once a month to patients who cannot absorb it from their diet.
   b. Preferred agent for long-term use: **cyanocobalamin**

IV. Hematopoietic Growth Factors

A. Role of hematopoietic growth factors
- These growth factors control the proliferation and differentiation of pluripotent stem cells.

B. Causes of bone marrow failure (see Table 17-1)

C. Drugs used to treat bone marrow failure

1. Epoetin alfa (erythropoietin)
- Erythropoietin is a glycoprotein that **stimulates RBC production.**

   a. Used in patients with **chronic renal failure,** those with cancer who are receiving chemotherapy, and those with AIDS
   b. Used illegally by athletes for its performance-enhancing properties

2. Sargramostim
- Recombinant **granulocyte-macrophage colony-stimulating factor** (GM-CSF)

   a. Promotes myeloid recovery in patients with non-Hodgkin's lymphoma, acute lymphoblastic leukemia, and Hodgkin's disease who are undergoing **bone marrow transplantation**
   b. Promotes myeloid recovery after standard-dose chemotherapy
   c. Treats drug-induced **bone marrow toxicity** or **neutropenia** associated with AIDS

3. Filgrastim
- **Granulocyte colony-stimulating factor** (G-CSF)

   a. Prevents and treats **chemotherapy-related febrile neutropenia**
   b. Promotes **myeloid recovery** in patients undergoing bone marrow transplantation

SECTION V

Analgesics

18

Nonsteroidal Anti-inflammatory Drugs and Other Nonopioid Analgesic-Antipyretic Drugs

Target Topics

- Aspirin
- Other NSAIDs
- COX-2 inhibitors
- Acetaminophen

I. General Considerations

A. **Nonsteroidal anti-inflammatory drugs** (NSAIDs) **inhibit the synthesis of eicosanoids from arachidonic acid** (Figure 18-1).

B. These drugs primarily **inhibit cyclooxygenase (COX)**, the enzyme responsible for the first step of prostaglandin synthesis.

- COX-1 is constituently expressed in many tissues, and COX-2 is induced in inflammatory cells.
- **Aspirin** is the **only irreversible inhibitor of COX.**

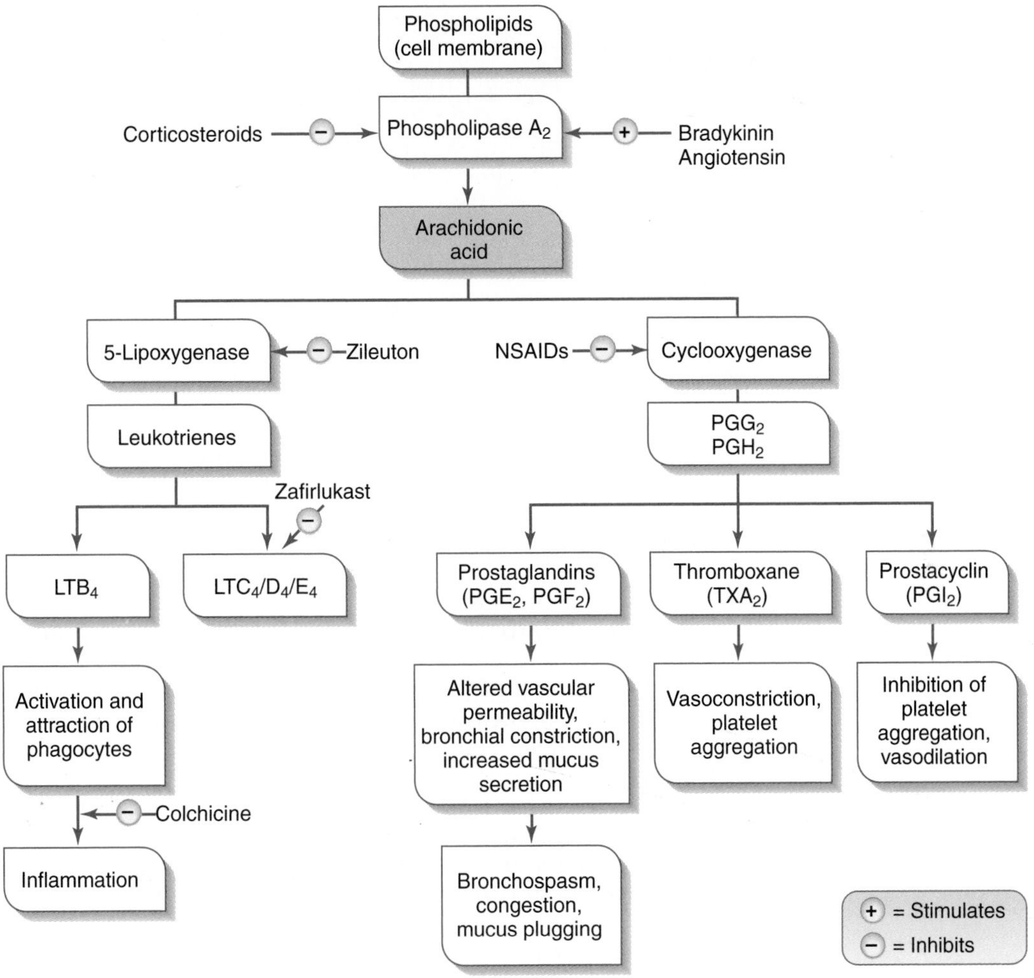

Figure 18-1 Schematic representation of the arachidonic acid pathway, which depicts the mediators formed from arachidonic acid, their biologic function, and drugs that stimulate or inhibit their formation. *NSAID,* Nonsteroidal anti-inflammatory drug.

II. NSAIDs (Box 18-1)

A. Aspirin and other salicylates

- Aspirin (acetylsalicylic acid), the **prototype NSAID,** is the standard against which all other NSAIDs are measured.

1. Mechanism of action

- Many effects of aspirin are due to **irreversible inhibition** of prostaglandin synthesis through acetylation of both COX-1 and COX-2.

Aspirin is an irreversible inhibitor of COX.

a. Antiplatelet effect: prolonged bleeding time but no change in the other coagulation indicators (e.g., prothrombin time, partial thromboplastin time)

b. Antithrombotic effect: inhibition of thromboxane syn-

BOX 18-1 Nonsteroidal Anti-inflammatory Drugs (NSAIDs) and Other Nonopioid Analgesics

NSAIDs	COX-2 Inhibitors (Selective NSAIDs)
Aspirin	Celecoxib
Diclofenac	Rofecoxib
Ibuprofen	*Nonopioid and Non-NSAID Analgesics*
Indomethacin	Acetaminophen
Ketoprofen	
Naproxen	
Oxaprozin	
Piroxicam	
Sulindac	

thesis (potent platelet aggregator and vasoconstrictor) via irreversible inhibition of platelet COX that lasts for the life span of platelets, or about 8 days (see Chapter 16)

2. Uses
   a. **Fever, acute rheumatic fever, headache, mild pain, dysmenorrhea**
   b. **Inflammatory conditions** such as osteoarthritis and rheumatoid arthritis
   c. **Prevention of platelet aggregation** in coronary artery disease, myocardial infarction, atrial fibrillation, postoperative deep vein thrombosis
3. Adverse effects
   a. **Gastric irritation**, gastrointestinal (GI) bleeding, peptic ulcer disease
      - Occurs to some degree with the use of all NSAIDs
   b. **Salicylism** (tinnitus, vertigo leading to deafness) with overdose (see Chapter 30)
      - Reversible with dosage reduction
   c. **Respiratory alkalosis** and **anion gap metabolic acidosis**
   d. **Renal failure**
      - Possibly due to decrease in prostaglandin E production, which leads to acute tubular necrosis
4. Contraindications
   a. **Hypersensitivity reactions**
      - Occurrence in patients with aspirin-induced nasal polyps leads to **urticaria** and **bronchoconstriction** (aspirin-induced asthma).
   b. **Hemophilia**
   c. Risk of **Reye's syndrome**
      - **Aspirin should *not* be given to children with viral infections;** use acetaminophen as an acceptable substitute.

Drug of choice in children with fever: acetaminophen

B. Other nonselective NSAIDs
- **Examples:** ibuprofen, naproxen, sulindac, piroxicam, indomethacin
- The major differences among these agents involve duration of action and potency.

1. **Mechanism of action**
   a. These NSAIDs **reversibly bind to both COX-1 and COX-2,** exhibiting antipyretic, analgesic, and anti-inflammatory effects that are similar to aspirin.
   b. **Antipyretic effects** involve blocking the production of prostaglandins in the central nervous system to reset the hypothalamic temperature control, facilitating heat dissipation by vasodilation.
2. **Uses**
   a. **Mild to moderate pain,** bone and joint trauma, inflammatory syndromes (e.g., rheumatoid arthritis, gout)
   b. **Fever**
3. **Adverse effects**
   a. **Gastric upset** and **GI bleeding,** due in part to inhibited synthesis of prostaglandins, which are protective in the GI tract
   b. Possibly **decreased renal function,** especially in patients with underlying renal disease, leading to renal failure (e.g., acute tubular necrosis)
   c. Risk of **premature closure of patent ductus arteriosus** in the fetus
      - **Use after 20 weeks of pregnancy is *not* recommended.**

C. **COX-2 inhibitors**
- **Examples:** celecoxib, rofecoxib

1. **Mechanism of action: selective inhibition** of COX-2
   - In contrast, most other NSAIDs are nonselective COX-1 or COX-2 inhibitors.
2. **Uses:** rheumatic arthritis, osteoarthritis, acute pain
3. **Adverse effects:** GI bleeding, renal failure
   - Compared with other NSAIDs, **COX-2 inhibitors have a lower incidence of adverse effects.**

III. Acetaminophen

- Acetaminophen has **no anti-inflammatory activity,** although it has analgesic and antipyretic effects similar to those of aspirin.

A. **Mechanism of action:** unknown

B. **Uses: osteoarthritis** (pain), **acute pain syndromes, fever**

C. **Adverse effects**
- Acetaminophen neither produces gastric irritation nor affects platelet function.

1. **Hepatic necrosis** is the most serious result of acute overdose.
2. **Acetylcysteine** is used to prevent hepatotoxicity after acute overdose (see Table 30-2).

19

Opioid Analgesics and Antagonists

Target Topics

- Strong opioid agonists
- Moderate opioid agonists
- Mixed opioid agonists-antagonists
- Opioid antagonists

I. Opioid Agonists (Box 19-1)

- Opioid agonists are classified into three categories: **strong, moderate**, and **weak.**

A. **General features**

1. **Mechanism of action**
   - The effects of endogenous opioid peptides (**endorphins** and **enkephalins**) and exogenous opioids result from activation of specific opioid receptors (Table 19-1).
   - The **major subtypes of opioid receptors**, delta (δ), kappa (κ), and mu (μ), have **varying effects** (Table 19-2).
2. **Pharmacologic actions of opioid agonists** (Box 19-2)
3. **Uses**
   - **a.** Relief of **severe pain**
   - **b. Sedation** and relief from anxiety (e.g., preoperatively)
   - **c. Cough suppression**
   - **d. Diarrhea suppression**
4. **Adverse effects** (primarily extensions of pharmacologic actions)
   - **a. Respiratory depression and coma**
   - **b. Sedation** and central nervous system (CNS) depression
   - **c.** Miosis

Respiratory and CNS depression: most important adverse effects of opioid analgesics

BOX 19-1 Opioid Agonists

Strong Opioid Agonists
Fentanyl
Meperidine
Methadone
Morphine

Moderate Opioid Agonists
Codeine
Hydrocodone
Oxycodone

Weak Opioid Agonists
Dextromethorphan
Diphenoxylate
Loperamide
Propoxyphene
Tramadol

TABLE 19-1 Effects of Representative Opioids on Opioid Receptor Subtypes

	Receptor Subtype		
Opioid	**Mu (μ)**	**Delta (δ)**	**Kappa (κ)**
Buprenorphine	Partial agonist		
Butorphanol	Antagonist		Weak agonist
Codeine	Weak agonist	Weak agonist	
Fentanyl	Agonist		
Meperidine	Agonist		
Morphine	Agonist	Weak agonist	Weak agonist
Nalbuphine	Antagonist		Agonist
Nalmefene	Antagonist	Antagonist	Antagonist
Naloxone	Antagonist	Antagonist	Antagonist
Naltrexone	Antagonist	Antagonist	Antagonist
Pentazocine	Partial agonist		Agonist

TABLE 19-2 Opioid Receptors and Their Associated Effects

Receptor	Effects of Activation
Mu (μ) receptor	Analgesia, euphoria, respiratory depression, miosis, decreased gastrointestinal motility, and physical dependence
Kappa (κ) receptor	Analgesia, miosis, respiratory depression, dysphoria, and some psychomimetic effects
Delta (δ) receptor	Analgesia (spinal and supraspinal)

BOX 19-2 Pharmacologic Actions of Opioid Agonists

Central Nervous System Effects
Analgesia
Euphoria or dysphoria
Inhibition of cough reflex
Miosis (pinpoint pupils)
Physical dependence
Respiratory depression (inhibit respiratory center in medulla)
Sedation

Cardiovascular Effects
Decreased myocardial oxygen demand
Vasodilation and orthostatic hypotension (histamine release)

Gastrointestinal and Biliary Effects
Decreased gastric motility and constipation (increased muscle tone leads to diminished propulsive peristalsis in colon)
Biliary colic from increased sphincter tone and pressure
Nausea and vomiting (from direct stimulation of chemoreceptor trigger zone)

Genitourinary Effects
Increased bladder sphincter tone
Increased urine retention

d. **Nausea and vomiting** (stimulation of chemosensitive trigger zone)
e. **Constipation**
f. Acute postural hypotension (histamine release)
g. **Elevated intracranial pressure**
- Increased CO_2 → vasodilation → increased cerebral blood flow → increased intracranial pressure

Miosis ("pinpoint pupil") is characteristic of opioid overdose.

h. **Abuse, physical and psychological dependence**
i. **Abstinence syndrome on withdrawal of the drug**
- Symptoms and treatment of opioid overdose (see Chapter 30)

B. Specific opioid agonists

1. Morphine
- Morphine is the **prototype** opioid agonist, the standard against which all other analgesics are measured.

Morphine: high first-pass effect

a. **Administration:** intravenous, intramuscular, or buccal (the drug is less effective orally)
b. **Primary use:** relief of **severe pain** associated with trauma, myocardial infarction (MI), or cancer
- Other use: **acute pulmonary edema** to reduce perception of shortness of breath, anxiety, and cardiac preload and afterload

2. Codeine
a. Relative to morphine: less potent and less likely to cause physical dependence
b. Primary use: **antitussive agent**

Codeine is the most constipating opioid.

- Other use: **analgesic** (mild to moderate pain; commonly given in combination with aspirin or acetaminophen)

3. Meperidine
- **a.** Uses
  - **(1) Obstetric analgesia** (may prolong labor)
  - **(2) Acute pain syndromes**, such as MI, neuralgia, painful procedures (short-term treatment)
- **b. Specific adverse effect: seizures** due to accumulation of a metabolite (**normeperidine**)

Use meperidine, rather than morphine, for pancreatitis; it produces less spasm of the sphincter of Oddi.

4. Methadone
- **a.** Relative to morphine: longer duration of action and milder withdrawal symptoms
- **b.** Uses
  - **(1) Maintenance therapy** for heroin addicts
  - **(2) Control of withdrawal symptoms** from opioids
  - **(3) Neuropathic pain**

5. Fentanyl and its derivatives
- Available as **long-acting transdermal patch** for continuous pain relief
- **a.** Relative to morphine: less nausea
- **b.** Uses
  - **(1) Anesthesia**, in some cases (cardiovascular surgery)
    - Other drugs for anesthesia: **alfentanil** and **sufentanil**
  - **(2) Neuroleptanalgesia** (combination of **fentanyl** and **droperidol**)
    - **(a)** General quiescence, reduced motor activity, and profound analgesia
    - **(b)** No complete loss of consciousness
    - **(c)** Calming effect for surgical or diagnostic procedures

6. Tramadol
- **a. Mechanism of action**
  - Tramadol is a **μ receptor agonist** that also inhibits neuronal reuptake of norepinephrine and serotonin.
- **b. Uses: acute and chronic pain syndromes**
- **c. Adverse effect: decreased seizure threshold**

7. Loperamide and diphenoxylate
- Drugs with minimal analgesic activity used in the treatment of **diarrhea**

8. Dextromethorphan
- Drug with minimal analgesic activity used as an **antitussive agent**

II. Mixed Opioid Agonists-Antagonists (Box 19-3)

A. General considerations
1. React with a particular receptor subtype (e.g., **strong κ but weak μ agonist**)
2. Effective analgesics
3. Respiratory depressant effects do not rise proportionately with increasing doses.

BOX 19-3 Mixed Opioid Agonists-Antagonists

Buprenorphine
Butorphanol
Nalbuphine
Pentazocine

BOX 19-4 Opioid Antagonists

Nalmefene
Naloxone
Naltrexone

4. Associated with a much **lower risk of drug dependence** than morphine

B. **Buprenorphine** (partial agonist on the μ receptor)
   1. Used for relief of **moderate or severe pain**
   2. Maintenance for **opioid-dependent patients**

C. **Butorphanol (κ agonist)**
   - **Uses: pain relief** (parenterally), **migraine headaches** (nasal spray)

D. **Nalbuphine (κ agonist, μ antagonist)**
   1. Used for relief of moderate to severe **pain associated with acute and chronic disorders** such as cancer, renal or biliary colic, and migraine or vascular headaches, as well as surgery
   2. Used as **obstetric analgesia** during labor and delivery

E. **Pentazocine (κ agonist):** oldest mixed opioid agonist-antagonist
   1. Used for **relief of moderate to severe pain**
   2. CNS effects **such as disorientation and hallucinations limit use.**

III. Opioid Antagonists (Box 19-4)

A. **Mechanism of action:** competition with opioid agonists for **μ receptors** to rapidly reverse the effects of morphine and other opioid agonists

B. **Uses**
   1. Treatment of **opioid overdose**
   2. Precipitation of a **withdrawal syndrome** when given to chronic users of opioid drugs

SECTION VI

Drugs That Affect the Respiratory and Gastrointestinal Systems and Used to Treat Rheumatic Disorders and Gout

20

Drugs Used in the Treatment of Asthma and Chronic Obstructive Pulmonary Disease

Target Topics

- Pharmacotherapy of asthma
- Use of anti-inflammatory drugs in the treatment of asthma and COPD
- Use of bronchodilators in the treatment of asthma and COPD

I. General Considerations

A. Asthma

- Asthma is an **obstructive airway disorder** resulting from smooth muscle hypertrophy, bronchospasm, increased mucus secretion, and mucosal edema.

1. Both **nonimmunogenic** (Box 20-1) and **immunogenic** factors (Figure 20-1) play a role in the pathogenesis of asthma.

BOX 20-1 Factors That May Cause Asthma

Viral Infections

Environmental Pollutants
Ozone
Nitrogen dioxide

Pharmacologic Stimuli
Aspirin
β-Adrenergic receptor antagonists
Dyes in food and medications

Occupational Factors
Metal salts
Wood, animal, and insect dust

Exercise

Emotional Stress

Immunogenic Factors

- Drug therapy, which includes anti-inflammatory agents and bronchodilators, affects these factors.

2. Clinical symptoms include **episodic bouts of coughing** associated with dyspnea, wheezing, and chest tightness.
3. A variety of drugs are used in the pharmacotherapy of asthma (Table 20-1).

B. Chronic obstructive pulmonary disease (COPD)

- This **progressive obstructive airway disorder**, which usually results from **smoking**, is marked by airway reactivity.

1. COPD involves **chronic bronchitis** and **emphysema.**
2. Clinical symptoms include **chronic cough** with **sputum production** and **dyspnea.**

II. Anti-inflammatory Agents Used to Treat Asthma (Box 20-2; see Figure 20-1)

A. Corticosteroids

1. Mechanism of action

- Corticosteroids generally inhibit the inflammatory response, thereby preventing bronchoconstriction and producing smooth muscle relaxation.

a. Inhibition of the release of arachidonic acid by increasing the synthesis of lipocortin, which inhibits phospholipase A_2 activity

b. Decreased synthesis of cyclooxygenase-2 (COX-2), an inducible form of COX in inflammatory cells

c. Inhibition of the production of cytokines involved in the inflammatory cascade (interferon-γ, interleukin-1, interleukin-2)

d. Effect on the concentration, distribution, and function of peripheral leukocytes, increasing the concentration

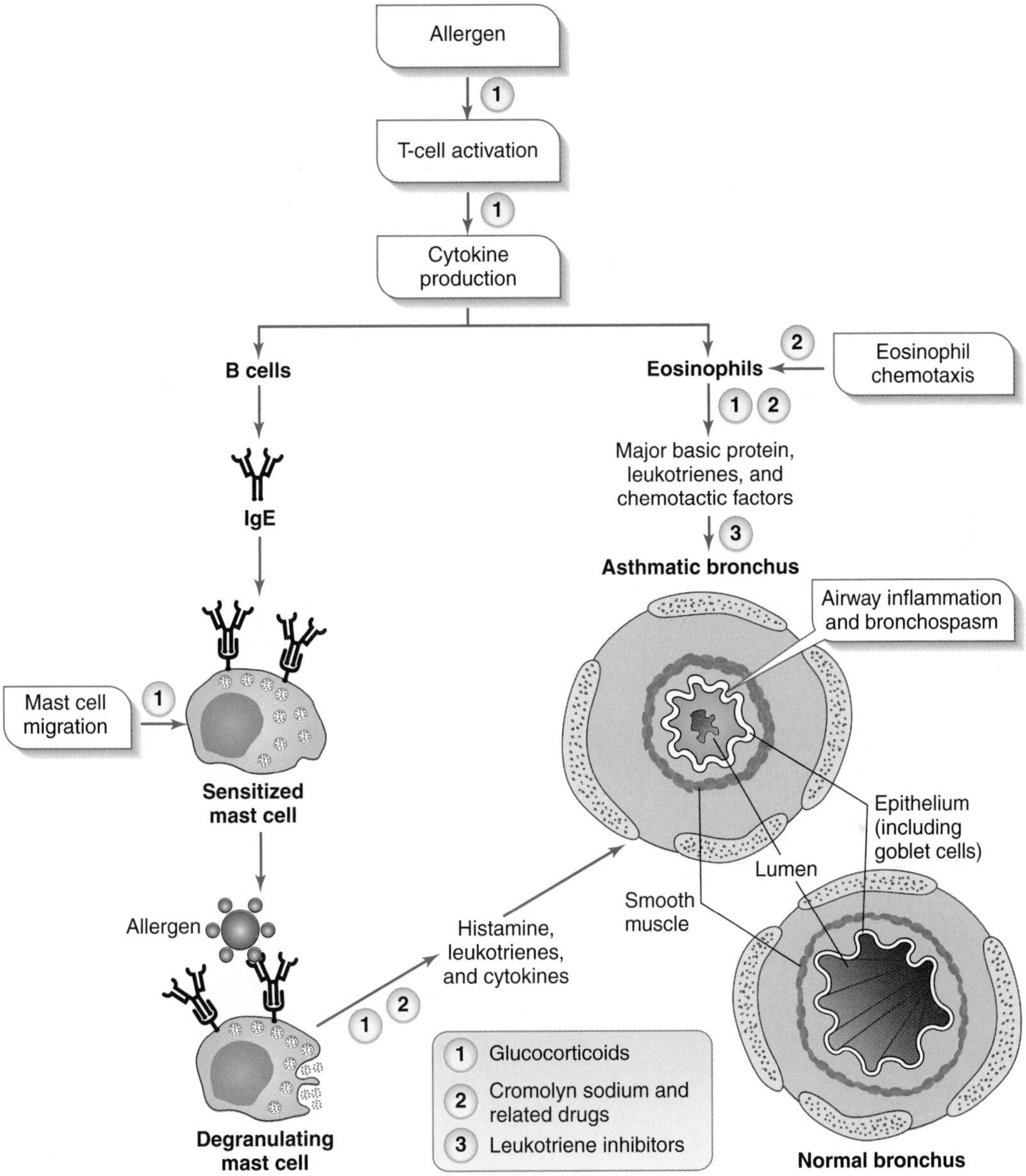

Figure 20-1 Sites of anti-inflammatory drug action in asthma. Cromolyn and related drugs prevent the release of mediators from mast cells and eosinophils. *IgE,* Immunoglobin E.

of neutrophils and decreasing the concentration of granulocytes, lymphocytes, and monocytes

2. Uses
   a. **Mild or moderate asthma or COPD (first-line therapy;** maintenance therapy)
      - **Inhaled** steroids
   b. **Severe airway obstruction** despite optimal bronchodilator therapy

Inhaled corticosteroids: fewer side effects than systemic corticosteroids

TABLE 20-1 Asthma Pharmacotherapy

Drug Type	Example	Use
Daily Medications for Long-Term Control		
Inhaled corticosteroids	Beclomethasone	First-line treatment
Systemic corticosteroids	Betamethasone	Used to gain prompt control when initiating long-term inhaled corticosteroids
Mast cell stabilizers	Cromolyn	May be initial choice in children Also used as prevention before exercise or allergen exposure
Long-acting β_2-receptor agonist	Salmeterol	Given concomitantly with anti-inflammatory agents Not used for acute symptoms
Methylxanthines	Theophylline	Adjunct to inhaled corticosteroids
Leukotriene inhibitors	Zafirlukast	Prophylaxis and long-term management (alone or in combination)
"Rescue" Medications Useful in Acute Episodes		
Short-acting β_2-receptor agonists	Albuterol	First choice for acute symptoms Prevention of exercise-induced bronchospasm Should be prescribed for all patients
Anticholinergic	Ipratropium	Additive benefit to inhaled β_2-receptor agonists in severe exacerbations Alternative for patients intolerant to β_2-receptor agonists

BOX 20-2 Anti-inflammatory Agents

Inhaled Corticosteroids
Beclomethasone
Flunisolide
Fluticasone

Oral Corticosteroids
Betamethasone
Methylprednisolone
Prednisone
Triamcinolone

Mast Cell Stabilizers
Cromolyn
Nedocromil

Leukotriene Pathway Inhibitors
Montelukast
Zafirlukast
Zileuton

- **Systemic** (oral or intravenous) steroids

c. **Asthma or COPD**
- **Combination therapy** with selective β_2-adrenergic receptor agonists such as salmeterol

d. **Emergency treatment** (parenteral) of severe asthma or COPD if bronchodilators do not resolve the airway obstruction
- See Chapter 22 for the discussion of the use of these agents in rheumatic disorders.

Taper the dose of oral corticosteroids in patients who have been taking the drug for > 1 week.

3. **Adverse effects:** iatrogenic Cushing's syndrome, diabetes mellitus, hypertension, peptic ulcer disease, hypomania, psychosis, adrenal insufficiency on abrupt cessation of therapy (see Chapter 22)

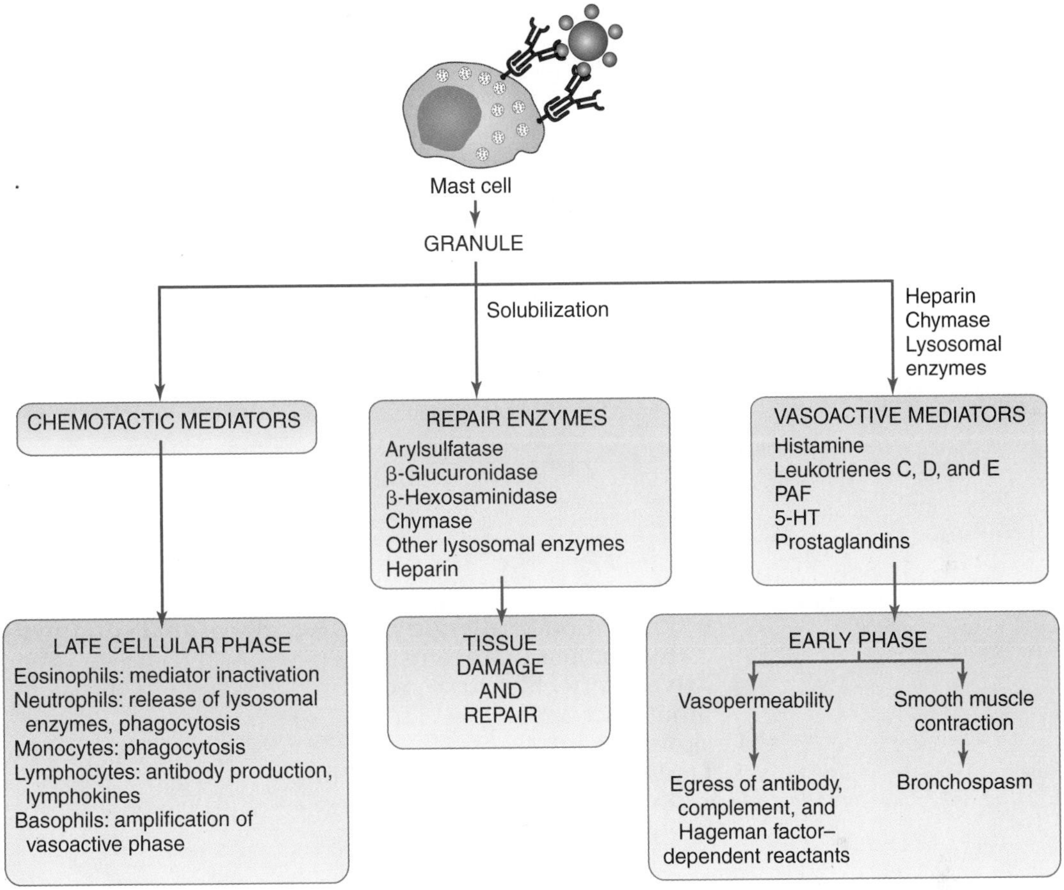

Figure 20-2 Early-phase and late-phase responses in asthma. *5-HT,* 5-Hydroxytryptamine; *PAF,* platelet activating factor.

- To prevent adrenal insufficiency, patients who have been receiving oral corticosteroid treatment for > 1 week should be given diminishing doses.

B. Mast cell stabilizers

- **Examples: cromolyn, nedocromil**

1. Pharmacokinetics

- Administration in the form of an **aerosol** before exposure to agents that trigger asthma

2. Mechanism of action (Figure 20-2)

a. Stabilize the plasma membranes of mast cells and eosinophils, preventing release of histamine, leukotrienes, and other mediators of airway inflammation

b. Decrease activation of airway nerves (nedocromil)

3. Uses

a. Prevention of asthmatic episodes, such as before exercise or in cold weather (primary use)

- Less effective in reducing bronchial reactivity in acute settings

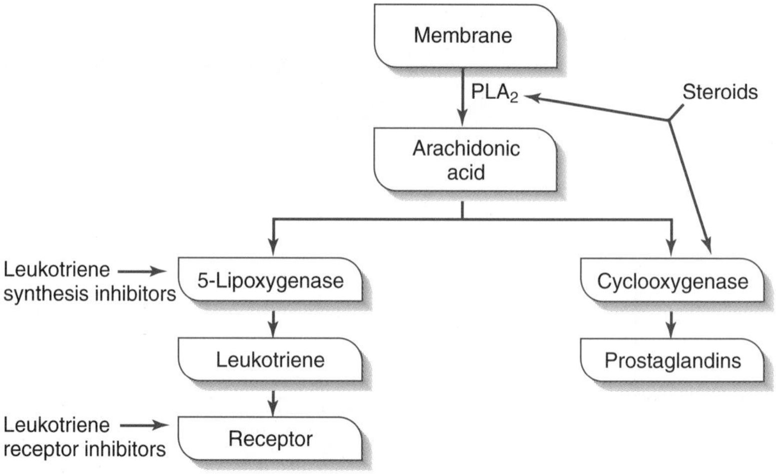

Figure 20-3 Role of prostaglandins and leukotrienes in asthma. Zileuton is a leukotriene synthesis inhibitor. Zafirlukast is a leukotriene receptor inhibitor. *PLA_2*, Phospholipase A_2.

b. Prevention of **allergic rhinitis** and **seasonal conjunctivitis** (*not* first-line agents)

4. **Adverse effects:** nausea, vomiting, dysgeusia (bad taste in mouth), cough

C. Leukotriene inhibitors

1. **Leukotriene synthesis inhibitor**
   - **Example: zileuton**

   a. **Pharmacokinetics**
   - **Oral** administration
   - **Rapid absorption** (enhanced by a high-fat diet)

   b. **Mechanism of action**
   - **Selective inhibitor of 5-lipoxygenase**, which catalyzes leukotriene formation (Figure 20-3; see Figure 20-1)
   - No effect on COX

   c. **Uses:** prevention and treatment of chronic asthma

   d. **Adverse effects**
   (1) **Flu-like syndrome** (chills, fever, fatigue, myalgia)
   (2) **Drowsiness**
   (3) **Elevated hepatic enzymes**

   e. **Drug interactions**
   - **Zileuton inhibits cytochrome P450 isozymes,** causing increased plasma concentrations of theophylline, warfarin, and other agents cleared by the liver.

Zileuton increases the $t_{1/2}$ of propranolol, theophylline, and warfarin.

2. **Leukotriene receptor antagonists**
   - **Examples: zafirlukast, montelukast**

   a. **Pharmacokinetics:** oral administration

   b. **Mechanism of action** (see Figures 20-1 and 20-3): **selective inhibition of binding of leukotrienes to their receptors,** reducing the airway inflammation that leads to edema, bronchoconstriction, and mucus secretion

BOX 20-3 Bronchodilators

Methylxanthines
Aminophylline
Theophylline

β_2-Adrenergic Receptor Agonists
Albuterol
Levalbuterol
Metaproterenol
Salmeterol
Terbutaline

Anticholinergic
Ipratropium

c. Uses
- **(1)** Control of **chronic asthma**
- **(2)** Not effective in acute bronchospasm

d. Adverse effects: headache, gastritis, upper respiratory tract symptoms (e.g., flu-like symptoms)

e. Drug interactions
- **Zafirlukast** inhibits the activity of the cytochrome P450 system.

III. Bronchodilators (Box 20-3)

A. β_2-Adrenergic receptor agonists: general considerations (see Chapter 5)
- **Examples: albuterol, terbutaline, salmeterol**

1. Pharmacokinetics

a. Administration: via a metered-dose **inhaler** or **nebulizer,** which has the greatest local effect on airway smooth muscle with the fewest systemic adverse effects

b. Duration of action
- Rapid-acting agents attain their **maximal effect in 30 minutes.**
- Action persists for 3–4 hours.

2. Mechanism of action (Figure 20-4)
- These **potent bronchodilators** (see Figure 20-1) relax smooth muscle by activation of adenylyl cyclase, increasing cyclic adenosine monophosphate (cAMP) levels by β receptors.

3. Uses

a. Treatment of acute asthma attacks

b. Prevention or treatment of bronchospasm caused by asthma or COPD

c. Asthma prophylaxis (oral albuterol, metaproterenol)

d. Emergency treatment of severe bronchospasm (subcutaneous terbutaline)

e. Delay of premature labor (terbutaline; see Chapter 26)

β_2-receptor agonists: the only bronchodilators used to counteract acute asthma attacks

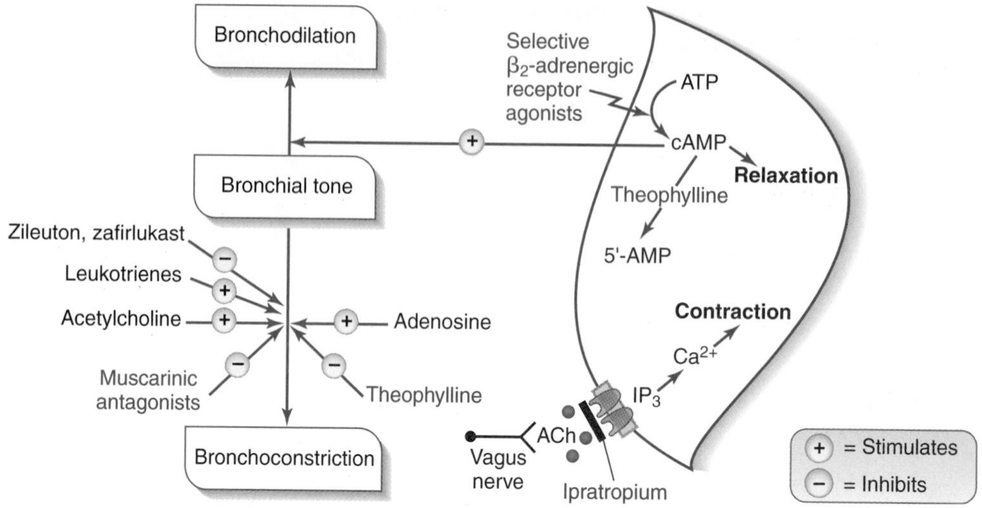

Figure 20-4 Mechanism of action of bronchodilators. *ACh,* Acetylcholine; *5′-AMP,* 5′-adenosine monophosphate; *ATP,* adenosine triphosphate; *cAMP,* cyclic adenosine monophosphate; *IP_3,* inositol triphosphate.

4. **Adverse effects**
   - **Systemic adverse effects occur with overdose.**
   - Many of these systemic effects are related to activation of the **sympathetic nervous system,** such as tachycardia, palpitations, anxiety, excitability, tremor, hyperglycemia, and hypokalemia.

B. β_2-Adrenergic receptor agonists: specific drugs

Albuterol is a "rescue" medication.

1. **Salmeterol:** longer acting drug (12 hours)
   - Should *not* be used to treat acute asthma attacks
2. **Levalbuterol:** R-isomer and active form of racemic albuterol
   - Inhalant with fewer central nervous system (CNS) and cardiac side effects

C. Epinephrine
- Used in **emergency settings** as subcutaneous injection or microaerosol for rapid bronchodilation in severe airway obstruction (see Chapter 5)

D. Methylxanthines
- **Examples: theophylline, aminophylline**

1. **Pharmacokinetics**
   - Decreasing hepatic function and drugs that inhibit the cytochrome P450 system (e.g., β-blockers, erythromycin, fluoroquinolones) increase the half-life ($t_{1/2}$) of theophylline.
   - Drugs that induce the cytochrome P450 system (e.g., barbiturates, phenytoin, rifampin) hasten the elimination of theophylline.

$t_{1/2}$ of theophylline: decreased in adults who smoke and in children

2. **Mechanism of action** (see Figure 20-4)
   - a. **Antagonize adenosine receptors** and affect intracellular calcium in smooth muscle cells
   - b. **Inhibit phosphodiesterase,** an enzyme that catalyzes degradation of cAMP

- The inhibition of phosphodiesterase probably causes **bronchodilation.**

c. Other effects include **CNS stimulation, cardiovascular action,** and **diuresis** (slight).

3. Uses

a. Adjunctive treatment of **acute asthma**

b. Prevention of **bronchospasm** associated with asthma or COPD

4. Adverse effects: gastrointestinal (GI) irritation, headache, anxiety, diuresis, palpitations, premature ventricular contractions, seizures

5. Precautions: patients with heart disease, liver disorders, seizure disorders, peptic ulcer disease

Theophylline has a narrow therapeutic index; levels need to be monitored closely when therapy is initiated.

E. Anticholinergic agents

- **Example: ipratropium** (muscarinic receptor antagonist; see Chapter 4)

1. Pharmacokinetics

- Administration via **aerosol** to local muscarinic receptors in the airway

2. Mechanism of action: blockade of the effects of vagus nerve stimulation

3. Uses

a. Prevention of bronchoconstriction in COPD (often given in combination with β_2-adrenergic receptor agonists)

b. Treatment of **asthma** (less effective than β_2-adrenergic receptor agonists)

4. Adverse effects: airway irritation, anticholinergic effects, GI upset, xerostomia, urinary retention, increased ocular pressure

21

Drugs Used in the Treatment of Gastrointestinal Disorders

Target Topics

- Treatment of peptic disorders
- Treatment of diarrhea
- Prokinetic drugs
- Treatment of nausea and vomiting
- Treatment of inflammatory bowel disease
- Treatment of constipation

I. Peptic Disorders

- This group of disorders includes **ulcers** of the stomach, esophagus, and duodenum; **Zollinger-Ellison syndrome; gastroesophageal reflux disease** (GERD); **gastritis;** and **esophagitis.**
- Physiologic **stimulants** of gastric acid secretion include gastrin, acetylcholine, and histamine acting on histamine H_2-receptors.

II. Drugs That Decrease Gastric Acidity (Box 21-1)

A. Histamine H_2-receptor antagonists

1. Cimetidine

a. Mechanism of action

(1) **Blocks histamine action** at the H_2-receptor site on

parietal cells, thus inhibiting gastric acid secretion (Figure 21-1)
(2) **Decreases production of pepsin**
(3) **Inhibits postprandial** and **basal gastric acid secretion**

b. Uses
(1) Healing of **duodenal and gastric ulcers** and prevention of their recurrence

BOX 21-1 Drugs That Decrease Gastric Acidity

H_2-Receptor Antagonists
Cimetidine
Famotidine
Nizatidine
Ranitidine

Proton Pump Inhibitors
Lansoprazole
Omeprazole

Antacids
Aluminum hydroxide
Magnesium hydroxide

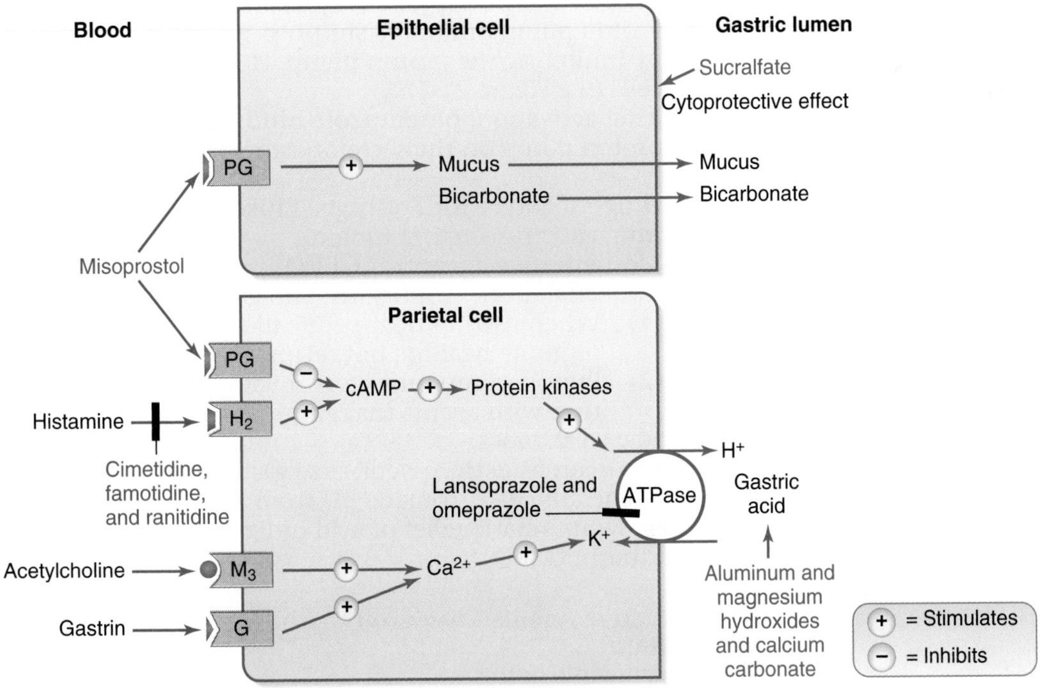

Figure 21-1 Gastric acid secretion and sites of drug action. *cAMP,* Cyclic adenosine monophosphate; *G,* gastrin receptor; *H_2,* histamine H_2 receptor; *M_3,* muscarinic M_3 receptor; *PG,* prostaglandin receptor.

- Intractable peptic ulcers may require higher doses or combination therapy.

(2) Control of secretory conditions such as **Zollinger-Ellison syndrome** and **GERD**

c. Adverse effects: antiandrogenic effects (**gynecomastia** and male sexual dysfunction)

d. Drug interactions: inhibition of liver microsomal metabolism of many drugs that utilize the cytochrome P450 system (e.g., β-blockers, benzodiazepines, calcium channel blockers, opioid agonists, tricyclic antidepressants)

Cimetidine extends the $t_{1/2}$ of many drugs that are metabolized in the liver.

2. Other H_2-receptor antagonists

- **Examples: ranitidine, famotidine, nizatidine**
- Therapeutic effects are similar to cimetidine.
- Drug interactions and antiandrogenic effects occur less commonly than with cimetidine.

a. Ranitidine: more potent than cimetidine

(1) Use: treatment of **duodenal ulcers associated with *Helicobacter pylori*** (given with a bismuth compound)

(2) Adverse effect: thrombocytopenia

b. Famotidine: most potent H_2-receptor antagonist

H_2-receptor blockade: > 90% reduction in basal, food-stimulated, and nocturnal gastric acid secretion

B. Proton pump inhibitors

- **Examples: omeprazole, lansoprazole**

1. Mechanism of action

a. Intragastric pH is higher and remains elevated longer than with H_2-receptor antagonist therapy.

b. Proton pump inhibitors **suppress gastric acid secretion** by inhibiting the proton pump, H^+/K^+/ATPase, in parietal cells (see Figure 21-1).

c. After activation, **omeprazole binds irreversibly** to the proton pump on the secretory surface of parietal cells.

2. Uses

a. Drugs of choice for **Zollinger-Ellison syndrome** resulting from gastrin-secreting tumors

b. Most effective agents for **GERD**

c. Duodenal ulcer, esophagitis, and gastric ulcer

(1) When used to treat peptic ulcer disease, these drugs promote healing, but relapse may occur.

(2) Proton pump inhibitors **must be given in combination** with agents that eliminate *H. pylori.*

Proton pump inhibitors are more effective than H_2-receptor blockers for treatment of peptic ulcer disease and GERD.

C. Antacids: weak bases

1. Mechanism of action: neutralize gastric hydrochloric acid and generally raise stomach pH from 1 to 3.0–3.5

2. Uses: symptomatic relief of acid indigestion, heartburn, GERD

III. Cytoprotective Agents (Box 21-2)

A. Sucralfate

1. Pharmacokinetics

a. Poorly soluble molecule that polymerizes in acid environment

BOX 21-2 Cytoprotective Drugs

Sucralfate

Prostaglandin Analogues
Misoprostol

Colloidal Bismuth Compounds
Bismuth subsalicylate

b. No significant absorption and no systemic effect

2. Mechanism of action

a. Selectively binds to necrotic ulcer tissue and **acts as barrier** to acid, pepsin, and bile, allowing duodenal ulcers time to heal

b. Stimulates synthesis of prostaglandins, which have cytoprotective effects on the gastrointestinal tract

3. Uses

a. Treatment of **active peptic ulcer disease**

b. Suppression of recurrence

B. Misoprostol: synthetic, oral prostaglandin E_1 analogue

1. Mechanism of action

a. Inhibits secretion of gastrin

b. Promotes secretion of mucus and bicarbonate

2. Use: prevention of nonsteroidal anti-inflammatory drug (NSAID)–induced gastric ulcers

3. Contraindication: pregnancy (can induce labor and uterine rupture)

Sucralfate requires acid pH for activation and should not be administered with antacids or H_2-receptor antagonists.

C. Colloidal bismuth compounds

- **Example: bismuth subsalicylate**

1. Mechanism of action: selective binding to ulcer coating, thereby protecting the ulcer from gastric acid

2. Uses

a. Control of **nonspecific diarrhea**

b. Prophylaxis of traveler's diarrhea, dyspepsia, and heartburn

c. Control of *H. pylori* (combination therapy)

IV. Drugs Used in the Treatment of *H. pylori* Infection

- *H. pylori* organisms can be identified in antral samples from most patients with duodenal and gastric ulcers.

A. Eradication requires **multiple drug therapy** to enhance the rate of ulcer healing, when compared with treatment with only H_2-receptor antagonists.

B. The **therapeutic regimen** usually includes a **proton pump inhibitor** in **combination** with two or more of the following drugs: amoxicillin, bismuth, clarithromycin, metronidazole, and tetracycline.

Triple drug therapy with metronidazole; a bismuth compound; and an antibiotic such as tetracycline, amoxicillin, or clarithromycin is recommended in some patients to overcome drug resistance.

V. Antidiarrheal Drugs (Box 21-3)

A. Inhibitors of acetylcholine (ACh) release

BOX 21-3 Antidiarrheal Drugs

Locally Acting Drugs
Bismuth subsalicylate
Kaolin-pectin
Polycarbophil

Opioids
Difenoxin
Diphenoxylate with atropine
Loperamide

- **Examples: diphenoxylate, difenoxin, loperamide**
- These drugs are also known as **opioid antidiarrheals** (see Chapter 19).

1. **Mechanism of action**
   a. These drugs **inhibit ACh release through presynaptic opioid receptors** in the enteric nervous system, disrupting peristalsis, decreasing intestinal motility, and increasing intestinal transit time.
   b. **Loperamide** does *not* cross the blood-brain barrier.
2. **Uses**
   a. Control and relief of **acute, nonspecific diarrhea**
   b. Treatment of **chronic diarrhea** associated with inflammatory bowel disease
3. **Contraindication: ulcerative colitis** (can induce toxic megacolon)

Loperamide produces less sedation and less abuse potential than diphenoxylate.

B. Locally acting agents

1. **Mechanism of action**
   a. **Inhibit intestinal secretions**
   b. Adsorb water and other substances
2. **Uses**
   a. **Bismuth:** management of infectious diarrhea, especially traveler's diarrhea
   b. **Adsorbents** (kaolin-pectin)
      - Can also bind potentially toxic substances

VI. Prokinetic Drugs

- **Example: metoclopramide**

A. Mechanism of action

1. Enhance **gastric motility** without stimulating gastric secretions
2. Augment cholinergic release of ACh from postganglionic nerve endings, sensitizing muscarinic receptors on smooth muscle cells
3. Block dopamine D_2 and 5-HT_3 receptors

B. Uses and clinical effects

1. **GERD:** reduced reflux and increased gastric emptying due to the decrease of the resting tone of the lower esophageal sphincter
2. **Nausea and vomiting:** antiemetic effect produced by **block-**

BOX 21-4 Antiemetics

Anticholinergic Drugs
Scopolamine

Antihistamines
Diphenhydramine
Meclizine

Dopamine D_2-Receptor Antagonists
Metoclopramide

Phenothiazines
Prochlorperazine
Promethazine

ade of dopamine D_2 receptors in the chemoreceptor trigger zone
3. **Gastroparesis:** promotion of motility

C. **Adverse effects:** extrapyramidal or dystonic reactions

VII. Antiemetic Drugs (Box 21-4)

A. **Physiology of emesis** (incompletely understood process)
1. Coordination of stimuli takes place in the **vomiting center,** located in the **reticular formation of the medulla.**
2. Input arises from the chemoreceptor trigger zone, vestibular apparatus, and afferent nerves.

B. Antiemetic drugs
1. **Serotonin 5-HT_3 receptor antagonists**
   - **Examples: ondansetron, granisetron**
   a. Safe and effective antiemetics
   b. Uses: **chemotherapy**-induced emesis, **postsurgery** nausea and vomiting
2. **Marijuana derivatives**
   - **Example: dronabinol**
   - **Use:** nausea and vomiting in patients with **AIDS or cancer**
3. **Metoclopramide:** dopamine D_2 receptor antagonist
4. **Antihistamines**
   - **Examples:** diphenhydramine, hydroxyzine
   - **Use:** nausea and vomiting associated with **motion sickness**
5. **Phenothiazines**
   - **Examples:** prochlorperazine, promethazine
   - Dopamine D_2 receptor antagonists

VIII. Drugs Used in the Treatment of Inflammatory Bowel Disease
- **Crohn's disease** and **ulcerative colitis** are often considered together as inflammatory bowel disease.

A. **Salicylates** (see Chapter 18)
1. **5-aminosalicylic acid** (5-ASA, mesalamine): active anti-inflammatory agent

a. **Mechanism of action:** inhibitor of cyclooxygenase (COX) pathway
b. **Uses:** ulcerative colitis, Crohn's disease (sometimes)
c. **Adverse effects:** abdominal pain, nausea, vomiting, headache

2. **Sulfasalazine**
   - Combination of sulfapyridine and mesalamine

   a. **Mechanism of action:** production of beneficial effects due to antibacterial action of sulfapyridine and **anti-inflammatory** (most important) properties of mesalamine
   b. **Uses:** ulcerative colitis, Crohn's disease (induce remission)
   c. **Adverse effects**
      (1) **Malaise**
      (2) **Nausea, abdominal discomfort**
      (3) **Headache**
      (4) Typical sulfonamide adverse effects (e.g., blood dyscrasias, skin reactions)

3. **Olsalazine**
   - Two 5-ASA molecules linked by a diazo bond (RN = NR′), cleaved by bacteria in colon
   - Used in the treatment of **ulcerative colitis**

B. **Immunosuppressive agents** (see Chapter 17)

1. **Hydrocortisone** and other glucocorticoids can induce remission of **ulcerative colitis** and **Crohn's disease.**
2. **Infliximab**, a monoclonal antibody to tumor necrosis factor-α, is used to treat moderate to severe **Crohn's disease.**

IX. **Laxatives** (Table 21-1)

A. **General considerations**

- Laxative abuse occurs frequently.
- **Contraindications** to these drugs include **unexplained abdominal pain** and **intestinal obstruction.**

B. **Types of laxatives** (Box 21-5)

1. **Bulk-forming laxatives:** psyllium, methylcellulose
   - Natural and semisynthetic polysaccharides and cellulose derivatives (similar to dietary fiber)
2. **Osmotic laxatives**
   - The osmotic effect of these laxatives increases water in the colon.

   a. **Saline cathartics:** magnesium salts, sodium phosphate
      - Used when prompt, complete evacuation is necessary

   b. **Other osmotic drugs:** lactulose, sorbitol
3. **Stool softeners: surfactants** (e.g., docusate) and **lubricants** (e.g., mineral oil)
4. **Stimulant laxatives:** castor oil, cascara, senna, phenolphthalein, bisacodyl
   - **Castor oil,** a primary irritant, increases intestinal motility.

TABLE 21-1 Effects of Common Laxatives

Type	Site of Action	Mechanism	Uses	Adverse Effects
Bulk-forming				
Psyllium	Small and large intestines	Increase bulk and moisture content in stool, stimulating peristalsis	Prevent straining during defecation	Esophageal or bowel obstruction if taken with insufficient liquid Flatulence
Osmotic				
Lactulose	Colon	Retain ammonia in colon, producing osmotic effect that stimulates bowel evacuation	Prevent and treat portal systemic encephalopathy Treat constipation	Abdominal discomfort Flatulence
Saline cathartics, magnesium citrate	Small intestine	Induce cholecystokinin release from duodenum, producing osmotic effect that produces distention, promoting peristalsis	Evacuate colon before diagnostic examination or surgery Accelerate excretion of parasites or poisons from GI tract	Electrolyte disturbance
Stimulant				
Senna	Colon	Act directly on intestinal smooth muscle to increase peristalsis	Facilitate defecation in diminished colonic motor response Evacuate colon before diagnostic examination or surgery	Urine discoloration Abdominal cramping Fluid and electrolyte depletion
Stool Softener				
Docusate	Small and large intestine	Lower surface tension Facilitate penetration of fat and water into stool	Short-term treatment of constipation Evacuate colon before diagnostic examination or surgery Prevent straining during defecation Modify fluid from ileostomy, colostomy	GI cramping

GI, Gastrointestinal.

BOX 21-5 Laxatives

Bulk-forming Laxatives
Methylcellulose
Psyllium

Osmotic Laxatives
Lactulose
Saline cathartics
(magnesium citrate, magnesium hydroxide, sulfate phosphate, sodium phosphate)
Sorbitol

Stimulants
Bisacodyl
Cascara sagrada
Castor oil
Phenolphthalein
Senna

Stool Softeners
Docusate
Mineral oil

22

Drugs Used in the Treatment of Rheumatic Disorders and Gout

Target Topics

- NSAIDs and COX-2 inhibitors in the treatment of arthritic disease
- Disease-modifying antirheumatic drugs (DMARDs)
- Drugs used in the treatment of gout

I. Antiarthritic Drugs (Box 22-1)
- The drugs used to treat **rheumatoid arthritis** act at various sites (Figure 22-1).

A. **Nonsteroidal anti-inflammatory drugs (NSAIDs) and cyclooxygenase-2 (COX-2) inhibitors** (see Chapter 18)
- NSAIDs and COX-2 inhibitors primarily provide **symptomatic relief** in the **initial therapy** of rheumatoid arthritis, rheumatic fever, and other inflammatory joint conditions, as well as treatment of acute pain syndromes.

B. Corticosteroids
- **Example: prednisone**

1. **Mechanism of action**
   a. **Decrease phospholipase** A_2 **and COX-2 activity** (see Chapter 23)
   b. Decrease immune component
2. **Use:** acute episodes of rheumatoid arthritis

BOX 22-1 Antiarthritic Drugs

Nonsteroidal Anti-inflammatory Drugs (NSAIDs)
Diclofenac
Diflunisal
Indomethacin
Oxaprozin
Piroxicam
Sulindac
Tolmetin

Cyclooxygenase-2 (COX-2) Inhibitors
Celecoxib
Rofecoxib

Corticosteroids
Prednisone

Disease-modifying Antirheumatic Drugs (DMARDs)
Antimetabolites
Methotrexate

Immunologic Drugs
Etanercept
Infliximab
Leflunomide

Antimalarial Drugs
Hydroxychloroquine

Gold Salts
Auranofin
Aurothioglucose

Chelators
Penicillamine

- Steroids result in dramatic improvement but do not arrest the disease process.

C. Disease-modifying antirheumatic drugs (DMARDs)
- **Examples:** methotrexate, immunosuppressive drugs, antimalarial drugs, gold salts, penicillamine

1. General characteristics
   - **a. Suppress proliferation and activity of lymphocytes** and polymorphonuclear neutrophils (PMNs)
   - **b. Counteract joint inflammation and destruction**
   - **c.** Slow progression of joint erosion in rheumatoid arthritis and systemic lupus erythematosus (SLE)

2. Methotrexate
   - **a. Mechanism of action:** inhibition of human folate reductase, lymphocyte proliferation, and production of cytokines and rheumatoid factor
   - **b. Uses:** rheumatoid arthritis, immunosuppression, cancer chemotherapy (see Chapter 29)
     - **More effective when used in combination** with other drugs, such as etanercept and infliximab

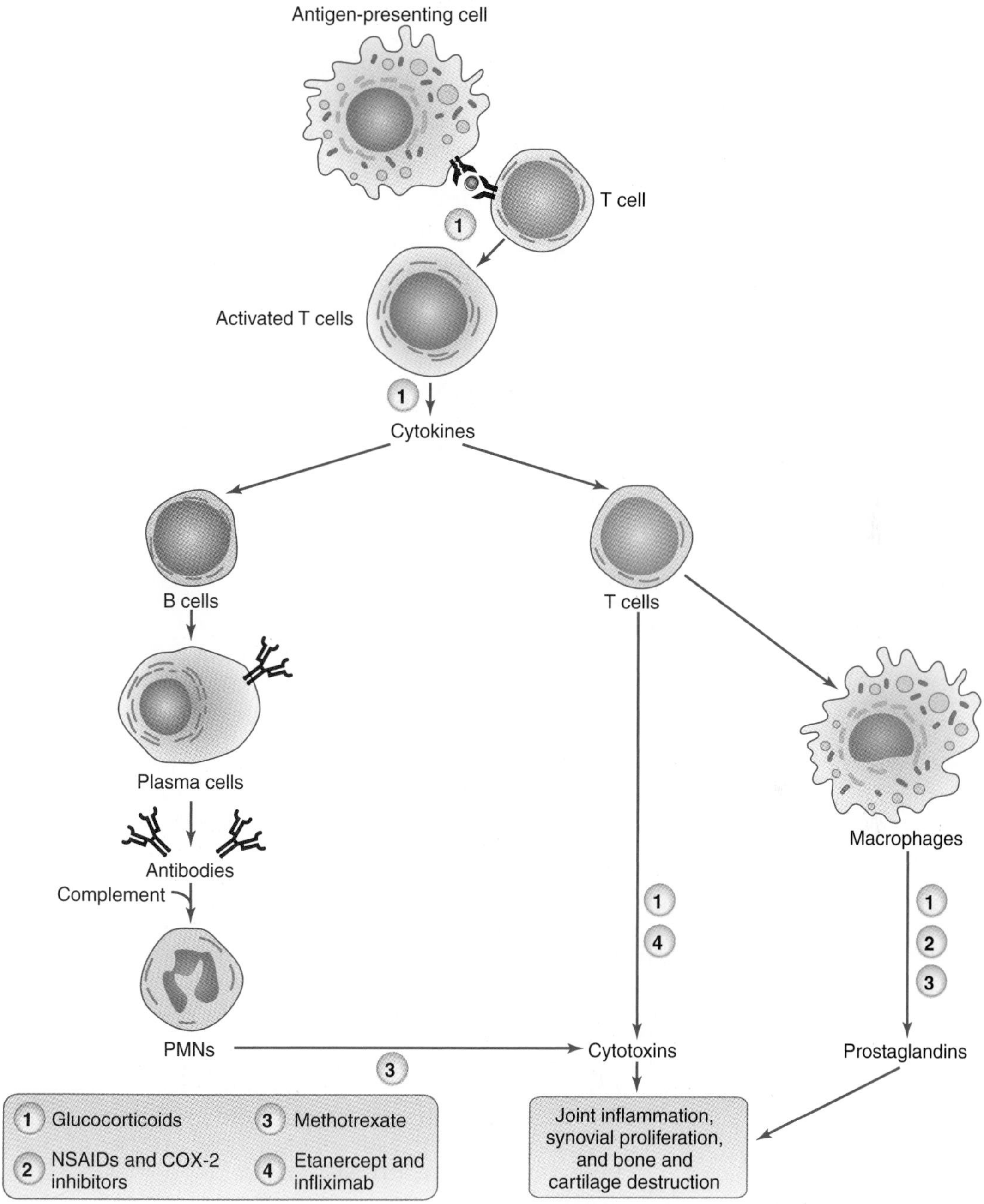

Figure 22-1 Pathogenesis of rheumatoid arthritis and sites of action of drugs. Etanercept and infliximab work by inactivating tumor necrosis factor. *COX-2,* Cyclooxygenase-2; *NSAID,* nonsteroidal anti-inflammatory drug; *PMN,* polymorphonuclear neutrophil.

- **c. Adverse effects**
    - **(1) Macrocytic anemia** (caused by folate deficiency)
    - **(2) Bone marrow suppression**
    - **(3)** Pulmonary fibrosis
    - **(4)** Teratogenic activity
- **3. Immunosuppressive drugs**
    - **a. Mechanism of action**
        - **(1) Leflunomide** inhibits mononuclear and T-cell proliferation.
        - **(2) Etanercept** and **infliximab** inhibit tumor necrosis factor-α.
    - **b. Uses:** Crohn's disease, rheumatoid arthritis
    - **c. Adverse effects:** headache, nausea and vomiting, serum sickness–like reaction
- **4. Antimalarial drugs** (see Chapter 28)
    - **Example: hydroxychloroquine**
    - **a. Mechanism of action** (unclear): may inhibit lymphocyte function and chemotaxis of PMNs
    - **b. Use** (other than malaria prophylaxis and treatment): **adjunct to NSAIDs** in the treatment of rheumatoid arthritis, juvenile chronic arthritis, Sjögren's syndrome, and SLE
    - **c. Adverse effects:** retinal degeneration, dermatitis
- **5. Gold compounds**
    - **Examples: aurothioglucose, auranofin**
    - **a. Mechanism of action:** alter morphology and function of macrophages, which may be a major mode of action
    - **b. Use:** early stages of adult and juvenile rheumatoid arthritis
    - **c. Adverse effects**
        - **(1) Cutaneous reactions** such as erythema and exfoliative dermatitis
        - **(2)** Blood dyscrasias
        - **(3) Renal toxicity**
- **6. Penicillamine: oral chelating agent**
    - **a. Mechanism of action:** chelates heavy metals
        - Penicillamine **should not be used in combination with gold compounds** to treat rheumatoid arthritis.
    - **b.** Uses
        - **(1) Wilson's disease**
        - **(2) Cystinuria**
        - **(3) Resistant cases of rheumatoid arthritis**
    - **c. Adverse effects:** aplastic anemia, renal disease (membranous glomerulonephritis)
- **7. Sulfasalazine**
    - **Uses:** rheumatoid arthritis, ankylosing spondylitis, ulcerative colitis (see Chapter 21)

II. Drugs Used in the Treatment of Gout (Box 22-2)

A. Types of gout

- **Gout** is a disorder of **uric acid metabolism** that results in deposition of monosodium urate in joints and cartilage (Figure 22-2).

1. **Primary gout** is caused by **overproduction** (from increase in de novo synthesis) or **underexcretion** (e.g., diabetes, starvation states) of uric acid.
2. **Secondary gout** is caused by **accumulation** of uric acid due to one of the following factors:
   a. Disease, such as leukemia

BOX 22-2 Drugs Used in the Treatment of Gout

Acute Therapy
Colchicine
COX-2 inhibitors
Indomethacin and other NSAIDs

Prevention
Allopurinol
Probenecid
Sulfinpyrazone

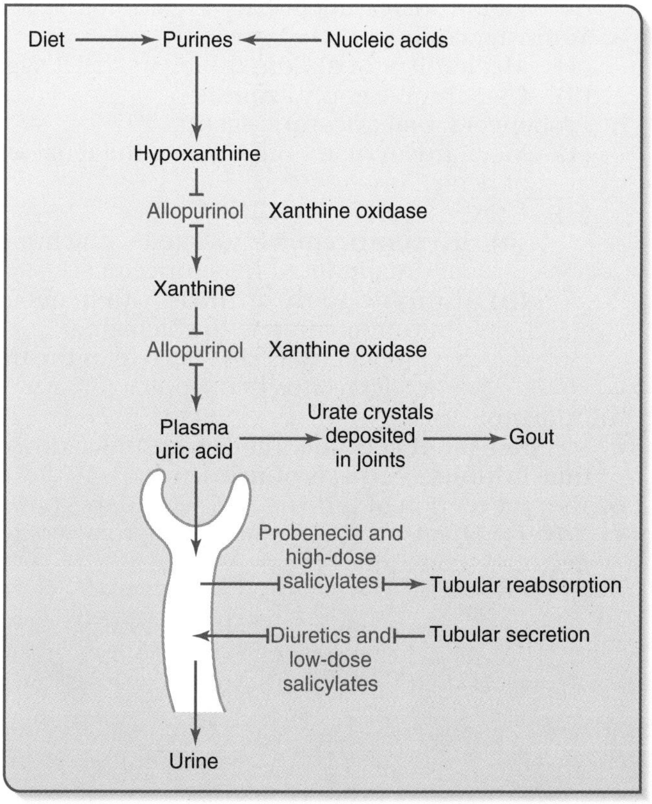

Figure 22-2 Sites of action of drugs that affect uric acid metabolism and excretion.

b. Drugs that interfere with uric acid disposition, such as diuretics (e.g., thiazides, furosemide, ethacrynic acid)

B. Treatment of acute attacks

1. Colchicine

a. Mechanism of action: binds to microtubule and inhibits leukocyte migration and phagocytosis, thereby blocking the ability to inflame the joint

- Colchicine is *not* an analgesic.

b. Use: reduction of pain and inflammation of **acute attacks of gouty arthritis**

c. Adverse effects: diarrhea, nausea and vomiting

2. Indomethacin and other NSAIDs or COX-2 inhibitors

a. All of these drugs are effective in the relief of pain and inflammation due to acute gouty arthritis (see Chapter 18).

b. Additional uses for indomethacin

(1) Ankylosing spondylitis and osteoarthritis of the hip

(2) Patent ductus arteriosus

C. Prevention of acute attacks

- The goal is to prevent gouty attacks by **decreasing the serum concentration of uric acid** (see Figure 22-2).

1. Uricosuric drugs

- These drugs block active reabsorption of uric acid in proximal tubule, increasing urinary excretion of uric acid.

a. Sulfinpyrazone

(1) Mechanism of action: inhibits platelet aggregation

(2) Use: chronic gouty arthritis

Probenicid can aggravate inflammation from gout if administered during the initial stages of an acute attack.

b. Probenecid: oral uricosuric agent

(1) Mechanism of action: inhibits the renal excretion of penicillins

(2) Uses

(a) Hyperuricemia associated with chronic gout or drug-induced hyperuricemia

(b) Chronic gouty arthritis with frequent attacks (in combination with colchicine)

- Probenecid is *not* effective in the treatment of acute attacks of gout.

Allopurinol should NOT be used in acute attacks of gout; it exacerbates symptoms.

2. Allopurinol

a. Mechanism of action: inhibits xanthine oxidase and thus **inhibits synthesis of uric acid**

b. Use: prevention of primary and secondary gout

c. Adverse effects: maculopapular rash, toxic epidermal necrolysis, vasculitis

SECTION VII

Drugs That Affect the Endocrine and Reproductive Systems

23

Drugs Used in the Treatment of Hypothalamic, Pituitary, Thyroid, and Adrenal Disorders

Target Topics

- Drugs used in the diagnosis and treatment of hypothalamic and pituitary disorders
- Drugs used in the treatment of thyroid disorders
- Glucocorticoids and mineralocorticoids
- Drugs used to treat disorders of adrenal function

I. General Considerations

- A hormone is a substance secreted by one tissue or gland that is transported via the circulation to a site where it exerts its effects on different tissues.

TABLE 23-1 Relationships Among Hypothalamic, Pituitary, and Target Gland Hormones

Hypothalamic	Pituitary	Target Organ	Target Organ Hormones
GHRH (+), SRIH (–)	GH (+)	Liver	Somatomedins
CRH (+)	ACTH (+)	Adrenal cortex	Glucocorticoids Mineralocorticoids Androgens
TRH (+)	TSH (+)	Thyroid	T_4, T_3
GnRH or LHRH (+)	FSH (+) LH (+)	Gonads	Estrogen Progesterone Testosterone
Dopamine (–) PRH (+)	Prolactin (+)	Breast	—

+, Stimulant; –, inhibitor.
ACTH, Adrenocorticotropic hormone; *CRH,* corticotropin-releasing hormone; *FSH,* follicle-stimulating hormone; *GH,* growth hormone; *GHRH,* growth hormone–releasing hormone; *GnRH* or *LHRH,* gonadotropin-releasing hormone; *LH,* luteinizing hormone; *PRH,* prolactin-releasing hormone; *SRIH,* somatotropin-releasing inhibiting hormone; *TRH,* thyrotropin-releasing hormone; *TSH,* thyroid-stimulating hormone.

- **A. Uses for hormones and synthetic analogues**
  - **1. Diagnostic tools** in endocrine disorders
  - **2. Replacement therapy** in endocrine disorders
  - **3. Treatment of nonendocrine disorders**
- **B. Interactions among the hypothalamic, pituitary, and peripheral glands** (Table 23-1; Figure 23-1)

II. Hypothalamic Hormones and Related Drugs (Box 23-1)

- **A. Sermorelin (growth hormone–releasing hormone)**
  - **1. Mechanism of action:** causes rapid elevation of growth hormone in the blood
  - **2. Use:** assessment of responsiveness and treatment of growth hormone deficiency
- **B. Somatostatin (growth hormone–inhibiting hormone)**
  - • **Octreotide** (synthetic analogue)
  - **1. Mechanism of action:** inhibits release of pituitary and gastrointestinal hormones
  - **2. Uses**
    - **a.** Symptomatic **treatment of hormone-secreting tumors,** including pituitary tumors, carcinoid tumors, insulinomas, vasoactive intestinal peptide tumors (VIPomas)
    - **b. Esophageal varices** (octreotide)
  - **3. Adverse effects:** abdominal pain, diarrhea, nausea and vomiting
- **C. Protirelin (thyrotropin-releasing hormone; TRH)**
  - **1. Mechanism of action:** stimulates synthesis and release of thyrotropin and prolactin from the anterior pituitary
  - **2. Use:** assessment of thyroid function in patients with pituitary or hypothalamic dysfunction
- **D. Corticotropin-releasing hormone (CRH; corticorelin)**
  - **1. Mechanism of action:** stimulates release of corticotropin and β-endorphin from the anterior pituitary

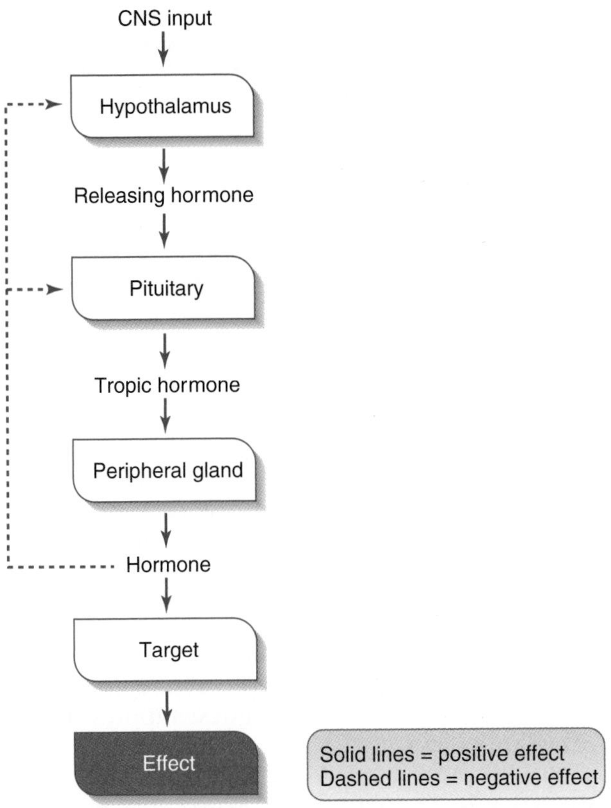

Figure 23-1 Regulation of hormone synthesis and secretion. A negative feedback mechanism is an example of a negative effect. *CNS,* Central nervous system.

BOX 23-1 Hypothalamic Hormones and Related Drugs

Corticorelin
Gonadorelin
Leuprolide
Nafarelin
Octreotide
Protirelin
Sermorelin
Somatostatin

2. **Use:** differentiation between hypothalamic and pituitary causes of corticotropin deficiency or excess

E. Gonadotropin-releasing hormone (GnRH)–related preparations

- **Leuprolide,** nafarelin, gonadorelin

1. **Mechanism of action**
   a. **Stimulate secretion of** follicle-stimulating hormone

BOX 23-2 Anterior Pituitary Hormones and Related Drugs

$ACTH_{1-24}$
Corticotropin
Cosyntropin
Human chorionic gonadotropin
Menotropins
Prolactin
Somatrem
Somatropin (recombinant human growth hormone)
Thyrotropin
Urofollitropin

(**FSH**) and luteinizing hormone (**LH**): pulsatile intravenous administration every 1–4 hours
   - **b. Inhibit gonadotropin release:** continuous administration of longer-lasting synthetic analogues
2. Uses
   - **a. Shorter-acting preparations:** treatment of delayed puberty, induction of ovulation in women with hypothalamic amenorrhea, stimulation of spermatogenesis in men with hypogonadotropic hypogonadism (infertility)
   - **b. Long-acting GnRH analogues:** suppression of FSH and LH in polycystic ovary syndrome, endometriosis, precocious puberty, prostate cancer
3. **Adverse effects:** menopausal symptoms, amenorrhea, testicular atrophy

III. Anterior Pituitary Hormones and Related Drugs (Box 23-2)

A. Growth hormone–related preparations

- Somatropin, somatrem, recombinant human growth hormone (rhGH)
- Growth hormone is required for stimulating normal growth in children and adolescents as well as for controlling metabolism in adults.
- Disorders characterized by an **excess of growth hormone** include **gigantism** (*before* puberty) and **acromegaly** (*after* fusion of epiphyseal plates of the long bones).
- Disorders characterized by a **deficiency** of growth hormone include **dwarfism.**

Excess growth hormone production results in gigantism and acromegaly; deficiency results in dwarfism.

1. **Mechanism of action**
   - **a. Increase production of somatomedins** in the liver and other tissues
   - **b. Oppose the actions of insulin**
2. **Uses:** hypopituitary dwarfism, cachexia, Turner's syndrome (single X chromosome)
3. **Adverse effects**
   - **a. Impaired glucose tolerance** may develop over long periods.
   - **b.** Only synthetic growth hormone is used today

(Creutzfeldt-Jakob disease resulted from the use of cadaveric growth hormone).

B. Thyrotropin (thyroid-stimulating hormone; TSH)
- **1. Mechanism of action**
  - **a. Stimulates growth of thyroid gland**
  - **b.** Stimulates the **synthesis** and **release** of **thyroid hormones**
- **2. Use:** diagnosis of hypothyroidism

C. Adrenocorticotropin (ACTH)–related preparations
- **Corticotropin, $ACTH_{1-24}$, cosyntropin**
- **1. Regulation of secretion**
  - **a.** Corticotropin levels undergo daily cyclic changes (**circadian rhythms**).
    - **Peak plasma levels** occur about **6:00 AM**, and the **lowest levels** occur about **12:00 AM.**
  - **b. Stress increases the release of corticotropin.**
- **2. Mechanism of action**
  - **a. Stimulate growth of the adrenal gland**
  - **b. Stimulate the production and release of glucocorticoids, mineralocorticoids, and androgens from the adrenal cortex**
- **3. Use:** differentiation between primary (adrenal malfunction) and secondary (pituitary malfunction) adrenocortical insufficiency
- **4. Adverse effects** (corticotropin or glucocorticoids): **Cushing's syndrome**
  - **a. General:** weight gain, cushingoid appearance ("moon face"), sodium retention, edema
  - **b. Musculoskeletal:** osteoporosis, myopathy, growth retardation (children)
  - **c. Ophthalmic:** cataracts, glaucoma
  - **d. Other:** diabetes mellitus, peptic ulcer disease, psychosis, decreased resistance to infection

ACTH and glucocorticoids cause iatrogenic Cushing's syndrome.

D. Urofollitropin (follicle-stimulating hormone; FSH)
- **1. Mechanism of action:** stimulates ovarian follicle growth (females) and spermatogenesis (males)
- **2. Uses:** infertility, polycystic ovary syndrome
- **3. Adverse effects:** multiple births, ovarian enlargement

E. Prolactin and related preparations
- **1. Prolactin**
  - **a. Regulation of secretion**
    - **(1) Stress, suckling, phenothiazines** (dopamine antagonists), and **TRH stimulate** the release of prolactin.
    - **(2) Dopamine and dopamine agonists** in the central nervous system (CNS), such as bromocriptine, tonically **inhibit** the release of prolactin.
  - **b. Mechanism of action:** stimulates milk production
  - **c. Use:** not available for clinical use
- **2. Inhibitors of prolactin release** (bromocriptine, pergolide)
  - **Uses:** prevention of breast tenderness and engorgement in women who are not breastfeeding; inhibition of

BOX 23-3 Posterior Pituitary Hormones and Related Drugs

Desmopressin
Oxytocin

lactation; treatment of amenorrhea and galactorrhea associated with hyperprolactinemia due to pituitary adenomas

IV. Posterior Pituitary Hormones and Related Drugs

- These hormones are **produced** in the **hypothalamus** and are transported to the posterior pituitary (neurohypophysis), where they are stored and released into the circulation (Box 23-3).

A. Vasopressin (antidiuretic hormone; ADH)

1. General considerations

- The synthetic analogue is **desmopressin.**

a. Disorders characterized by an **absence of ADH** include diabetes insipidus (severe polyuria, hypernatremia).

b. Disorders characterized by an **excess of ADH** include syndrome of inappropriate antidiuretic hormone (SIADH), water retention, hyponatremia, and possible pulmonary disease.

2. Regulation of secretion

a. Increases in plasma osmolality (e.g., **dehydration) result in increased secretion of ADH.**

b. Decreases in blood pressure (e.g., due to **hemorrhage) increase ADH secretion.**

Excess ADH results in SIADH, water retention, hyponatremia, and possible pulmonary disease; absence of ADH results in diabetes insipidus.

3. Mechanism of action

a. Modulates renal tubular reabsorption of water, increasing permeability of the distal tubule and collecting ducts to water

- This effect is mediated by an **increase in cAMP** associated with stimulation of the **V_2 receptor.**

b. At high concentrations, **causes vasoconstriction** (helps maintain blood pressure during hemorrhage)

- This effect occurs via the stimulation of the **V_1 receptor.**

4. Uses

a. Central (neurogenic) diabetes insipidus

- **Thiazide diuretics** are used to treat **nephrogenic diabetes insipidus** because they paradoxically cause a reduction in the polyuria of patients with diabetes insipidus.

b. Esophageal variceal bleeding and **colonic diverticular bleeding** (some cases)

c. Ventricular fibrillation or pulseless ventricular tachycardia

5. Adverse effects: overhydration, hypertension

6. Drugs that affect the secretion or action of ADH

BOX 23-4 Thyroid Hormones and Related Drugs

β-Adrenergic receptor antagonists
Iodide (radioactive iodine)
Levothyroxine
Liothyronine
Methimazole
Propylthiouracil

a. Diuretics, carbamazepine, morphine, tricyclic antidepressants increase ADH release.

b. Ethanol decreases ADH release.

- **Lithium** and **demeclocycline**, which reduce the action of ADH at the collection ducts of the nephron, are used to treat **SIADH.**

B. Oxytocin

- This substance, which is secreted by the supraoptic and paraventricular nuclei on the hypothalamus, is used to **induce labor** and **stimulate uterine contractions** (see Chapter 26).

V. Thyroid Hormones and Related Drugs (Box 23-4)

- Thyroid hormones are required for normal growth and development.
- These substances play a role in metabolism (calorigenic activity).

A. Thyroxine (T_4)- and triiodothyronine (T_3)-related preparations

- T_3 is less tightly bound than T_4 to the transport protein, thyroxine-binding globulin (TBG).
- T_3 is approximately four times more potent than T_4.

1. Regulation of thyroid function

a. Thyrotropin (TSH) from the anterior pituitary stimulates the synthesis and secretion of T_4 and T_3.

b. Iodine deficiency results in decreased thyroid hormone synthesis, leading to increased TSH release and goiter.

2. Drugs that affect thyroid function (Table 23-2)

3. Levothyroxine (T_4)

a. Pharmacokinetics

(1) Slow-acting: 1–3 weeks required for full therapeutic effect

(2) Half-life ($t_{1/2}$): 9–10 days in hyperthyroid patients

b. Uses: thyroid replacement and suppression therapy

c. Adverse effects: cardiotoxicity, excessive thermogenesis, increased sympathetic activity, insomnia, anxiety, tension

Thyroid hormone may cause hyperthyroid symptoms and allergic skin reactions.

4. Triiodothyronine (T_3), liothyronine (synthetic T_3)

- Faster acting than T_4, but not usually used because T_4 is converted to T_3 in the body

TABLE 23-2 Drugs That Affect Thyroid Function

Drug	Effect on Thyroid Gland
Amiodarone	Altered thyroid synthesis, causing hyperthyroidism
Androgens	Decreased TBG, causing decrease in T_4
Carbamazepine	Induced cytochrome P450 system, causing hypothyroidism
Estrogens	Increased TBG, causing increase in T_4
Glucocorticoids	Decreased TBG, causing decrease in T_4
Iodides	Altered thyroid synthesis, causing hyperthyroidism
Levodopa	Altered thyroid synthesis, causing hypothyroidism
Lithium	Altered thyroid synthesis, causing hypothyroidism
Phenobarbital	Induced cytochrome P450 system, causing hypothyroidism
Phenytoin	Induced cytochrome P450 system, causing hypothyroidism
Rifampin	Induced cytochrome P450 system, causing hypothyroidism
Salicylates	Displaced from TBG, causing hyperthyroidism
Tamoxifen	Increased TBG, causing increase in T_4

T_4, Thyroxine; *TBG,* thyroxine-binding globulin.

B. Antithyroid agents

1. Thioamides

- **Examples: propylthiouracil, methimazole**

a. Mechanism of action: inhibit synthesis of T_3 and T_4

(1) Prevent oxidation of iodide to iodine

(2) Inhibit coupling of two iodotyrosyl residues (iodinated tyrosine molecules) to form T_3 or T_4

b. Uses: hyperthyroidism, thyrotoxicosis

Propylthiouracil inhibits conversion of peripheral T_4 to T_3.

c. Adverse effects: hypothyroidism, hepatotoxicity, leukopenia, agranulocytosis

2. Iodide (sodium or potassium iodide, intravenous or oral)

a. Mechanism of action: rapidly inhibits release of T_3 and T_4 in pharmacologic doses

b. Uses

(1) Preparation for **surgical thyroidectomy** (decreases size and vascularity of gland)

(2) Treatment of **thyrotoxicosis**

c. Adverse effects: blocked uptake of radioactive iodine, induction of **hyperthyroidism**

- Iodide should be avoided if therapy with radioactive iodine is necessary.

3. Radioactive iodine (^{131}I)

- ^{131}I, the radioactive isotope of iodine, is **administered orally.**

a. Mechanism of action: trapped by the thyroid gland and incorporated into thyroglobulin

- Emission of beta radiation destroys the cells of the thyroid gland.

b. Use: hyperthyroidism

c. Adverse effects: bone marrow suppression, angina, radiation sickness

4. β-Adrenergic receptor antagonists (see Chapter 5)

- **Use:** reduction of symptoms of thyrotoxicosis, such as

BOX 23-5 Adrenal Hormones and Related Drugs

Glucocorticoids
Short- to Medium-acting
Cortisone
Hydrocortisone (cortisol)
Prednisolone
Prednisone

Intermediate-acting
Fluprednisolone
Triamcinolone

Long-acting
Betamethasone
Dexamethasone

Mineralocorticoids
Desoxycorticosterone
Fludrocortisone

Glucocorticoid Antagonists and Synthesis Inhibitors
Aminoglutethimide
Ketoconazole
Metyrapone
Mifepristone
Mitotane

Mineralocorticoid Antagonists
Spironolactone

tremor, palpitations, anxiety, heat intolerance, tachycardia, and arrhythmias

VI. Adrenocorticosteroids (Box 23-5)
A. **Glucocorticoids**
- **Examples:** cortisol, hydrocortisone

1. **Synthesis and secretion**
    a. **Synthesized from cholesterol**
        - Adrenocorticosteroids are not stored by the adrenal gland but are released as soon as they are produced.

    b. **Regulated by ACTH** and exhibits a similar circadian rhythm
2. **Mechanism of action:** suppression of the release of arachidonic acid from phospholipids by inhibiting phospholipase A_2 and expressing COX-2, resulting in an **anti-inflammatory action** (see Chapter 2 for signaling mechanism)
3. **Uses**
    a. Substitution therapy in adrenocortical insufficiency
    b. **Nonendocrine disorders** (Table 23-3)
    c. **Diagnostic functions**
        - Adrenocorticosteroids suppress ACTH production to identify the source of a particular hormone or estab-

TABLE 23-3 Nonadrenal Disorders Treated with Corticosteroids

Nature of the Condition	Disorder
Allergic reactions	Angioedema, anaphylaxis
Bone and joint disorders	Rheumatoid arthritis, systemic lupus erythematosus
Collagen vascular disorders	Systemic lupus erythematosus
Eye diseases	Iritis, keratitis, chorioretinitis
Gastrointestinal disorders	Crohn's disease, ulcerative colitis
Hematologic disorders	Idiopathic cytopenic purpura
Neurologic disorders	Acute spinal cord injury, multiple sclerosis flare, increased intracranial pressure
Organ transplants	Kidney transplant
Pulmonary diseases	COPD or asthma flares
Renal disease	Glomerulonephropathies (Goodpasture's syndrome)
Skin disorders	Psoriasis, dermatitis, eczema
Thyroid diseases	Malignant exophthalmos, subacute thyroiditis

COPD, Chronic obstructive pulmonary disease.

lish whether production of a hormone is influenced by secretion of ACTH.
- Urine levels of steroid metabolites are of diagnostic value.

4. Adverse effects

a. Adrenal suppression due to negative feedback mechanisms

(1) The degree of suppression is a function of the **dose** and **length of therapy**.

(2) When therapy is discontinued, the **dose must be tapered.**

b. Iatrogenic **Cushing's syndrome**

c. Metabolic effects

(1) **Hypokalemic alkalosis** due to the mineralocorticoid effects of the glucocorticoid

(2) **Glycosuria** due to the effect on glucose metabolism

d. Edema due to Na^+ and fluid retention

e. Increased susceptibility to infection

f. Peptic ulcer disease

g. Musculoskeletal effects

(1) **Myopathy:** skeletal muscle weakness

(2) **Osteoporosis**

h. Behavioral disturbances: psychosis, euphoria, insomnia, restlessness

i. Ophthalmic effects: permanent visual impairment, exophthalmos, retinopathy, cataracts

B. Mineralocorticoids

- **Aldosterone:** naturally occurring hormone
- **Fludrocortisone:** oral synthetic adrenocorticosteroid with both mineralocorticoid and glucocorticoid activity (only mineralocorticoid effects at usual doses)

1. Synthesis and secretion

- **Angiotensin II** is the primary stimulus.

2. Mechanism of action
   a. Increase the retention of Na^+ and water
   b. Increase the excretion of K^+ and H^+
3. Use: adrenocortical insufficiency (administered with glucocorticoids)

C. Antagonists of adrenocortical agents
1. Glucocorticoid antagonists and synthesis inhibitors
   a. Metyrapone
      (1) Mechanism of action: inhibits 11 β-hydroxylase, thus inhibiting production of cortisol
      (2) Uses
         (a) Diagnostic test for the production of ACTH
         (b) Treatment of **Cushing's syndrome**
   b. Aminoglutethimide
      (1) Mechanism of action: inhibits enzymatic conversion of cholesterol to pregnenolone, leading to reduced synthesis of all **adrenocortical hormones**
      (2) Use: Cushing's syndrome
   c. Ketoconazole
      • **Antifungal agent**
      (1) Mechanism of action: inhibits mammalian synthesis of glucocorticoids and steroid hormones by inhibiting the cytochrome P450 system and 11 β-hydroxylase
      (2) Use: Cushing's syndrome
   d. Mifepristone (RU 486)
      • Glucocorticoid receptor antagonist and progesterone antagonist (see Chapter 26)
   e. Mitotane: adrenocortical cytotoxic antineoplastic agent
      • Use: adrenocortical carcinoma
2. Mineralocorticoid antagonists
   • **Example: spironolactone** (see Chapter 15)
   a. Mechanism of action: competitive inhibitor of aldosterone
   b. Uses
      (1) Hypertension (in combination with thiazide diuretics as a potassium-sparing diuretic)
      (2) Primary hyperaldosteronism (treatment and diagnosis)
      (3) Hirsutism (women)
      (4) Ascites associated with cirrhosis
      (5) Severe congestive heart failure

24

Drugs Used in the Treatment of Diabetes Mellitus and Errors of Glucose Metabolism

Target Topics

- Insulins
- Oral hypoglycemic agents
- Metformin
- Thiazolidinediones ("insulin sensitizers")
- Glucagon

I. General Considerations (Table 24-1)
   A. **Types of diabetes mellitus**
      1. **Type 1:** an autoimmune disease characterized by a **loss of pancreatic β cells**
      2. **Type 2:** a disease characterized by **β cells that are desensitized to a glucose challenge and peripheral tissues that are resistant to insulin**
   B. Complications
      - **Chronic hyperglycemia** results in neuropathy, retinopathy, nephropathy, peripheral vascular disease, and coronary artery disease.
   C. **Drugs that impair glucose tolerance** include corticosteroids, thiazide diuretics, and combination oral contraceptives.

TABLE 24-1 Characteristics of Type 1 and Type 2 Diabetes Mellitus

	Type 1	Type 2
Age of onset	Usually < 25 years	Usually > 40 years
Acuteness of onset	Usually sudden	Usually gradual
Presenting features	Polyuria, polydipsia, polyphagia, acidosis	Often asymptomatic
Body habitus	Often thin	Usually overweight
Control of diabetes	Difficult	Easy
Ketoacidosis	Frequent	Seldom, unless under stress
Insulin requirement	Always	Often unnecessary
Control by oral agents	Never	Frequent
Control by diet alone	Never	Frequent
Complications	Frequent	Frequent

BOX 24-1 Drugs Used in the Treatment of Diabetes Mellitus

Insulins
Lente
Lispro
NPH
Regular
Ultralente

Sulfonylureas
Chlorpropamide
Glipizide
Glyburide
Tolbutamide

Biguanide
Metformin

α-Glucosidase Inhibitors
Acarbose

Thiazolidinediones
Pioglitazone
Rosiglitazone

NPH, Neutral Protamine Hagedorn.

II. Hypoglycemic Agents (Box 24-1)

A. Insulin

1. Synthesis and secretion

- Insulin, a **polypeptide hormone,** is composed of two chains joined together by disulfide linkages.

a. Synthesis: by **β cells of the pancreas** and by **proteolytic enzymes** into insulin and C peptide

b. Release: regulated by blood glucose levels

Use C peptide levels to differentiate between exogenous insulin (overdose) and endogenous insulin (overproduction/insulinoma).

2. Physiologic action

a. Promotion of glucose uptake by the liver, muscle cells, and adipocytes, resulting in **decreased serum glucose levels**

b. Translocation of the glucose transporter to the cell surface

3. Insulin preparations

- Different insulin preparations have different effects on plasma glucose use (Figure 24-1; Table 24-2).
- Beef insulin is no longer used in the United States.

a. Human insulin is produced using recombinant DNA technology.

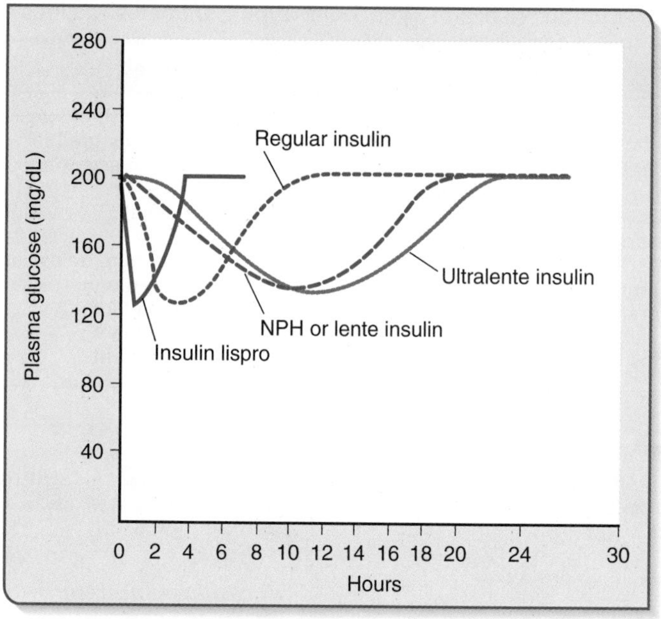

Figure 24-1 Effects of various insulin preparations on plasma glucose levels in a fasting individual.

TABLE 24-2 Therapeutic Time Course of Insulin Preparations

Preparation	Onset of Action	Duration of Action	Peak Effect
Rapid-acting Insulin			
Insulin lispro	0–15 minutes	< 5 hours	30–90 minutes
Short-acting Insulin			
Insulin injection (regular insulin)	30–45 minutes	5–7 hours	2–4 hours
Intermediate-acting Insulins			
Insulin zinc suspension (lente insulin) or isophane insulin suspension (neutral protamine Hagedorn insulin; NPH)	1–4 hours	18–24 hours	6–14 hours
Long-acting Insulin			
Extended insulin zinc suspension (ultralente insulin)	4–6 hours	≥ 30 hours	18–26 hours

b. **Pork insulin** is more immunogenic than human insulin.

4. **Uses: diabetes mellitus, hyperkalemia**
5. **Adverse effects: hypoglycemia, lipodystrophy** (change in the subcutaneous fat at the site of injection)

B. Oral hypoglycemic agents

1. **Sulfonylureas**
   - **First-generation drugs:** chlorpropamide, tolbutamide

- **Second-generation drugs:** glipizide, glyburide

a. Mechanism of action

(1) Stimulate the release of insulin from the functional β cells of the pancreas

(2) Bind to ATP-sensitive potassium-channel receptors on the β cells, depolarizing the membrane

b. Use: type 2 diabetes mellitus

c. Adverse effects

(1) Hypoglycemia

(2) Disulfiram-like reaction after ingestion of ethanol (most prominent with chlorpropamide)

- Ethanol also **inhibits gluconeogenesis;** thus, hypoglycemia can occur more readily in patients receiving oral hypoglycemic drugs.

Sulfonamide hypersensitivity: cross hypersensitivity with sulfonamides, thiazides, furosemide

2. Biguanides

- **Example: metformin**

a. Mechanism of action

(1) Do *not* stimulate insulin release

(2) Improve glucose tolerance

(a) Increase peripheral utilization of glucose

(b) Decrease hepatic gluconeogenesis

(3) Do *not* induce weight gain

(4) Reduce macrovascular complications of type 2 diabetes mellitus

b. Use: type 2 diabetes mellitus

c. Adverse effects: lactic acidosis, especially in patients who have cardiac, renal, or hepatic disease

3. Thiazolidinediones ("insulin sensitizers")

- **Examples: rosiglitazone, pioglitazone** (troglitazone removed from the market)

a. Mechanism of action

(1) Decrease hepatic gluconeogenesis

(2) Enhance uptake of glucose by skeletal muscle cells

(3) Act via the **peroxisome proliferator-activated receptor-γ,** a nuclear receptor that alters gene transcription

b. Use: type 2 diabetes mellitus, especially in patients with insulin resistance

c. Adverse effects: elevated hepatic enzymes, hepatic failure

4. α-Glucosidase inhibitors

- **Example: acarbose**

a. Mechanism of action: inhibitor of α-glucosidases in enterocytes of the small intestine, resulting in delayed carbohydrate digestion and reduced absorption

b. Use: type 2 diabetes mellitus

- α-Glucosidase inhibitors effectively **lower postprandial serum glucose** but have minimal effects on fasting glucose.

c. Adverse effects: abdominal pain, diarrhea, flatulence

Metformin may cause lactic acidosis.

III. Hyperglycemic Agent: Glucagon

A. Regulation of secretion

- Glucagon is synthesized by the **α cells of the pancreas.**

1. **Stimulators:** α-adrenergic agents, amino acids
2. **Inhibitors:** glucose, secretin, somatostatin, free fatty acids

Endogenous hormones that counter-regulate insulin: glucagon, cortisol, epinephrine

B. Physiologic actions

- Glucagon increases blood glucose by **stimulating glycogenolysis** and **gluconeogenesis** in the liver.
- Many of the actions of glucagon oppose those of insulin (e.g., hyperglycemia, increased gluconeogenesis).

Treat hypoglycemia with IV glucose or glucagon.

C. Uses

1. **Severe hypoglycemia in unconscious patients (emergency use)**
2. **Diagnostic uses**
   a. **Radiologic and contrast procedures** (reduction of gastrointestinal spasms)
   b. **Glycogen storage disease**
   c. **Pheochromocytoma** and insulinoma
   d. **Growth hormone dysfunction**
3. Treat overdoses of β-blockers.

25

Drugs Used in the Treatment of Bone and Calcium Disorders

Target Topics

- Parathyroid hormone
- Vitamin D and calcitonin
- Bisphosphonates
- Estrogens and raloxifene

I. General Considerations
- **Parathyroid hormone (PTH)** and **vitamin D** play a role in the **regulation of calcium and phosphorus** (Figure 25-1; Table 25-1).

A. PTH

1. **Regulation of secretion:** stimulated by hypocalcemia
2. **Use:** no therapeutic use at present
   - PTH may be used in the treatment of osteoporosis in the future.

B. Disorders of parathyroid function

1. **Hypoparathyroidism**
   - Often occurs after accidental damage to or removal of the parathyroid gland during thyroid surgery
   - Leads to a **decrease in serum calcium** and an **increase in serum phosphate**
2. **Hyperparathyroidism**
   - May be seen with **adenomas** or **carcinomas** of the parathyroid gland or occur as a result of a compensatory

Regulators of calcium and phosphorous: PTH, vitamin D, calcitonin

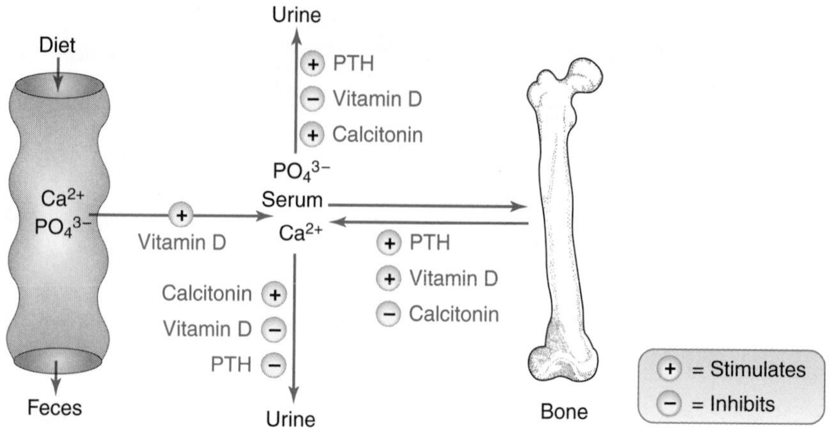

Figure 25-1 The effects of vitamin D, parathyroid hormone *(PTH),* and calcitonin on serum calcium *(Ca^{2+})* and phosphate *(PO_4^{3-})* on bone mineral homeostasis.

TABLE 25-1 Actions of Parathyroid Hormone and Vitamin D on Intestine, Kidney, and Bone

	Parathyroid Hormone	Vitamin D
Intestine	↑ Calcium and phosphate absorption by ↑ $1,25(OH)_2D$ production	↑ Calcium and phosphate absorption by $1,25(OH)_2D$
Kidney	↓ Calcium excretion ↑ Phosphate excretion	Calcium and phosphate excretion may be ↓ by 25(OH)D and $1,25(OH)_2D$
Bone	↑ Calcium and phosphate resorption in high doses Low doses may ↑ bone formation	↑ Calcium and phosphate resorption by $1,25(OH)_2D$ Bone formation may be ↑ by $24,25(OH)_2D$
Net effect on serum levels	↑ Serum calcium ↓ Serum phosphate	↓ Serum calcium ↓ Serum phosphate

mechanism when chronic hypocalcemia (malabsorption, vitamin D deficiency) is present

II. Drugs That Affect Calcium Levels (Box 25-1)

A. Calcitonin

- This peptide is produced by the **parafollicular cells of the thyroid gland.**

1. **Regulation of secretion:** stimulation of release by hypercalcemia
2. **Mechanism of action:** inhibits bone resorption and increases kidney excretion, thereby lowering serum calcium and phosphate levels
3. **Uses**
   a. Administered parenterally to treat **hypercalcemia**
   b. **Paget's disease**
   c. **Postmenopausal osteoporosis (intranasal)**

BOX 25-1 Drugs That Affect Calcium Levels

Drugs That Increase Calcium Levels
Calcium
Parathyroid hormone
Vitamin D (dihydrotachysterol, calcitriol)

Drugs That Decrease Calcium Levels
Bisphosphonates (etidronate, pamidronate, alendronate, risedronate)
Calcitonin
Estrogens and raloxifene
Phosphate
Plicamycin (cytotoxic antibiotic)

B. Vitamin D
- Vitamin D deficiency causes **rickets** in children and **osteomalacia** in adults.

Vitamin D deficiency: rickets (children) and osteomalacia (adults)

1. **Sources and formation**
   a. Sterols are converted by sunlight to **ergocalciferol** (vitamin D_2) and **cholecalciferol** (vitamin D_3) in the skin.
      - **Dihydrotachysterol:** ergocalciferol analogue
   b. Sterols are **metabolized by the liver and kidney** to active forms of vitamin D (see Table 25-1).
      (1) **Calcitriol:** $1,25(OH)_2D_3$
      (2) **Secalcifediol:** $24,25(OH)_2D_3$
2. **Uses**
   a. **Rickets:** prevention; given with calcium to supplement the diet of infants
   b. **Hypoparathyroidism:** given with calcium supplements
   c. **Osteoporosis:** prevention and treatment
   d. **Chronic renal disease**
3. **Hypervitaminosis D**
   a. **Hypercalcemia**
   b. **Fatigue**
   c. **Nephrocalcinosis**, calcification of soft tissues

Hypervitaminosis D: hypercalcemia, fatigue, nephrocalcinosis, calcification of soft tissues

C. Calcium
1. **Pharmacokinetics:** limited gastrointestinal absorption (< 30%)
2. **Uses**
   a. **Bone and normal growth**
   b. **Osteoporosis:** prevention and treatment
   c. **Hypocalcemia**
   d. **Chronic renal disease**
3. **Adverse effects:** constipation

D. Phosphate
- Quickly lowers serum calcium levels when given intravenously

E. Bisphosphonates
- **Examples: etidronate, pamidronate, alendronate, risedronate**

1. **Mechanism of action:** bind to hydroxyapatite in bone, inhibiting osteoclast activity
2. Uses
   - **a. Postmenopausal bone loss**
   - **b. Hypercalcemia due to malignancy**
   - **c. Osteoporosis and compression fractures**
   - **d. Paget's disease**
3. **Adverse effects: reflux esophagitis** (gastroesophageal reflux disease; GERD)
   - To avoid this condition, patients should:
   - **a.** Take these drugs on an **empty stomach, with at least 8 oz water**, immediately upon awakening
   - **b.** Remain in an **upright position for at least 30 minutes after taking drug**
   - **c.** *Not* drink or eat anything for **30 minutes after taking drug**

F. Estrogens and raloxifene (selective estrogen receptor modulator; SERM)

Drugs used in the treatment of postmenopausal prevention of osteoporosis: estrogens with or without progestins, bisphosphonates, raloxifene

1. **Mechanism of action:** reduces bone resorption
2. **Uses: postmenopausal osteoporosis** (reduces bone loss)
   - *Cannot* restore bone

G. Plicamycin (cytotoxic antibiotic)

1. **Mechanism of action:** inhibits osteoclast activity
2. **Use: hypercalcemia** (intravenous), especially associated with cancer (e.g., breast cancer)

26

Drugs Used in Reproductive Endocrinology

Target Topics

- Oxytocin and prostaglandins
- Estrogens and progestins
- Oral contraceptives
- Androgens and antiandrogens

I. Drugs That Act on the Uterus (Box 26-1)

A. Oxytocin

- This peptide hormone is synthesized in the hypothalamus and stored in the posterior pituitary until it is needed.
- It plays a facilitatory role in **parturition** and is an essential element in the **milk-ejection reflex**; suckling → oxytocin release → milk "let-down."

1. **Mechanism of action**
   - **a.** Stimulates **contraction of uterine muscle**
   - **b.** Stimulates **smooth muscles of mammary glands**
2. **Uses**
   - **a. Induction of labor** (administered intravenously)
   - **b. Control of postpartum hemorrhage** (administered intravenously)
   - **c. Promotion of milk ejection** (administered intranasally)
3. **Adverse effects:** uterine rupture, water intoxication, hypertension, fetal death

BOX 26-1 Drugs That Act on the Uterus

Cause Contraction
Ergot alkaloids: ergonovine, methylergonovine
Oxytocin
Prostaglandins: dinoprostone (PGE_2), carboprost ($PGF_{2\alpha}$)

Cause Relaxation
β_2-Adrenoceptor agonist: terbutaline
Magnesium sulfate
NSAIDs

4. Contraindications
    a. **Fetal distress**
    b. Prematurity
    c. Abnormal fetal presentation
    d. Cephalopelvic disproportion

B. Prostaglandins
- **Examples: dinoprostone** (PGE_2), **carboprost** ($PGF_{2\alpha}$)

1. **Mechanism of action:** potent stimulation of uterine tissue
2. Uses
    a. Induction of abortion
    b. Softening of the cervix before induction of labor (administered intravaginally)
    c. Facilitation of labor
3. Adverse effects
    a. **Prolonged vaginal bleeding**
    b. Severe uterine cramps

C. Ergot alkaloids and related compounds
- **Examples:** ergonovine, methylergonovine

1. **Mechanism of action:** increase the motor activity of the uterus, resulting in forceful, prolonged contractions
2. **Use:** prevention of postpartum bleeding
3. **Adverse effects:** nausea, vomiting, abdominal pain, prolactin suppression

Ergot alkaloids should only be used postpartum.

D. Other drugs that affect the uterus
1. **Nonsteroidal anti-inflammatory drugs (NSAIDs)**
    a. **Mechanism of action:** inhibit prostaglandin synthesis
    b. **Use:** relief of cramps associated with menstruation (**dysmenorrhea**)
        - The therapeutic effect is attributed to **blocking** of the increased endometrial synthesis of **prostaglandins** during menstruation.
2. **β_2-Adrenoceptor agonist (terbutaline)**
    a. **Mechanism of action:** mediate relaxation of uterine smooth muscle
    b. **Use:** prevention of premature labor (tocolytic agent)
3. **Magnesium sulfate**
    a. **Mechanism of action:** relax uterine muscle
    b. **Uses:** prevention of premature labor (tocolytic agent); treatment of preeclampsia and eclampsia

BOX 26-2 Gonadal Hormones and Inhibitors

Estrogens
Conjugated estrogens
Estradiol
Ethinyl estradiol

Selective Estrogen Receptor Modulators (SERMs)
Clomiphene
Raloxifene
Tamoxifen

Progestins
Norethindrone
Norgestimate
Norgestrel
Progesterone

Antiprogestins
Danazol
Mifepristone

Androgens
Methyltestosterone
Testosterone

Antiandrogens
Bicalutamide
Finasteride
Flutamide
GnRH analogues
Ketoconazole

II. Estrogens and Related Drugs (Box 26-2)

A. Estrogens

1. **Synthesis and secretion**
   a. Formation in ovarian follicles: controlled by **follicle-stimulating hormone** (FSH)
   b. Major secretory product of the ovary: **estradiol**
2. **Physiologic actions**
   a. Necessary for the normal maturation of females
   b. Important for the proliferation of endometrial tissue and normal menstrual cycling
3. **Pharmacokinetics:** metabolized by the liver
4. **Uses**
   a. **Oral contraception**
   b. **Estrogen replacement therapy** (ERT) in individuals with primary hypogonadism and in postmenopausal women
   c. **Osteoporosis:** prevention and treatment
   d. Suppression of ovulation in women with intractable **dysmenorrhea** or excessive ovarian androgen secretion
   e. **Androgen-dependent cancers** (e.g., carcinoma of the prostate gland)
5. **Adverse effects**
   a. Postmenopausal bleeding during ERT
   b. Nausea
   c. Breast tenderness
   d. Increased incidence of **migraine headaches**, cholestasis, **hypertension**, gallbladder disease, **thrombophlebitis, thromboembolism**, increased platelet aggregation, and accelerated blood clotting
6. **Contraindications**
   a. **Estrogen-dependent neoplasms** (e.g., endometrial carcinoma)

Women who smoke should not use estrogens.

b. **Known or suspected carcinoma of the breast**
c. **Liver disease**
d. History of **thromboembolic disorders**
e. **Smoking**

B. Selective estrogen receptor modulators (SERMs)
- Agonists in some tissues and antagonists in other tissues
- Sometimes called partial agonists

1. **Clomiphene**
   a. **Mechanism of action:** blocks estrogen negative feedback, causing an **increase in FSH and luteinizing hormone (LH)**
   b. **Uses:** to stimulate ovulation in the treatment of infertility
   c. **Adverse effects:** multiple pregnancies (incidence: 5–10%)
2. **Tamoxifen**
   a. **Mechanism of action:** acts as an estrogen receptor antagonist in the breast
   b. **Uses:** breast cancer (receptor positive): prophylaxis and treatment
   c. **Adverse effects:** hot flashes, nausea and vomiting (incidence: 25%)
3. **Raloxifene** (see Chapter 25)
   - Partial agonist in bone but does not stimulate the endometrium or breast

C. Progestins
- **Progesterone** is the most important progestin in humans.

1. **Synthesis and secretion**
   a. **Synthesis:** ovary, testes, adrenal cortex, placenta
   b. **Synthesis and secretion:** corpus luteum stimulated by LH
2. **Physiologic actions**
   a. Contributes to the development of a **secretory endometrium**
   b. **Suppresses uterine contractility**, especially during pregnancy
3. **Uses**
   a. Hormonal **contraception**
   b. Dysmenorrhea, endometriosis, uterine bleeding disorders
   c. Hirsutism
   d. Hormonal replacement therapy (estrogens and progestins)

D. Antiprogestins
1. **Mifepristone** (RU 486): postcoital contraceptive agent
2. **Danazol**
   - Weak progestational, androgenic, and glucocorticoid drug

   a. **Mechanism of action:** decreases secretion of FSH and LH
   b. **Uses**
      (1) **Endometriosis**
      (2) Fibrocystic disease of the breast
      (3) Hereditary angioedema
   c. **Adverse effects:** androgenic effects, weight gain, seborrhea, hirsutism, edema, alopecia

III. Oral Contraceptives

A. Types

1. **Estrogen-progestin combination contraceptives**
   - **Estrogen** (**ethinyl estradiol** or **mestranol**) and **progestin** (**norethindrone, norgestrel,** or **norgestimate**)

   a. **Monophasic combination tablets:** same combination of estrogen and progestin given for 20–21 days and stopped for 7–8 days

   b. **Biphasic combination:** same estrogen dose for 21 days, with a higher progestin dose in the last 10 days

   c. **Triphasic combination:** generally the same estrogen dose for 21 days, with a varying progestin dose over the 3 weeks of administration
2. **Continuous progestins**

   a. **Daily progestin tablets:** for patients for whom estrogen administration is undesirable

   b. **Implantable progestin preparation**
   - The **Norplant system,** a subcutaneous implant of **levonorgestrel,** allows secretion of progestin in the blood for up to 5 years.
   - Capsules are implanted under the skin and can be removed at any time.

B. Mechanism of action

1. **Combination contraceptives:** selectively inhibit pituitary function (LH and FSH release), thus blocking ovulation
2. **Progestin-only contraceptives:** affect ovarian function and cervical mucus

C. Uses: **contraception**, endometriosis

D. Adverse effects: venous thrombolic disease, myocardial infarction, cerebrovascular disease, cholestatic jaundice

IV. Androgens and Inhibitors (see Box 26-2)

- Testosterone is the most important androgen in humans.

A. Androgens

1. **Synthesis and secretion**
   - Stimulated by **LH**

   a. Produced primarily by **testes** (Leydig cells) in males and by **ovaries** and **adrenal cortex** in females

   b. Converted to 5α-dihydrotestosterone (DHT) by the enzyme 5α-reductase in some tissues (e.g., prostate, skin)
2. **Physiologic actions**

   a. **Stimulates libido** (increased sex drive) in both males and females

   b. Accounts for the major changes that occur in males at puberty

   c. Has **anabolic activity**
3. **Uses**

   a. Replacement therapy in **hypogonadism** or hypopituitarism

   b. Acceleration of growth in childhood

Finasteride is extremely teratogenic.

c. **Anabolic agent** (especially in debilitating diseases such as AIDS-associated wasting syndrome and breast cancer and in geriatric patients)

4. **Adverse effects**
   a. **Masculinization** (in women)
   b. **Azoospermia**, decrease in testicular size
5. **Abuse potential**
   - Because androgens stimulate muscle growth, some athletes misuse these agents in attempts to improve athletic performance.

B. Androgen suppression and antiandrogens

1. **Androgen suppression**
   - Gonadotropin-releasing hormone (GnRH) analogues such as leuprolide and goserelin produce gonadal suppression when blood levels are continuous rather than pulsatile.
2. **Finasteride**
   a. **Mechanism of action:** inhibits the androgen-metabolizing enzyme 5α-reductase, thus inhibiting formation of DHT and androgen necessary for prostate growth and function
   b. **Uses: benign prostatic hyperplasia** (BPH), male pattern baldness
   c. **Adverse effects**
      (1) **Teratogenic properties**
         - Pregnant women are cautioned about working with finasteride because breathing the dust could result in teratogenesis.
         - It is recommended that double condoms be used during intercourse if the man is taking this drug.

      (2) Impotence, decreased libido
3. **Receptor antagonists**
   a. **Flutamide, bicalutamide**
      - **Uses:** carcinoma of the prostate

   b. **Cyproterone**
      - **Uses:** hirsutism (women), excessive libido (men)
4. **Ketoconazole**
   a. **Mechanism of action:** decreases testosterone synthesis (males)
   b. **Use:** carcinoma of the prostate (experimental)

SECTION VIII

Anti-infective Drugs

27

Antimicrobial Drugs

Target Topics

- Cell wall synthesis inhibitors
- Protein synthesis inhibitors
- Inhibitors of folate metabolism
- DNA gyrase inhibitors

I. General Considerations

- Antibacterial drugs exhibit **selective toxicity** by destroying pathogenic microorganisms yet causing minimal side effects in the host.
- It is important to reach and maintain adequate blood levels to destroy microorganisms and prevent development of microbial resistance.

A. Mechanism of action

- Antibacterial drugs act at a number of different sites (Figure 27-1).

B. Mechanisms of microbial resistance

- Resistance often correlates with the frequency of antimicrobial use, the total quantity of drug dispensed, the location of the patient when receiving the medication, and the immune status of the patient.

1. Pathogens or cells fail to absorb the drug, or they inactivate or remove it (i.e., pump it out).
2. The target receptors are modified or the production of target molecules is increased.
3. Altered metabolic pathways bypass the drug target.

Drugs that cause hepatotoxicity: tetracyclines, isoniazid, erythromycin, clindamycin, sulfonamides, amphotericin B

Drugs that cause renal toxicity: cephalosporins, vancomycin, aminoglycosides, sulfonamides, amphotericin B

4. Multidrug resistance is often transmitted by plasmids.

C. Functions
1. **Antibacterial action** (Table 27-1)
   a. **Bactericidal:** kill disease-causing microorganisms
   b. **Bacteriostatic:** prevent bacterial growth and multiplication
2. **Prophylaxis** (Table 27-2)

D. Adverse effects
1. **Organ-directed toxicity**
   a. **Ototoxicity:** aminoglycosides, vancomycin, minocycline
   b. **Hematopoietic toxicity:** chloramphenicol, sulfonamides
   c. **Hepatotoxicity:** tetracyclines, isoniazid, erythromycin, clindamycin, sulfonamides, amphotericin B
   d. **Renal toxicity:** cephalosporins, vancomycin, aminoglycosides, sulfonamides, amphotericin B
2. **Idiosyncrasies** (unexpected individual reactions)
   a. **Hemolytic anemias:** sulfonamides, nitrofurantoin
   b. **Photosensitivity:** tetracyclines, fluoroquinolones
3. **Hypersensitivity reactions**
   - These reactions are most notable with penicillins and sulfonamides but can occur with most antimicrobial drugs.
4. **Superinfections**
   a. **Candidiasis**
      - **Treatment:** oral **nystatin** or **amphotericin B**
   b. **Pseudomembranous colitis** caused by *Clostridium difficile*
      - **Treatment:** oral **metronidazole** or **vancomycin**
   c. **Staphylococcal enterocolitis**
      - **Treatment:** oral **vancomycin**

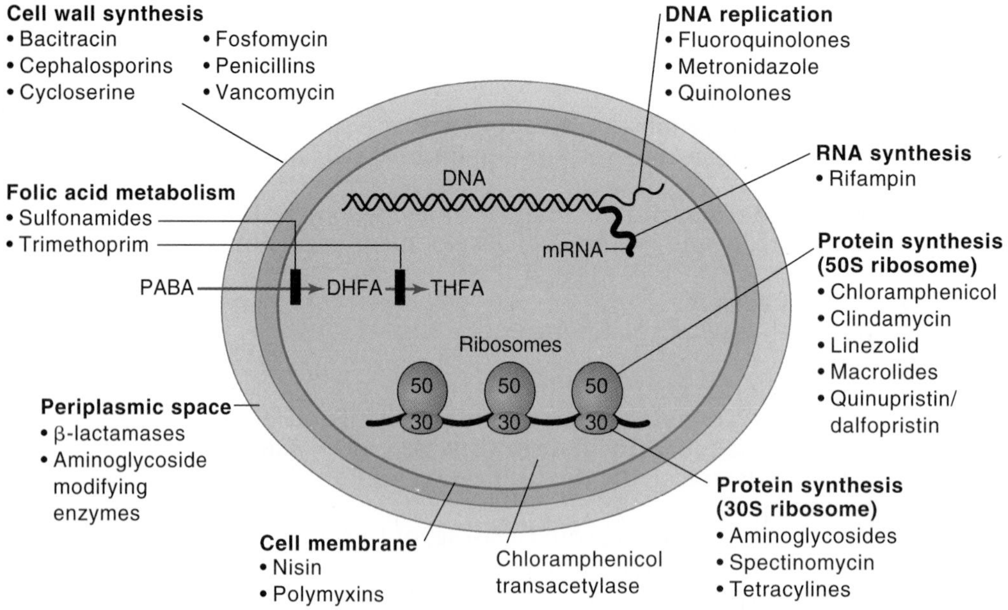

Figure 27-1 Sites of action of antimicrobial drugs and enzymes that inactivate these drugs. *DHFA,* Dihydrofolic acid; *PABA, p*-aminobenzoic acid; *THFA,* tetrahydrofolic acid.

TABLE 27-1 Antibiotics of Choice for Various Infections

Drug	Organism (Disease)
Amoxicillin, clarithromycin (omeprazole*)	*Helicobacter pylori* (peptic ulcer)
Ampicillin	*Listeria* (meningitis)
Ceftriaxone	*Neisseria gonorrhoeae* (gonorrhea)
Cephalosporins (third-generation)	*Haemophilus influenzae* (pneumonia, meningitis) *Klebsiella* (meningitis)
Doxycycline	*Borrelia burgdorferi* (Lyme disease) Rickettsiae (Rocky Mountain spotted fever)
Erythromycin	*Legionella* (legionnaires' disease)
Fluconazole or nystatin	*Candida* (candidiasis)
Isoniazid, rifampin, ethambutol, pyrazinamide	*Mycobacterium tuberculosis* (tuberculosis)
Macrolides	*Mycoplasma pneumoniae* (atypical pneumonia) *Legionella* (legionnaires' disease) *Corynebacterium diphtheriae* *Chlamydia*
Metronidazole	*Trichomonas* (trichomoniasis)
Penicillin G	*Neisseria meningitidis* (meningitis) *Treponema pallidum* (syphilis) Infections caused by streptococci, pneumococci, other meningococci, *Bacillus anthracis, Clostridium, Bacteroides* (except *B. fragilis*)
Quinolones	*Campylobacter* (diarrhea)
Tetracycline	*Vibrio cholerae* (cholera)
Other tetracyclines	*Chlamydia* (pneumonia, lymphogranuloma venereum)
Trimethoprim-sulfamethoxazole	*Salmonella, Shigella* (diarrhea)
Metronidazole or vancomycin (oral)	*Clostridium difficile* (diarrhea)

*Omeprazole is not an antibiotic but is used in combination with antibiotics for treatment of *H. pylori.*

TABLE 27-2 Prophylactic Use of Anti-infective Drugs

Drug	Use
Cefazolin	Surgical procedures
Ampicillin or penicillin	Group B streptococcal infections
Trimethoprim-sulfamethoxazole	*Pneumocystis carinii* pneumonia UTIs
Rifampin	*Haemophilus influenzae* type B Meningococcal infection
Chloroquine	Malaria
Isoniazid	Tuberculosis
Azithromycin	*Mycobacterium avium* complex in patients with AIDS
Ampicillin or azithromycin	Dental procedures in patients with valve abnormalities

AIDS, Acquired immunodeficiency syndrome; *UTI,* urinary tract infection.

BOX 27-1 β-Lactam Drugs and Other Cell Wall Synthesis Inhibitors

Penicillins
Amoxicillin
Ampicillin
Mezlocillin
Nafcillin
Oxacillin
Penicillin G
Penicillin V
Piperacillin
Ticarcillin

Cephalosporins
First-Generation Drugs
Cefazolin
Cephalexin
Cephalothin (prototype; no longer available in the United States)
Cephradine

Second-Generation Drugs
Cefaclor
Cefotetan
Cefoxitin

Third-Generation Drugs
Cefoperazone
Ceftazidime
Ceftriaxone

Fourth-Generation Drugs
Cefepime

Other β-Lactam Drugs
Aztreonam
Imipenem-cilastatin
Meropenem

Other Cell Wall Synthesis Inhibitors
Bacitracin
Fosfomycin
Vancomycin

II. Cell Wall Synthesis Inhibitors (Box 27-1)

- These drugs inhibit various intracellular or extracellular steps in the synthesis of the cell wall (see Figure 27-1).
- **β-Lactam antibiotics are most often used.**

A. Penicillins

- **Key characteristics:** β-lactam ring, penicillinase sensitivity, acid labile, inhibition of cell wall synthesis, hypersensitivity

1. Pharmacokinetics

a. Absorption

- May be destroyed by gastric acid
- Acid-resistant **penicillin V:** oral administration

b. **Distribution:** poor movement across the noninflamed blood-brain barrier
c. **Excretion:** unchanged in urine by tubular secretion, which is inhibited by probenecid

2. **Pharmacodynamics**
   a. **Mechanism of action**
      (1) **Bind to specific penicillin-binding proteins (PBPs)** located inside the bacterial cell wall, thus inhibiting the cross-linking in bacterial cell wall synthesis
      (2) Inhibit transpeptidase enzymes
   b. **Causes of resistance**
      (1) **Inactivation by β-lactamases** (most common)
      (2) Alteration in target PBPs
      (3) Permeability barrier, preventing drug penetration
         - Contributes to the resistance of many gram-negative bacteria

Alterations in PBPs: responsible for methicillin resistance in staphylococci and penicillin resistance in pneumococci

3. **Uses**
   a. **Penicillin G**
      (1) **Pharyngitis** (hemolytic streptococcus)
      (2) **Syphilis** (*Treponema pallidum*)
      (3) **Pneumonia** (pneumococcus, streptococcus)
      (4) **Meningitis** (meningococcus, pneumococcus)
   b. **Benzathine penicillin G**
      - Intramuscular injection: low blood levels for up to 3 weeks
      - Useful in situations in which organisms are very sensitive (e.g., *T. pallidum* in syphilis)
   c. **Ampicillin and amoxicillin**
      (1) **Urinary tract infections** (UTIs) (*Escherichia coli*)
      (2) **Infectious diarrhea** (*Salmonella*)
      (3) **Otitis media or sinusitis** (*Haemophilus*)
      (4) **Meningitis** (*Listeria*)
      (5) **Endocarditis** (prevention)
   d. **Ticarcillin:** potent against **nosocomial *(Pseudomonas)* infections**
      - Usually combined with an aminoglycoside
   e. **Piperacillin**
      - More active against *Pseudomonas* than ticarcillin
   f. **Penicillinase-resistant β-lactam antibiotics (nafcillin, oxacillin)**
      - Used against penicillinase-producing microorganisms
      (1) **Endocarditis**
      (2) **Osteomyelitis** (staphylococci)

Primary use of penicillin: infections with gram (+) bacteria

4. **Adverse effects: allergic reactions** (most serious)

Antistaphylococcal penicillins (e.g., nafcillin): ineffective against infections with MRSA

B. Cephalosporins
- **Key characteristics:** β-lactam ring, increased resistance to penicillinases, inhibition of cell wall synthesis, acid resistance (some agents), nephrotoxicity

1. **Mechanism of action:** similar to penicillins but penicillinase-resistant

Ampicillin rash: nonallergic rash in patients with mononucleosis who take ampicillin

2. Uses
   a. **First-generation (cefazolin)**
      - **Cephalothin**, the prototype first-generation cephalosporin, *is no longer available in the United States.*
      - **Cefazolin** has good activity against **gram-positive bacteria** and modest activity against gram-negative bacteria.
      (1) **Cellulitis** (staphylococcus, streptococcus)
      (2) **Surgical prophylaxis**
   b. **Second-generation (cefaclor, cefoxitin, cefotetan, cefuroxime)**
      - Increased activity against **gram-negative bacteria** (*E. coli, Klebsiella, Proteus, Haemophilus influenzae, Moraxella catarrhalis*)
      (1) Pelvic inflammatory disease, diverticulitis, surgical prophylaxis
      (2) Pneumonia, bronchitis (*H. influenzae*)
   c. **Third-generation (ceftriaxone, cefotaxime)**
      - Decreased activity against gram-positive bacteria but increased activity against **gram-negative bacteria** (*Enterobacter, Serratia*)
      - Activity against *Pseudomonas aeruginosa* in a subset of drugs (**ceftazidime, cefoperazone**)
      (1) **Meningitis** (*Neisseria gonorrhoeae*)
      (2) **Gonorrhea**, community-acquired pneumonia, Lyme disease, meningitis, osteomyelitis (**ceftazidime**)

Many third-generation cephalosporins that penetrate into the CNS are useful in meningitis.

   d. **Fourth-generation (cefepime)**
      - Extensive **gram-positive and gram-negative** activity and increased resistance to β-lactamases
      - **Use:** neutropenic fever
3. **Adverse effects**
   - Disulfiram-like effect with alcohol (some second- and third-generation cephalosporins)
   - **Dose-dependent nephrotoxicity**, especially when used with other nephrotoxic drugs (e.g., aminoglycosides)

Cross-sensitivity to cephalosporins: less than 5% of patients with penicillin allergy

C. **Other β-lactam drugs**
1. **Aztreonam**
   - This monobactam, which is given intravenously, has no activity against gram-positive or anaerobic bacteria.
   a. **Use:** infections with **gram-negative rods**, including *Serratia, Klebsiella,* and *Pseudomonas*
   b. **Adverse effects**: pseudomembranous colitis, candidiasis
2. **Carbapenems**
   - **Examples: imipenem, meropenem**
   a. **Meropenem:** not inactivated by dehydropeptidases
   b. **Imipenem**
      (1) Rapidly inactivated by renal tubule dehydropeptidases
      (2) **Must be given with cilastatin**, a dehydropeptidase inhibitor

Imipenem must be given with cilastatin to prevent inactivation by renal tubule dehydropeptidases.

   c. **Uses:** broad-spectrum activity, including anaerobes

BOX 27-2 Drugs That Affect the Cell Membrane

Nisin
Polymyxin

d. **Adverse effects:** nausea, vomiting, pseudomembranous colitis, confusion, myoclonia, seizures (not with meropenem)

3. **Clavulanic acid:** β-lactamase inhibitor
   - Other β-lactamase inhibitors: sulbactam and tazobactam
   a. Given in combination with β-lactamase–sensitive penicillins, such as **ampicillin, amoxicillin**, ticarcillin, and piperacillin
   b. Not active against methicillin-resistant *Staphylococcus aureus* (MRSA)

D. Other cell wall synthesis inhibitors

1. **Vancomycin**
   a. **Mechanism of action**
      - Prevents chain elongation and cross-linking by binding to the D-ala-D-ala terminus of the peptidoglycan peptide, thus **inhibiting cell wall synthesis**
   b. **Uses**
      - Active against only **gram-positive bacteria**
      (1) Infections caused by penicillin-resistant *S. aureus* and MRSA, enterococci, and other gram-positive bacteria in penicillin-allergic patients
      (2) *C. difficile*–caused diarrhea
         - **Oral administration** results in poor gastrointestinal (GI) absorption.
   c. **Adverse effects**
      (1) **Ototoxicity**
      (2) **Nephrotoxicity**
      (3) **"Red man syndrome"** (flushing from histamine release when given too quickly)
2. **Fosfomycin**
   a. **Mechanism of action:** inhibits cell wall synthesis
   b. **Uses**
      (1) Uncomplicated lower UTIs in women
      (2) Infections caused by gram-positive (enterococci) and gram-negative bacteria
   c. **Adverse effects:** asthenia, diarrhea, dizziness
3. **Bacitracin** (Box 27-2)
   - **Given in combination with polymyxin or neomycin** ointments for prophylaxis of superficial infections
   a. **Mechanism of action:** inhibits the transmembrane transport of peptidoglycan units
   b. **Uses:** skin and ocular infections (gram-positive cocci) (topical applications)

BOX 27-3 Protein Synthesis Inhibitors

Inhibitors of the 30S Ribosomal Subunit
Aminoglycosides
Amikacin
Gentamicin
Streptomycin
Tobramycin

Tetracyclines
Demeclocycline
Doxycycline
Minocycline
Tetracycline

Inhibitors of the 50S Ribosomal Subunit
Macrolides
Azithromycin
Clarithromycin
Erythromycin

Other Antibiotics
Chloramphenicol
Clindamycin
Linezolid
Quinupristin-dalfopristin

Other Protein Synthesis Inhibitors
Mupirocin

III. Drugs That Affect the Cell Membrane

A. Polymyxin B

1. **Mechanism of action:** bactericidal
   - Interacts with specific lipopolysaccharide component of the outer cell membrane, increasing permeability to polar molecules
2. **Use:** infections with gram-negative bacteria (topical)

B. Nisin (under study)

- 34-Amino acid peptide produced by *Lactococcus*

1. **Mechanism of action**
   - Interacts with and perturbs the cell membrane by forming ion channels
2. **Uses:** vancomycin-resistant enterococcus (VRE), *C. difficile*

IV. Protein Synthesis Inhibitors (Box 27-3)

- These drugs reversibly or irreversibly **bind to the 30S or 50S ribosomal subunit** (see Figure 27-1).

A. Aminoglycosides

- **Examples: amikacin, gentamicin, streptomycin, tobramycin**
- **Key characteristics:** irreversible binding to the 30S ribosomal subunit; bactericidal action; several mechanisms of resistance; adverse effects: nephrotoxicity, ototoxicity, and neuromuscular junction blockade

1. **Pharmacokinetics**
   a. Usually given by **intramuscular or intravenous injection** (poorly absorbed from the GI tract)
   b. Dosage monitoring using plasma levels
   c. Often used for once-a-day dosing
   d. Eliminated by glomerular filtration
2. **Pharmacodynamics**
   a. **Mechanism of action: bactericidal**
      (1) Undergo active transport across cell membrane via an **oxygen-dependent** process after crossing the outer membrane via a **porin** channel
      (2) Once bound to **specific 30S ribosome proteins,** inhibit protein synthesis
         (a) Interfere with the "initiation complex" of peptide formation
         (b) **Misread mRNA,** causing the incorporation of incorrect amino acids into the peptide
         (c) **Synergy with β-lactam antibiotics**
   b. **Causes of resistance**
      (1) **Adenylation, acetylation,** or **phosphorylation** (occurs via plasmids) as the result of the production of an enzyme by the inactivating microorganism
      (2) Alteration in porin channels or proteins involved in the oxygen-dependent transport of aminoglycosides
      (3) Deletion or alteration of the receptor on the 30S ribosomal subunit that binds the aminoglycosides
3. Uses

Aminoglycosides: treatment of gram (–) infections

   - Infections with **aerobic gram-negative bacteria** (*E. coli, Proteus, Klebsiella, Serratia, Enterobacter*)
   - Infection with ***P. aeruginosa*** (in combination with antipseudomonal penicillins, such as piperacillin)

   a. **Streptomycin:** tuberculosis
   b. **Amikacin, gentamicin, tobramycin:** gram-negative coverage often in combination with penicillin or cephalosporin
   c. **Neomycin:** skin and eye infections (topical), GI peristalsis (oral)
4. **Adverse effects**
   a. Ototoxicity
   b. **Nephrotoxicity (acute tubular necrosis)**
   c. **Neuromuscular junction blockade** (high doses; see Chapter 6)

B. Tetracyclines
- **Examples: minocycline, doxycycline**
- **Key characteristics:** chelation; bacteriostatic action; inhibition of protein synthesis; broad spectrum of action; multiple drug resistance; adverse effects: GI toxicity, tooth discoloration, and photosensitivity

1. **Pharmacokinetics**
   a. **Absorption:** decreased by chelation with divalent and trivalent cations (e.g., metals, especially calcium)

b. **Distribution:** high concentration in the bones, teeth, kidneys, and liver

c. **Excretion**

(1) **Tetracycline:** cleared by the **kidney**

(2) **Minocycline, doxycycline:** cleared more by the **liver**

2. **Pharmacodynamics**

a. **Mechanism of action (bacteriostatic)**

- Tetracyclines bind reversibly to the 30S subunit of the ribosome, blocking binding of aminoacyl-tRNA to the acceptor site (A site) on the mRNA-ribosome complex, thus inhibiting protein synthesis

b. **Causes of resistance**

(1) Decreased intracellular accumulation caused by **impaired influx** or **increased efflux** via an active transport protein pump (encoded on a plasmid)

(2) Ribosomal protection by synthesis of proteins that interfere with the binding of tetracyclines to the ribosome

(3) Enzymatic inactivation of tetracyclines

3. **Uses**

Tetracyclines: antibiotic of choice for chlamydial infection, brucellosis, mycoplasma pneumonia, rickettsial infections, some spirochetes (Lyme disease)

- Infections with **gram-positive and gram-negative bacteria**, including *Mycoplasma pneumoniae, Chlamydia,* and *Vibrio cholerae*

a. Rocky Mountain spotted fever (*Rickettsia*)

b. Lyme disease (doxycycline)

c. Syndrome of inappropriate antidiuretic hormone (SIADH) (demeclocycline)

d. Syphilis and gonorrhea (alternative treatment)

4. **Adverse effects**

a. **Nausea**, diarrhea (*C. difficile*)

b. **Inhibition of bone growth** (fetuses, infants, and children)

c. **Discoloration of teeth**

d. Superinfections (e.g., candidiasis)

e. **Photosensitivity**

C. Macrolides

- **Examples: erythromycin, clarithromycin, azithromycin**
- **Key characteristics:** bacteriostatic or bactericidal inhibitors of protein synthesis, elimination by biliary secretion

1. **Mechanism of action**

a. Bind reversibly to the **50S ribosomal unit**

b. **Block peptidyl transferase** and **prevent translocation from the aminoacyl site to the peptidyl site**

2. **Causes of resistance**

a. Plasma-encoded reduced permeability

b. Intracellular metabolism of the drug

c. Modification of the ribosomal binding site

3. **Uses**

Macrolides: used to treat gram (+) infections

- **Secondary drugs** for infections caused by **gram-positive bacteria in penicillin-sensitive patients**

a. **Erythromycin:** legionnaires' disease, *Mycoplasma* pneumonia, neonatal genital or ocular infections, chlamydial infections
b. **Azithromycin:** *Mycobacterium avium* complex prophylaxis in patients with advanced HIV; sinusitis and otitis media (*H. influenzae, M. catarrhalis*); chlamydial infections
c. **Clarithromycin:** infection caused by *Helicobacter pylori* in addition to the uses for azithromycin

4. **Adverse effects**
   - **Erythromycin**, a potent **inhibitor of the cytochrome P450 system**, increases the effects of carbamazepine, clozapine, cyclosporine, digoxin, midazolam, quinidine, and the protease inhibitors.

   a. **GI effects:** anorexia, nausea, vomiting, diarrhea
   b. **Hepatotoxicity:** cholestatic hepatitis
   c. Pseudomembranous colitis

D. Other protein synthesis inhibitors

1. **Chloramphenicol**
   a. **Mechanism of action**
      - Inhibits protein synthesis at the **50S ribosome;** bacteriostatic
      - Inhibits peptidyl transferase

   b. **Uses**
      (1) *Salmonella* infections (typhoid)
      (2) **Ampicillin-resistant** *H. influenzae* meningitis

   c. **Adverse effects**
      (1) **Aplastic anemia** and bone marrow toxicity
      (2) **Gray baby syndrome (deficiency of glucuronyl transferase)**

Chloramphenicol: inhibitor of microsomal oxidation that increases blood levels of phenytoin, tolbutamide, and warfarin.

Chloramphenicol: potential to cause lethal aplastic anemia

2. **Clindamycin**
   a. **Mechanism of action:** inhibits protein synthesis at the 50S ribosome; bacteriostatic
   b. **Uses:** severe gram-positive **anaerobic infections** (*Bacteroides* and others; aspiration pneumonia)
   c. **Adverse effects:** severe diarrhea, pseudomembranous colitis (*C. difficile*)

3. **Linezolid**
   a. **Mechanism of action:** binds to the 50S ribosome, interfering with protein synthesis
   b. **Uses:** infections caused by MRSA or VRE
   c. **Adverse effects:** diarrhea, nausea, vomiting, headache
      - Patients should **avoid consuming tyramine-containing foods** (e.g., aged cheese, red wine), because linezolid inhibits monoamine oxidase.

4. **Quinupristin-dalfopristin**
   a. **Mechanism of action:** interferes with protein synthesis; bactericidal
   b. **Uses:** infections caused by MRSA, enterococcus
      (1) Severe bacteremia
      (2) Pneumonia
   c. **Adverse effects:** nausea, vomiting, diarrhea

5. Mupirocin
  - **a. Mechanism of action:** interferes with protein synthesis
  - **b. Uses:** impetigo, nasal colonization by MRSA (eradication)
  - **c. Adverse effects:** nasal irritation, pharyngitis

V. Antimetabolites Used for Microorganisms (Box 27-4)

- These antimicrobials **interfere with the metabolism of folic acid** (see Figure 27-1).

A. Sulfonamides

- **Key characteristics:** competitive inhibition of *p*-aminobenzoic acid (PABA); synergistic action with trimethoprim; primary use is for UTIs; adverse effects: acute hemolytic anemia, crystalluria

BOX 27-4 Antimetabolites

Sulfonamides
Sulfamethoxazole
Sulfasalazine
Sulfisoxazole

Dihydrofolate Reductase Inhibitors
Co-trimoxazole (trimethoprim-sulfamethoxazole)
Trimethoprim

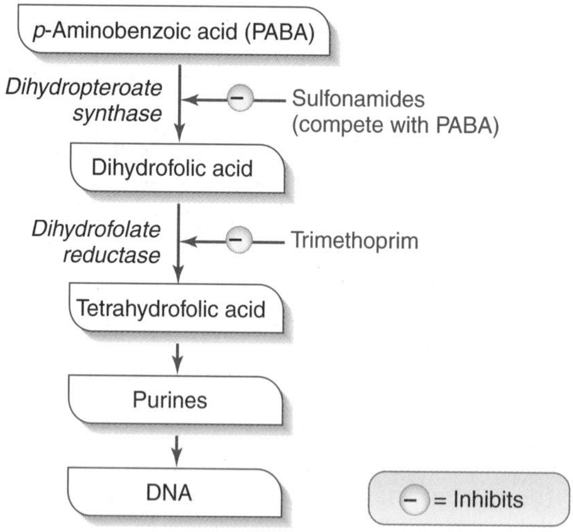

Figure 27-2 Sequential inhibition of tetrahydrofolic acid synthesis. Dihydropteroate is inhibited by sulfonamides and sulfones (dapsone). Dihydrofolate reductase is inhibited by trimethoprim (bacteria, protozoa); pyrimethamine (protozoa); and methotrexate (mammals). Trimethoprim is used in the treatment of certain infections; pyrimethamine is used in the treatment of malaria; and methotrexate is used as an anticancer and immunosuppressive agent.

1. **Pharmacodynamics**
   a. **Mechanism of action:** bacteriostatic
      - Competitively **inhibit dihydropteroate synthetase** (Figure 27-2)
      - Have a synergistic action when given with trimethoprim, causing a sequential blockade of the formation of tetrahydrofolate
   b. **Resistance**
      - Mutations cause **excess production of PABA.**
2. Uses
   - Usually given in combination with other drugs such as **trimethoprim**
   - Infections with *Nocardia, Chlamydia trachomatis,* and some protozoa
   - Infections caused by many gram-positive and gram-negative bacteria, especially enteric bacteria such as *E. coli, Salmonella, Shigella,* and *Enterobacter*
   a. **UTIs (trimethoprim-sulfamethoxazole)**
   b. Respiratory infections
   c. Ulcerative colitis **(sulfasalazine)**
   d. Burn therapy (**silver sulfadiazine**; good for *P. aeruginosa*)

Primary use for sulfonamides: UTIs

3. **Adverse effects**
   a. **Blood dyscrasias:** agranulocytosis, leukemia, aplastic anemia
   b. Crystalluria and hematuria
   c. **Hypersensitivity reactions:** Stevens-Johnson syndrome
4. Contraindications
   a. **Relative contraindications:** preexisting bone marrow suppression, blood dyscrasias, megaloblastic anemia secondary to folate deficiency
   b. **Absolute contraindications:** Glucose-6-phosphate dehydrogenase (G6PD) deficiency, megaloblastic anemia, porphyria, neonatal period

B. Trimethoprim
1. **Mechanism of action:** inhibits dihydrofolate reductase
2. Uses
   a. **Prostatitis**
   b. **Vaginitis**

BOX 27-5 DNA Gyrase Inhibitors: Fluoroquinolones

Ciprofloxacin
Gatifloxacin
Levofloxacin
Lomefloxacin
Norfloxacin
Ofloxacin
Sparfloxacin
Trovafloxacin

c. **Otitis media** and **bronchitis** (in combination with sulfonamide)

3. **Adverse effects:** similar to those of sulfonamides

C. **Combination product** (co-trimoxazole; trimethoprim-sulfamethoxazole)
- Agent of choice for *P. carinii* pneumonia, symptomatic *Shigella* enteritis, symptomatic *Salmonella* infections resistant to ampicillin and chloramphenicol, UTIs, upper respiratory infections

VI. Inhibitors of DNA Gyrase: Fluoroquinolones (Box 27-5)

- Fluoroquinolones interfere with bacteria DNA synthesis (see Figure 27-1).
- **Examples:** ciprofloxacin, norfloxacin, ofloxacin, levofloxacin

A. **Mechanism of action:** bactericidal by inhibition of DNA gyrase, the enzyme responsible for counteracting the excessive supercoiling of DNA during replication or transcription

B. **Resistance:** due to a change in the gyrase enzyme or decreased permeability

C. **Uses**
- Infections with aerobic gram-negative rods, including Enterobacteriaceae, *Pseudomonas,* and *Neisseria*
- Infections caused by *Campylobacter jejuni, Salmonella, Shigella,* and *Mycobacterium avium* complex

1. **Sinusitis, bronchitis, pneumonia**
2. **UTIs**
3. **Neutropenic fever** (ciprofloxacin)

D. **Adverse effects**

1. **Nausea**
2. **Interactions with other drugs**
   - Patients taking fluoroquinolones should avoid calcium, theophylline, and caffeine.
3. **Interference with collagen synthesis**
   a. Causes tendon rupture
   b. Should be avoided during pregnancy

Ciprofloxacin may cause rupture of the Achilles tendon.

28 Other Anti-infective Drugs

Target Topics

- Treatment of tuberculosis
- Treatment of viral infections
- Treatment of parasitic infections
- Treatment of fungal infections

I. Antimycobacterial Drugs (Box 28-1)
- The management of tuberculosis is summarized in Table 28-1.

A. Isoniazid (INH)

1. Pharmacokinetics
- Metabolism occurs by **acetylation** (*N*-acetyltransferase; NAT), which is under genetic control.
- Individuals are either "fast" or "slow" acetylators.

2. Mechanism of action: bactericidal
- **Inhibits synthesis of mycolic acids**, thus inhibiting mycobacterial cell wall synthesis

3. Use: tuberculosis (*Mycobacterium tuberculosis*)

a. Prophylaxis in tuberculin converters (**positive skin test**)

b. Treatment with rifampin, ethambutol, pyrazinamide, or streptomycin (see Table 28-1)

4. Adverse effects

a. Hepatic damage (especially in individuals > 35 years of age)

b. Peripheral neuritis (reversed by pyridoxine; more prominent in "slow" acetylators)

B. Rifampin

1. Mechanism of action
- Binds to the β-subunit of **bacterial DNA-dependent RNA**

polymerase, inhibiting binding of the enzyme to DNA and blocking RNA transcription

2. **Uses**
   a. **Tuberculosis** (*M. tuberculosis*)
      (1) Prophylaxis in cases of INH resistance or in individuals who are older than 35 years of age
      (2) Treatment in combination with other drugs (see Table 28-1)
   b. Prophylaxis in contacts of *Neisseria meningitidis* and *Haemophilus influenzae* type B

BOX 28-1 Antimycobacterial Drugs

Dapsone
Ethambutol
Isoniazid
Pyrazinamide
Rifabutin
Rifampin
Streptomycin

TABLE 28-1 Management of Tuberculosis

Therapeutic Goal and Drug-Related Patient Features	Initial Drug Treatment	Subsequent Drug Treatment
Prevention of Tuberculosis		
Not resistant to isoniazid	Isoniazid (6 months)	None
HIV-negative; resistant to isoniazid	Rifampin (6 months)	None
HIV-positive	Rifampin* or rifabutin (12 months)	None
Treatment of Tuberculosis		
Not resistant to isoniazid	Combination of isoniazid, rifampin, ethambutol, and pyrazinamide for 2 months	Combination of isoniazid and rifampin (4 more months if HIV-negative or 7 more months if HIV-positive)
Possibly resistant to isoniazid	Combination of isoniazid, rifampin, pyrazinamide, and either ethambutol or streptomycin (6 months)	Individualized therapy based on microbial susceptibility testing
Resistant to multiple drugs†	Combination of at least four drugs believed to be active in patient population (6 months)	Individualized therapy based on microbial susceptibility testing

*In HIV-infected patients, substitution of rifabutin for rifampin minimizes drug interactions with protease inhibitors and nucleoside reverse transcriptase inhibitors.

†Patients suspected of having multidrug resistance include those from certain demographic populations, those who have failed to respond to previous treatment, and those who have experienced a relapse of tuberculosis.

- **c. Legionnaires' disease** (in combination with azithromycin)
- **d.** Leprosy (*Mycobacterium leprae*) (combination therapy)

3. Adverse effects
- **a.** Red-orange **discoloration of urine, tears, saliva**
- **b. Hepatotoxicity**
- **c. Drug interactions**
  - Rifampin, a potent inducer of the cytochrome P450 hepatic enzyme systems, can reduce the plasma concentrations of many drugs.

Treatment with rifampin often results in permanent discoloration of soft contact lenses.

Rifampin: potent inducer of cytochrome P450 hepatic enzymes

C. Ethambutol

1. Mechanism of action: unknown; possibly inhibits RNA synthesis

2. Use: tuberculosis (combination therapy; see Table 28-1)

3. Adverse effects: optic neuritis, reduction in red-green visual acuity
- **Annual eye examination is necessary.**

D. Pyrazinamide

1. Mechanism of action: unknown

2. Use: tuberculosis (combination therapy; see Table 28-1)

3. Adverse effects: hyperuricemia, hepatotoxicity, photosensitivity

E. Rifabutin
- Rifabutin is a less potent inducer of cytochrome P450 hepatic enzymes than is rifampin.

1. Mechanism of action: inhibition of mycobacterial RNA polymerase

2. Uses
- **a.** Substitute for rifampin in the treatment of **tuberculosis in HIV-infected patients**
- **b.** Prevention and treatment of ***Mycobacterium avium* complex**

F. Dapsone

1. Mechanism of action: bacteriostatic inhibitor of folic acid synthesis

2. Use: leprosy (*M. leprae*)

3. Adverse effects
- **a. Optic neuritis, neuropathy**
- **b. Glucose-6-phosphate dehydrogenase (G6PD) deficiency**, which leads to hemolytic anemia

II. Antiviral Drugs (Box 28-2)
- The mechanism of viral replication and the effects of antiviral drugs are shown in Figure 28-1.

A. Drugs used in the prevention and treatment of influenza

1. Amantadine and rimantadine

a. Mechanism of action
- Blocks the uncoating of the virus particle and the subsequent release of viral nucleic acid into the host cell
- May also interfere with penetration of the cell wall by absorbed virus

b. Uses

BOX 28-2 Antiviral Drugs

Drugs Used in the Treatment and Prophylaxis of Influenza
Amantadine
Oseltamivir
Rimantadine
Zanamivir

Antiherpes Drugs
Acyclovir
Foscarnet
Ganciclovir

Interferons
Interferon alfa
Interferon beta

Antiretroviral Drugs
Nucleoside Reverse Transcriptase Inhibitors
Didanosine (ddI)
Lamivudine (3TC)
Stavudine (d4T)
Zalcitabine (ddC)
Zidovudine (AZT)

Nonnucleoside Reverse Transcriptase Inhibitors
Delavirdine
Nevirapine

Protease Inhibitors
Indinavir
Nelfinavir
Ritonavir
Saquinavir

Other Antiviral Drugs
Ribavirin

(1) **Influenza A** (prophylaxis)
(2) **Parkinson's disease** (see Chapter 11)
c. **Adverse effects:** dizziness, anxiety, impaired coordination

2. **Oseltamivir and zanamivir**
   a. **Mechanism of action:** inhibit viral neuraminidase
   b. **Use:** influenza (prevention and treatment of symptoms)
   c. **Adverse effects:** nausea, vomiting, bronchitis

B. Interferons
1. **Mechanism of action:** inhibit viral penetration and uncoating along with peptide elongation
2. **Uses**
   a. **Interferon alfa** (systemic): hairy-cell leukemia, AIDS-related Kaposi's sarcoma, condyloma acuminatum, chronic hepatitis B and hepatitis C
   b. **Interferon beta:** multiple sclerosis
3. **Adverse effects:** neutropenia, anemia, influenza symptoms

C. Ribavirin

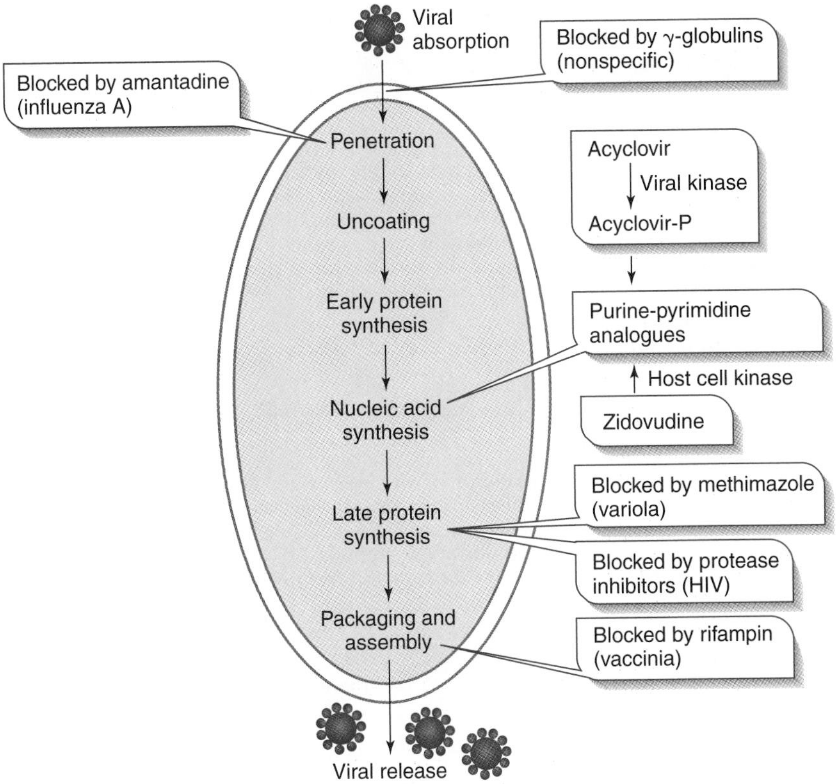

Figure 28-1 Mechanism of viral replication and the site of action of antiviral drugs.

- The antiviral action of this synthetic nucleoside **requires intracellular phosphorylation.**

1. **Mechanism of action:** selectively inhibits viral DNA and RNA synthesis
2. **Use:** inhalation therapy in respiratory syncytial virus (RSV) infections and influenza
3. **Adverse effects:** respiratory depression, hemolytic anemia

D. Antiherpes drugs

1. **Acyclovir and ganciclovir**
   - **a. Mechanism of action**
     - These drugs are **phosphorylated by viral thymidine kinases;** the phosphorylated metabolites inhibit viral DNA polymerase.
   - **b. Resistance** involves loss of thymidine kinase activity.
   - **c. Uses:** herpes simplex, herpes genitalis, herpes zoster, varicella zoster, cytomegalovirus (ganciclovir)
   - **d. Adverse effects:** nephrotoxicity, confusion, coma, encephalopathy
2. **Foscarnet**
   - **a. Mechanism of action**
     - No dependence on thymidine kinase, with no phosphorylation necessary.

TABLE 28-2 Adverse Effects of Antiretroviral Agents

Drug	Adverse Effect(s)
Nucleoside Reverse Transcriptase Inhibitors	
Didanosine (ddI)	Peripheral neuropathy, pancreatitis (dose-dependent)
Lamivudine (3TC)	Headache, elevated hepatic enzymes, hyperbilirubinemia (dose reduction is necessary in renal disease)
Stavudine (d4T)	Peripheral sensory neuropathy
Zalcitabine (ddC)	Peripheral sensory neuropathy, esophageal ulcers
Zidovudine (AZT)	Bone marrow suppression, anemia
Nonnucleoside Reverse Transcriptase Inhibitors	
Delavirdine	Rash, pruritus
Nevirapine	Rash, elevated hepatic enzymes
Protease Inhibitors	
Indinavir	Hyperbilirubinemia, nephrolithiasis
Nelfinavir	Diarrhea, anaphylactoid reactions, inhibition of metabolism of many drugs
Ritonavir	Multiple drug interactions
Saquinavir	Gastrointestinal disturbance, rhinitis

- Selective inhibition of the viral-specific DNA polymerases

b. Uses: cytomegalovirus, herpes simplex virus, varicella zoster virus

c. Adverse effects: renal impairment, headache, seizures

E. Antiretroviral drugs

- These drugs may have serious side effects (Table 28-2).

1. Nucleoside reverse transcriptase inhibitors

- **Zidovudine (AZT), didanosine (ddI), lamivudine (3TC), stavudine (d4T), zalcitabine (ddC)**

a. Mechanism of action: inhibit viral RNA–directed DNA polymerase (reverse transcriptase) following phosphorylation

b. Use: HIV infection (treatment and prevention)

2. Nonnucleoside reverse transcriptase inhibitors

- **Delavirdine, nevirapine**

a. Mechanism of action

- Directly inhibit reverse transcriptase, with no activation required
- Not incorporated into viral DNA

b. Use: HIV infection

3. Protease inhibitors

Combination therapy (reverse transcriptase inhibitor and protease inhibitor): successful delay of the emergence of resistance in HIV-positive individuals

- **Indinavir, nelfinavir, ritonavir, saquinavir**

a. Mechanism of action: competitively inhibit HIV protease

(1) Indinavir and **ritonavir:** inhibit the cytochrome P450 system

(2) Saquinavir: metabolized by the cytochrome P450 system but **does not inhibit the enzyme**

b. Use: HIV infection

BOX 28-3 Antiparasitic Drugs

Antimalarial Drugs
Chloroquine
Mefloquine
Primaquine

Antihelmintic Drugs
Ivermectin
Mebendazole
Praziquantel
Pyrantel pamoate
Thiabendazole

Other Antiprotozoal Drugs
Metronidazole
Pentamidine

III. Antiparasitic Drugs (Box 28-3)
  A. Antimalaria drugs
    1. Chloroquine
      a. Pharmacokinetics
        (1) **Extensive tissue binding**, with a very large volume of distribution (13,000 L)
        (2) Slow release from the tissues
        (3) Liver metabolism, renal excretion
      b. Mechanism of resistance: membrane P-glycoprotein pump that expels chloroquine from the parasite
      c. Uses: clinical cure and prophylaxis (all species of *Plasmodium*)
        - Treatment of infections caused by *Plasmodium vivax* and *Plasmodium ovale* requires use of chloroquine in combination with primaquine.
      d. Adverse effects: visual impairment, hearing loss, tinnitus, aplastic anemia

Chloroquine should be avoided or used cautiously in patients with ocular, hematologic, neurologic, or hepatic diseases.

    2. Mefloquine
      - **Use:** chloroquine-resistant and multidrug-resistant **falciparum malaria** (prophylaxis and treatment)
    3. Primaquine
      a. Mechanism of action: active against **late hepatic stages** (hypnozoites and schizonts) of ***P. vivax*** and ***P. ovale***
      b. Uses
        (1) **Malaria** (in combination with chloroquine)
        (2) ***Pneumocystis carinii*** **pneumonia** (PCP) (alternative therapy; in combination with clindamycin)
      c. Adverse effects: anorexia, weakness, hemolytic anemia, leukopenia

Individuals with G6PD deficiency who take primaquine are susceptible to hemolytic anemia.

  B. Other antiprotozoal drugs
    1. Metronidazole
      a. Uses
        (1) **Urogenital trichomoniasis** (*Trichomonas vaginalis*),

giardiasis (*Giardia*), **amebiasis** (*Entamoeba histolytica*)
(2) **Aspiration pneumonia**
(3) **Anaerobic infections** (including *Clostridium difficile, Bacteroides fragilis*)

Metronidazole: patients who are taking this drug should *not consume alcohol.*

b. Adverse effects: metallic taste, disulfiram-like effect

2. Pentamidine
- **Uses:** PCP in HIV-infected individuals, *Trypanosoma gambiense*

C. Antihelmintic drugs

1. Praziquantel

a. Mechanism of action
- **Increases calcium permeability**, depolarizing cells
- Results in contraction followed by **paralysis of worm musculature**

b. Uses
(1) **Schistosomiasis**
(2) Infections with **flukes** (trematodes) and **tapeworms** (cestodes)

c. Adverse effects
(1) Headaches, dizziness, drowsiness
(2) Gastrointestinal (GI) disturbances

2. Thiabendazole and **mebendazole**

a. Mechanism of action: block microtubule formation

b. Uses
(1) **Thiabendazole:** strongyloidiasis, cutaneous larva migrans (alternative drug)
(2) **Mebendazole:** ascariasis, trichuriasis, hookworm, pinworm (*Enterobius vermicularis*), cysticercosis (*Taenia solium*), *Echinococcus* infestations

c. Adverse effects: abdominal pain, diarrhea

3. Pyrantel pamoate

a. Mechanism of action
- Acts as a **depolarizing neuromuscular blocking agent on the nicotinic receptor**
- Increases the effects of acetylcholine and **inhibits cholinesterase** in the worm

b. Uses: ascariasis, pinworm (*E. vermicularis*), hookworm, whipworm (*Trichuris trichiura), Trichostrongylus*

c. Adverse effects: nausea, vomiting, diarrhea, anorexia

4. Ivermectin

a. Mechanism of action: increases chloride permeability, thus polarizing cells, which leads to paralysis

b. Uses: strongyloidiasis, onchocerciasis

IV. Antifungal Drugs (Box 28-4)

- Antifungal agents are commonly used in **debilitated and immunosuppressed patients** with conditions such as leukemia, lymphoma, immunodeficiencies, and diabetes.
- The mechanisms of action of some antifungal agents are shown in Figure 28-2.

A. Amphotericin B (polyene antibiotic)

1. **Pharmacokinetics**
   - The drug is given **intravenously or intrathecally;** it is *not* absorbed orally.
   - Placement of the active drug in a **lipid delivery system** (liposomal amphotericin B) results in **increased efficacy** and **decreased toxicity.**
2. **Mechanism of action**
   - **Binds to ergosterol** in fungal cell membranes, causing an **increase in membrane permeability**
3. **Use:** severe systemic fungal infection (**drug of choice**)
4. **Adverse effects**
   a. **Nephrotoxicity**
   b. **Pancytopenia, anemia**
   c. **Hepatotoxicity**

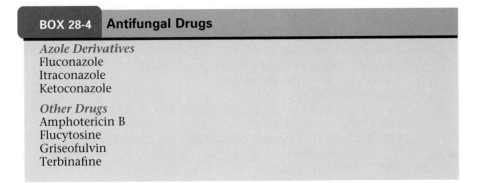

BOX 28-4 Antifungal Drugs

Azole Derivatives
Fluconazole
Itraconazole
Ketoconazole

Other Drugs
Amphotericin B
Flucytosine
Griseofulvin
Terbinafine

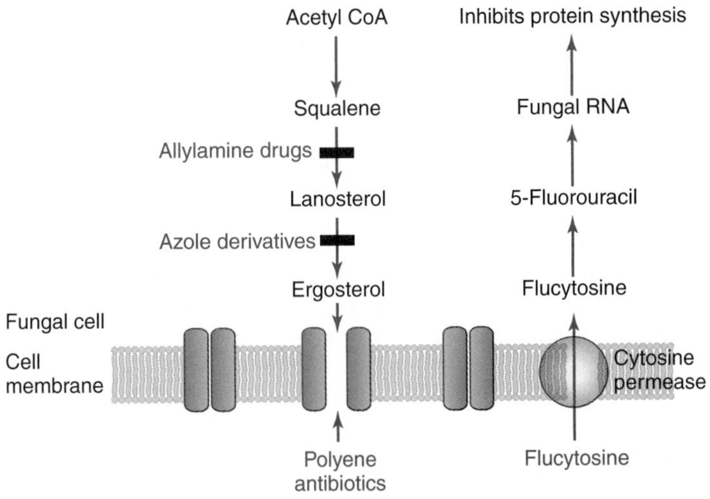

Figure 28-2 Mechanism of action of some antifungal drugs. Amphotericin B and nystatin are polyenes; terbinafine is an allylamine; and ketoconazole, fluconazole, and itraconazole are azoles. *CoA,* Coenzyme A.

B. **Flucytosine**

1. **Mechanism of action: conversion to fluorouracil** (an antimetabolite) only in fungal cells
   - Competes with uracil by interfering with pyrimidine metabolism and disrupting both RNA and protein synthesis
2. **Uses:** systemic fungal infections due to *Candida* species, including *C. glabrata,* and *Cryptococcus neoformans*
3. **Adverse effects:** nausea, vomiting, diarrhea, bone marrow suppression

C. **Azole drugs**

- **Examples: ketoconazole, itraconazole, fluconazole**

1. **Pharmacokinetics**
   - The three drugs listed as examples are absorbed orally.
   - **Fluconazole** is the only azole antifungal agent with good central nervous system (CNS) penetration.
2. **Mechanism of action**
   - Azoles **inhibit ergosterol synthesis** by preventing conversion of lanosterol to ergosterol (essential component of the fungal cell membrane) (see Figure 28-2).
3. **Uses**
   - **a.** **Mucocutaneous candidiasis** and nonmeningeal coccidioidomycosis
   - **b.** Cryptococcal meningitis (**fluconazole**)
   - **c.** *Aspergillus* (**itraconazole**)
4. **Adverse effects**
   - **a.** Elevation of serum transaminase levels
   - **b.** **Gynecomastia** (blocks adrenal steroid synthesis)
   - **c.** Inhibition of cytochrome P450 enzymes (especially ketoconazole)

Azole derivatives: inhibition of cytochrome P450 enzymes

D. **Griseofulvin**

1. **Mechanism of action**
   - Decreases microtubule function, disrupting the mitotic spindle structure of the fungal cell and causing an arrest of the M phase of the cell cycle
   - Concentrates in keratinized tissue, so selectively localizes in the skin, with an affinity for diseased skin
2. **Uses: dermatophytic infections** such as ringworm and athlete's foot (*Microsporum, Trichophyton*)

E. **Terbinafine**

1. **Mechanism of action**
   - **a.** Inhibits the fungal enzyme squalene epoxidase
   - **b.** Interferes with ergosterol biosynthesis (like azoles)
   - **c.** Concentrates in keratinized tissue (like griseofulvin)
2. **Use:** dermatophytosis, especially **onychomycosis** (replaces griseofulvin)
3. **Adverse effects** (rare): headache, GI upset

SECTION IX

Drugs Used in the Treatment of Cancer

29

Chemotherapeutic Drugs

Target Topics

- Alkylating agents
- Antimetabolites
- Antibiotics
- Plant alkaloids
- Hormones

I. General Considerations (Box 29-1)

- Cancer is a disease in which the cellular control mechanisms that govern proliferation and differentiation are changed.

A. Drugs used in cancer chemotherapy target important **biosynthetic processes in proliferating cells** (Figure 29-1).

B. The goal of cancer chemotherapy is to **destroy cancer cells selectively** with as few effects on normal cells as possible.

C. Adverse effects of chemotherapeutic drugs (Table 29-1)

- Individual drugs have "signature" side effects.

1. **Bone marrow suppression**
2. **Toxicity to mucosal cells of the gastrointestinal tract,** which leads to nausea, ulcers, and diarrhea
3. **Toxicity to skin and hair follicles,** which results in hair loss
4. **Teratogenic effects**

Ondansetron is used to treat the nausea and vomiting associated with anticancer drugs.

BOX 29-1 Chemotherapeutic Drugs

Drugs That Alter DNA
Alkylating Drugs
Busulfan
Carboplatin
Carmustine
Cisplatin
Cyclophosphamide
Lomustine
Melphalan

Antibiotics
Bleomycin
Dactinomycin
Daunorubicin
Doxorubicin

Antimetabolites
Folic Acid Antagonist
Methotrexate

Purine Antagonists
6-Mercaptopurine
6-Thioguanine

Pyrimidine Antagonists
Cytarabine
5-Fluorouracil

Mitotic Inhibitors
Paclitaxel
Vinblastine
Vincristine

Podophyllotoxins
Etoposide

Hormones and Hormone Regulators
Hormones
Androgens
Diethylstilbestrol
Estrogens
Prednisone

Modulators of Hormone Release and Action
Aminoglutethimide
Leuprolide
Tamoxifen

5. **Sterility**
6. **Immunosuppression**

II. Drugs That Alter DNA

A. Alkylating drugs

1. **Cyclophosphamide**
   - Prodrug that requires activation by the cytochrome P450 system
   - a. **Mechanism of action:** cell cycle–nonspecific
     - Cross-links DNA strands, stopping DNA processing
   - b. **Uses**
     - (1) **Chronic lymphocytic leukemia (CLL), non-Hodgkin's lymphoma, multiple myeloma**
     - (2) **Breast, ovarian, and lung cancers**

"Signature" adverse effect of cyclophosphamide: hemorrhagic cystitis

2. **Busulfan**
   - a. **Mechanism of action:** cell cycle–nonspecific, bifunctional alkylating agent
   - b. **Use: chronic granulocytic leukemia** (drug of choice)
3. **Carmustine and lomustine:** nitrosourea drugs
   - a. **Mechanism of action:** cell cycle–nonspecific
   - b. **Use: primary and metastatic brain tumors**
4. **Cisplatin and carboplatin**
   - a. **Mechanism of action**
     - Cross-links to any nucleic acid or protein structure

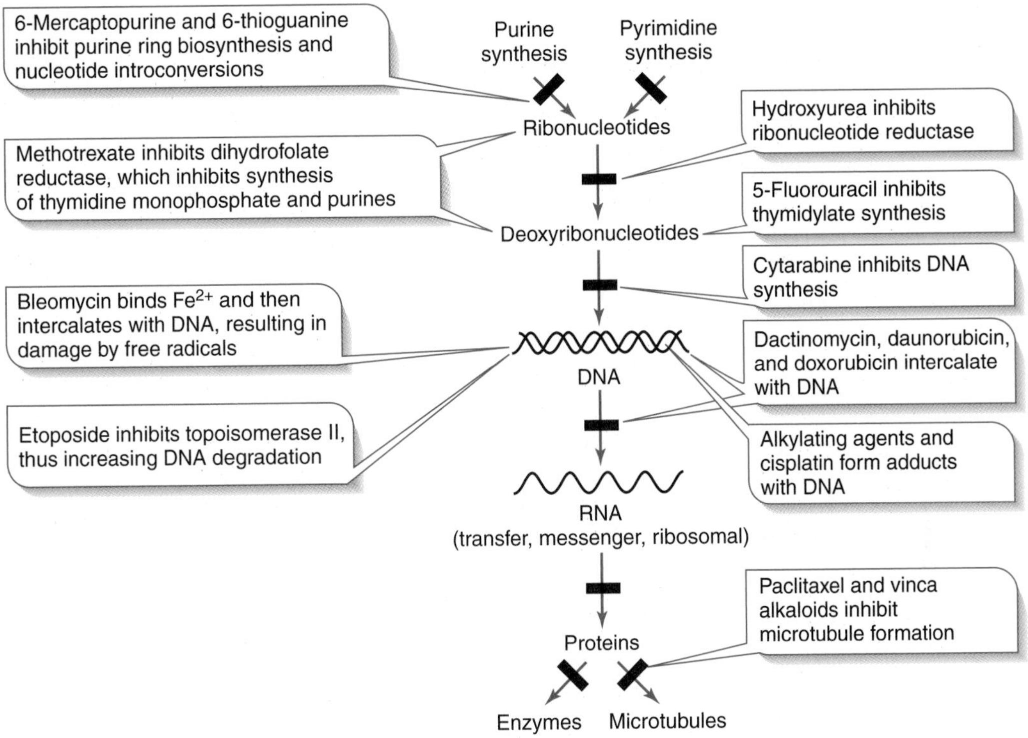

Figure 29-1 Sites of action of chemotherapeutic drugs.

that forms irreversible covalent bonds, thereby **inhibiting DNA replication, RNA transcription, and protein synthesis**

b. Uses
- **(1)** **Genitourinary cancers:** testicular (in combination with **vinblastine** and **bleomycin**), ovarian, urinary bladder
- **(2)** **Non–small cell lung cancer**

Severe nephrotoxicity may occur with cisplatin therapy.

5. Melphalan
- **Uses: breast and ovarian cancers, multiple myeloma**

B. Intercalating agents: antibiotics

1. Dactinomycin (actinomycin D)

a. Mechanism of action: cell cycle–nonspecific
- Intercalates between base pairs of DNA, preventing DNA and RNA synthesis

b. Uses
- **(1)** **Trophoblastic tumors**
- **(2)** **Wilms' tumor** in combination with surgery and vincristine
- **(3)** **Ewing's sarcoma**

2. Daunorubicin and doxorubicin

a. Mechanism of action: cell cycle–nonspecific
- **(1)** Intercalate between base pairs of DNA
- **(2)** Inhibit topoisomerase II, causing faulty DNA repairs

TABLE 29-1 Therapeutic Uses and Adverse Effects of Drugs Used in Cancer Chemotherapy

Drug	Use: Type(s) of Cancer*	Important Adverse Effect(s)
Aminoglutethimide	Breast, prostate	Adrenal suppression, dizziness, rash
Bleomycin	Testicular, ovarian, cervical, thyroid	Pulmonary fibrosis; very little bone marrow toxicity
Busulfan	CML, polycythemia vera	Interstitial pulmonary fibrosis
Carmustine/lomustine	Brain	Leukopenia, thrombocytopenia, hepatotoxicity
Cisplatin	Head and neck, lung, testicular, cervical, thyroid, ovarian	Ototoxicity, severe nephrotoxicity, *mild* bone marrow suppression
Cyclophosphamide	Leukemias/lymphomas	Hemorrhagic cystitis, alopecia
Cytarabine	Leukemias	Bone marrow suppression, CNS toxicity, immunosuppression
Dactinomycin	Wilms' tumor	Hepatotoxicity
Daunorubicin/doxorubicin	Acute leukemia, Hodgkin's disease, breast and lung	Cardiomyopathy (daunorubicin)
Diethylstilbestrol	Prostate	Teratogenic (cervical adenocarcinoma in offspring)
Etoposide	Lung, testicular	Bone marrow suppression
5-Fluorouracil	Colon, stomach, prostate, breast	Bone marrow suppression, GI toxicity
Leuprolide	Prostate, breast	Hot flashes
Melphalan	Multiple myeloma	Bone marrow suppression
6-Mercaptopurine	Leukemias	Bone marrow suppression
Methotrexate	Wilms' tumor, choriocarcinoma, leukemias	Bone marrow suppression, oral and GI tract ulceration, diarrhea, hepatotoxicity†
Paclitaxel (Taxol)	Breast, ovarian	Bone marrow suppression
Tamoxifen	Breast	Hot flashes
Vinblastine	Lymphomas	Bone marrow suppression
Vincristine	ALL	Neurotoxicity/peripheral neuropathy, low bone marrow suppression

ALL, Acute lymphocytic leukemia; *CML,* chronic myelogenous leukemia; *CNS,* central nervous system; *GI,* gastrointestinal.
*Not a complete list; for most cancers, drug combinations are used.
†Adverse effects, especially toxicity, may be reversed with **folic acid** ("leucovorin rescue").

Signature adverse effect of daunorubicin: cardiotoxicity (cardiomyopathy)

b. Uses

(1) **Daunorubicin:** acute granulocytic leukemia (AGL), acute lymphocytic leukemia (ALL)

(2) **Doxorubicin:** breast, endometrial, ovarian, testicular, thyroid, and lung cancers; sarcomas

3. Bleomycin

- Concentrates in skin and lungs

a. Mechanism of action: cell cycle–specific (most active during the G_2 and M phases)

- Causes formation of free radicals, which affects DNA

Most serious adverse effect of bleomycin therapy: pulmonary fibrosis

b. Uses

(1) **Squamous cell carcinoma of the head, neck, and skin**

(2) **Lymphomas**

(3) **Testicular cancer**

III. Antimetabolites

A. Folic acid antagonists: methotrexate (MTX)

1. **Mechanism of action:** cell cycle–specific
   - Inhibits conversion of folic acid to tetrahydrofolic acid (dihydrofolate reductase inhibitor)
2. **Uses**
   a. **Choriocarcinoma** (women)
   b. **ALL, non-Hodgkin's lymphoma**
   c. Tumors of the breast, testis, bladder, and lung
   d. Systemic lupus erythematosus, rheumatic arthritis, Crohn's disease

B. Purine antagonist: 6-mercaptopurine (6-MP)

1. **Mechanism of action:** cell cycle–specific
   - Inhibits purine synthesis
2. **Use:** ALL

C. Pyrimidine antagonists

1. **5-Fluorouracil (5-FU)**
   a. **Mechanism of action:** cell cycle–specific (most active during the S phase)
      - Active metabolite inhibits thymidylate synthase and interferes with DNA and RNA synthesis.
   b. **Uses:** gastric, breast, colorectal, and skin neoplasms
2. **Cytarabine (Ara-C)**
   a. **Mechanism of action:** cell cycle–specific (active during the S phase)
      - Active metabolite inhibits DNA polymerase, thus interfering with DNA synthesis.
   b. **Uses:** AGL, non-Hodgkin's lymphoma

IV. Mitotic Inhibitors

A. Vinca alkaloids

1. **Vinblastine**
   a. **Mechanism of action:** cell cycle–specific (active during the M phase; metaphase)
      - **Binds to tubulin** (microtubular protein) and prevents polymerization
   b. **Uses**
      (1) **Hodgkin's and non-Hodgkin's lymphomas**
      (2) **Testicular carcinoma** (in combination with **cisplatin** and **bleomycin**)
2. **Vincristine**
   a. **Mechanism of action:** similar to vinblastine
   b. **Uses:** same as for vinblastine, plus ALL and Wilms' tumor

B. Paclitaxel (Taxol)

1. **Mechanism of action:** cell cycle–specific (active during the G_2 and M phases)
   - **Binds to tubulin** and prevents depolarization
2. **Uses**
   a. **Refractory ovarian and breast cancers**
   b. **Non–small cell lung cancer**

Major adverse effect of vincristine (dose-limiting): neurotoxicity, such as peripheral neuropathy

V. Podophyllotoxin: Etoposide (VP-16)

A. Mechanism of action: cell cycle–specific (active during the G_2 phase)
- **Inhibits topoisomerase II**

B. Uses
1. **Non-Hodgkin's lymphoma**
2. **Testicular cancer**
3. **Small cell lung cancer**

VI. Hormones and Hormone Regulators

A. Hormones
1. **Corticosteroids (prednisone**; see Chapter 23)
   - **a. Mechanism of action:** inhibits cytokine production and T-cell production
   - **b. Uses:** often used in combination with other antineoplastic agents
     - (1) **ALL in children, CLL**
     - (2) **Multiple myeloma**
     - (3) **Hodgkin's and non-Hodgkin's lymphomas**
2. **Diethylstilbestrol** (synthetic **estrogen**)
   - **Uses:** breast, prostate, and endometrial cancers
   - Other **estrogens** are useful in prostate carcinoma and breast cancer (see Chapter 26).
3. **Androgens** (see Chapter 26)
   - **Use:** breast cancer in premenopausal women

B. Modulation of hormone release and action
1. **Aminoglutethimide**
   - **a. Mechanism of action:** blocks first step in adrenal steroid synthesis and inhibits estrogen synthesis (aromatase inhibitor)
   - **b.** Use: **metastatic breast cancer** (equivalent to tamoxifen but with more adverse effects)
2. **Tamoxifen**
   - **a. Mechanism of action**
     - (1) **Blocks estrogen receptors** in cancer cells that require estrogen for growth and development
     - (2) Acts as a **weak agonist at estrogen receptors** in other tissues
   - **b.** Uses
     - (1) **Breast and endometrial cancers**
     - (2) **Metastatic melanoma** (some effect)
3. **Leuprolide** (see Chapter 26)
   - **a. Pharmacokinetics**
     - Synthetic analogue of a naturally occurring gonadotropin-releasing hormone (GnRH)
     - Administered as an injection
   - **b.** Uses
     - (1) **Advanced prostate or breast cancers** (hormonal antagonist)
     - (2) **Endometriosis**

SECTION X

Toxicology

30 Toxicology and Drugs of Abuse

Target Topics

- Treatment of poisoning
- Teratogenic substances
- Substances of abuse

I. General Principles of Toxicology

- **Toxicology** is the **study of the hazardous effects of chemicals**, including drugs, on biologic systems.
- **Toxicity** is a reflection of **how much**, **how fast**, and **how long** an individual is exposed to a poison.

A. Primary determinants of toxicity

1. Dose and dose **rate**
2. **Duration of exposure**
3. **Route of exposure**

B. Factors that affect toxicity

1. **Biotransformation**
   - Methanol is converted to formaldehyde and formic acid (toxic metabolites).
2. **Genetic factors**
   - Individuals are "fast" or "slow" acetylators of isoniazid.
3. **Immune status:** hypersensitivity reactions such as penicillin hypersensitivity

TABLE 30–1 Symptoms and Treatment of Poisoning

Agent	Clinical Features	Treatment	Comments
Alkalies (hydroxides in soaps, cleansers, drain cleaners)	GI irritation	Supportive care H_2O	NO EMESIS OR LAVAGE More potent than strong acids
Bleach (sodium hypochlorite)	Irritation, delirium	Supportive care; milk, ice cream, or beaten eggs; antacids	NO EMESIS
Carbon monoxide	Headaches, dizziness, metabolic acidosis, retinal hemorrhage	Supportive care, oxygen	Cherry-red blood
Corrosives	GI irritation, seizures, weakness	Milk, antacids, calcium gluconate (antidote for oxalates); milk of magnesia (antidote for mineral acids)	NO EMESIS OR LAVAGE
Cyanide	Seizures, ECG changes	Amyl nitrite or sodium nitrite plus sodium thiosulfate	Rapid treatment necessary
Ethylene glycol	Renal failure; metabolic acidosis with anion gap	Ethanol IV or fomepizole (antidotes), sodium bicarbonate for acidosis, supportive care	Culprit: toxic metabolite (oxalic acid)
Heavy metals			
Arsenic	Vomiting, diarrhea, seizures, neuropathy, nephropathy	Chelation (dimercaprol or penicillamine)	Delayed reaction: white lines on fingernails (Mees' lines)
Iron	GI irritation, blood loss, acidosis	Deferoxamine	Keep away from children
Lead	Abdominal pain, lead lines on gums, basophilic stippling, weakness, behavioral changes, peripheral neuropathy, encephalopathy	Chelation (dimercaprol, EDTA, succimer, or penicillamine)	In old paints and glazes
Mercury	Renal failure, GI irritation, behavioral changes	Chelation (dimercaprol); milk or eggs	Delayed reaction: "mad as a hatter"
Hydrocarbons	Pulmonary infiltrates, CNS depression, seizures, tinnitus	Supportive care	NO EMESIS OR LAVAGE Delayed reaction: chemical pneumonitis
Methanol	Visual disturbance, metabolic acidosis, respiratory failure	Ethanol IV or fomepizole (antidotes), sodium bicarbonate for acidosis, supportive care	Culprit: toxic metabolite (formic acid)
Salicylates	Respiratory alkalosis, metabolic acidosis, increased temperature, tinnitus, respiratory failure, seizures	Supportive care, alkalinize urine, dialysis	Uncouple oxidative phosphorylation
Strychnine	Seizures, respiratory failure, rigidity	Supportive care, activated charcoal	Glycine antagonist in spinal cord, blocking nerve impulses

CNS, Central nervous system; *ECG*, electrocardiogram; *EDTA*, ethylenediamine-tetraacetate; *GI*, gastrointestinal; *IV*, intravenous.

TABLE 30–2 Specific Antidotes for Selected Drugs and Toxins

Antidote	Poison
Drugs That Chelate Metals	
Calcium disodium edetate (EDTA)	Lead
Deferoxamine	Iron
Dimercaprol	Arsenic, gold, mercury, lead
Penicillamine	Lead, copper, arsenic, gold
Succimer	Lead
Substances That Act Against Specific Drugs or Toxins	
Acetylcysteine	Acetaminophen
Amyl nitrite	Cyanide
Atropine	Cholinesterase inhibitor
Digoxin-specific FAB antibodies	Cardiac glycosides (e.g., digitalis)
Esmolol	Theophylline, caffeine, metaproterenol
Ethanol	Methanol or ethylene glycol
Flumazenil	Benzodiazepine
Fomepizole	Ethylene glycol
Glucagon	β-blockers
Naloxone	Opioids
Oxygen	Carbon monoxide
Physostigmine	Anticholinergics
Pralidoxime (2-PAM)	Organophosphates
Pyridoxine	Isoniazid
Sodium bicarbonate	Cardiac depressants (tricyclic antidepressants, quinidine)

4. **Photosensitivity:** skin photosensitivity due to demeclocycline
5. **Species differences**
   - Malathion is rapidly metabolized by humans but not by insects.
6. **Age**
   - Both toxicodynamic and toxicokinetic parameters vary with age.
7. **Gender**
   - Hormonal status affects both toxicodynamic and toxicokinetic parameters.
8. **Environmental factors**
9. **Nutritional status/protein binding**
10. **Drug interactions**
    - Interactions between drugs and between drugs and environmental chemicals may occur by both toxicokinetic and toxicodynamic mechanisms.

II. Treatment of Acute Poisoning (Tables 30-1 and 30-2)

A. **Obtain** important **historical information** and determine the severity of exposure.

B. **Check vital signs.**

C. **Remove stomach contents** if indicated.

1. **Gastric lavage**
   - Not recommended > 4 hours after poisoning

   a. **Contraindications**

   (1) **> 30 minutes after ingestion** of corrosive material

TABLE 30–3 Teratogenic Effects of Selected Drugs*

Drug	Adverse Effects
Alkylating agents and antimetabolites (anticancer drugs)	Cardiac defects; cleft palate; growth retardation; malformation of ears, eyes, fingers, nose, or skull; other anomalies
Carbamazepine	Abnormal facial features; neural tube defects, such as spina bifida; reduced head size; other anomalies
Diethylstilbestrol (DES)	Effects in female offspring: clear cell vaginal or cervical adenocarcinoma; irregular menses and reproductive abnormalities, including decreased rate of pregnancy and increased rate of preterm deliveries Effects in male offspring: cryptorchism, epididymal cysts, hypogonadism
Ethanol	Fetal alcohol syndrome (growth retardation; hyperactivity; mental retardation; microcephaly and facial abnormalities; poor coordination; other anomalies)
Phenytoin	Fetal hydantoin syndrome (cardiac defects; malformation of ears, lips, palate, mouth, and nasal bridge; mental retardation; microcephaly, ptosis, strabismus; other anomalies)
Retinoids (systemic)	Spontaneous abortions; hydrocephaly; malformation of ears, face, heart, limbs, and liver; microcephaly; other anomalies
Tetracycline	Hypoplasia of tooth enamel, staining of teeth
Thalidomide	Deafness; heart defects; limb abnormalities (amelia or phocomelia); renal abnormalities; other anomalies
Valproate	Cardiac defects; central nervous system defects; lumbosacral spina bifida; microcephaly
Warfarin anticoagulants	Fetal warfarin syndrome (chondrodysplasia punctata; malformation of ears and eyes; mental retardation; nasal hypoplasia; optic atrophy; skeletal deformities; other anomalies)

* *Other substances known to be teratogenic:* arsenic, cadmium, lead, lithium, methyl mercury, penicillamine, polychlorinated biphenyls, and trimethadione. *Other drugs that should be avoided during the second and third trimester of pregnancy:* angiotensin-converting enzyme inhibitors, chloramphenicol, indomethacin, prostaglandins, sulfonamides, and sulfonylureas. *Other drugs that should be used with great caution during pregnancy:* antithyroid drugs, aspirin, barbiturates, benzodiazepines, corticosteroids, fluoroquinolones, heparin, opioids, and phenothiazines.

(2) **Ingestion of hydrocarbon solvents** (aspiration pneumonia)

(3) Coma, stupor, delirium, or seizures (present or imminent)

b. Substance used to reduce absorption of poison

- **Activated charcoal** adsorbs many toxins if given immediately before or after lavage.

2. Induced emesis

a. Same contraindications as for gastric lavage

b. Makes use of **syrup of ipecac** (slow-acting oral emetic)

D. Provide symptomatic and supportive treatment.

E. Use specific **antidotes** when appropriate (see Table 30-2).

F. Increase the rate of excretion when appropriate.

- Use cathartics (e.g., **magnesium sulfate**); altered urine pH

The smaller the volume of distribution (V_d), the more effective the hemodialysis.

(e.g., **ammonium chloride** to acidify urine, **sodium bicarbonate** to alkanize urine; osmotic diuretics (e.g., **mannitol**); hemodialysis; peritoneal dialysis; and hemoperfusion.

1. **Acidification of urine:** increased excretion of weak organic bases
2. **Alkalinization of urine:** increased excretion of weak organic acids

III. Teratogenic Effects of Specific Drugs (Table 30-3)

IV. Dependence and Drugs of Abuse

- Repeated drug use may lead to dependence (Table 30-4).

A. Physical dependence

- **Examples:** ethanol (Table 30-5), barbiturates, opioids
- Repeated administration produces an altered or adaptive physiologic state in which signs and symptoms of withdrawal **(abstinence syndrome)** occur if the drug is not present.

Disulfiram discourages ethanol use.

B. Psychological dependence

- **Examples:** amphetamines, cocaine, lysergic acid diethylamide (LSD)
- Affected individuals use a drug repeatedly for personal satisfaction and engage in compulsive drug-seeking behavior.

C. Substance dependence (addiction)

- Chronic use of a drug results in a cluster of symptoms (e.g., craving, withdrawal symptoms, drug-seeking behavior) indicating that the individual continues to use the substance despite substance-related problems (e.g., medical, financial, social).

TABLE 30–4 Drugs of Abuse

Drug	Effect	Withdrawal	Treatment
Alcohol	Slurred speech, unsteady gait, nystagmus, lack of coordination, mood changes	Tremor, tachycardia, insomnia, seizures, delusions, hypertension	Clonidine, lorazepam, chlordiazepoxide, disulfiram
Amphetamines	Psychomotor agitation, pupil dilation, tachycardia, euphoria, hypertension, paranoia, seizures	Dysphoria, fatigue	Supportive care, labetalol
Barbiturates	Same as alcohol	Anxiety, seizures, hypertension, irritability	Same as alcohol
Benzodiazepines	CNS depression, respiratory depression	Anxiety, hypertension, irritability	Supportive care, flumazenil
Caffeine	CNS stimulation, hypertension	Lethargy, headache, irritability	Supportive care
Cocaine	CNS stimulation, arrhythmias, psychomotor agitation, pupil dilation, tachycardia, euphoria, paranoia (similar to amphetamines)	Dysphoria, fatigue (same as amphetamines)	Supportive care, labetalol
Lysergic acid diethylamide (LSD)	Anxiety, paranoia, pupil dilation, tremors, tachycardia, hallucinations	None	No specific treatment Severe agitation may respond to diazepam
Marijuana	Euphoria, dry mouth, increased appetite, conjunctival injection	Irritability, nausea	No specific treatment
Methylenedioxymethamphetamine (MDMA, ecstasy)	Amphetamine-like hyperthermia, hypertension	Dysphoria, fatigue, brain damage	Cool-down
Nicotine	CNS stimulation, increased GI motility	Anxiety, dysphoria, increased appetite	Bupropion, clonidine
Opioids	Pinpoint pupils, respiratory depression, hypotension	Dysphoria, nausea, diarrhea	Supportive care, naloxone, methadone, clonidine
Phencyclidine hydrochloride (PCP)	Aggressive behavior, horizontal-vertical nystagmus, ataxia, seizures, hallucinations	None	Life support, diazepam, haloperidol

CNS, Central nervous system; *GI*, gastrointestinal.

TABLE 30–5 Stages of Ethanol Poisoning*

Degree of Poisoning	Blood Alcohol (mg/dL)	Symptoms
Acute, mild	50–150	Decreased inhibitions, visual impairment, lack of muscular coordination, slowing of reaction time
Moderate	150–300	Major visual impairment, more pronounced symptoms of mild intoxication, slurred speech
Severe	300–500	Approaching stupor, severe hypoglycemia, seizures, death
Coma	> 500	Unconsciousness, slowed respiration, complete loss of sensations, death (frequent)

*Disulfiram inhibits acetaldehyde dehydrogenase, which causes acetaldehyde to accumulate in the blood, resulting in nausea and vomiting if alcohol is consumed.

Tests

COMMON LABORATORY VALUES

Test	Conventional Units	SI Units
Blood, Plasma, Serum		
Alanine aminotransferase (ALT, GPT at 30° C)	8-20 U/L	8-20 U/L
Amylase, serum	25-125 U/L	25-125 U/L
Aspartate aminotransferase (AST, GOT at 30° C)	8-20 U/L	8-20 U/L
Bilirubin, serum (adult) Total // Direct	0.1-1.0 mg/dL // 0.0-0.3 mg/dL	2-17 μmol/L // 0-5 μmol/L
Calcium, serum (Ca^{2+})	8.4-10.2 mg/dL	2.1-2.8 mmol/L
Cholesterol, serum	Rec: < 200 mg/dL	< 5.2 mmol/L
Cortisol, serum	8:00 AM: 6-23 μg/dL // 4:00 PM: 3-15 μg/dL	170-630 nmol/L // 80-410 nmol/L
	8:00 PM: ≤ 50% of 8:00 AM	Fraction of 8:00 AM: ≤ 0.50
Creatine kinase, serum	Male: 25-90 U/L	25-90 U/L
	Female: 10-70 U/L	10-70 U/L
Creatinine, serum	0.6-1.2 mg/dL	53-106 μmol/L
Electrolytes, serum		
Sodium (Na^+)	136-145 mEq/L	135-145 mmol/L
Chloride (Cl^-)	95-105 mEq/L	95-105 mmol/L
Potassium (K^+)	3.5-5.0 mEq/L	3.5-5.0 mmol/L
Bicarbonate (HCO_3^-)	22-28 mEq/L	22-28 mmol/L
Magnesium (Mg^{2+})	1.5-2.0 mEq/L	1.5-2.0 mmol/L
Estriol, total, serum (in pregnancy)		
24-28 wk // 32-36 wk	30-170 ng/mL // 60-280 ng/mL	104-590 // 208-970 nmol/L
28-32 wk // 36-40 wk	40-220 ng/mL // 80-350 ng/mL	140-760 // 280-1210 nmol/L
Ferritin, serum	Male: 15-200 ng/mL	15-200 μg/L
	Female: 12-150 ng/mL	12-150 μg/L
Follicle-stimulating hormone, serum/plasma (FSH)	Male: 4-25 mIU/mL	4-25 U/L
	Female: premenopause 4-30 mIU/mL	4-30 U/L
	midcycle peak 10-90 mIU/mL	10-90 U/L
	postmenopause 40-250 mIU/mL	40-250 U/L
Gases, arterial blood (room air)		
pH	7.35-7.45	$[H^+]$ 36-44 nmol/L
P_{CO_2}	33-45 mm Hg	4.4-5.9 kPa
P_{O_2}	75-105 mm Hg	10.0-14.0 kPa
Glucose, serum	Fasting: 70-110 mg/dL	3.8-6.1 mmol/L
	2 hr postprandial: < 120 mg/dL	< 6.6 mmol/L
Growth hormone–arginine stimulation	Fasting: < 5 ng/mL	< 5 μg/L
	provocative stimuli: > 7 ng/mL	> 7 μg/L
Immunoglobulins, serum		
IgA	76-390 mg/dL	0.76-3.90 g/L
IgE	0-380 IU/mL	0-380 kIU/L
IgG	650-1500 mg/dL	6.5-15 g/L
IgM	40-345 mg/dL	0.4-3.45 g/L

COMMON LABORATORY VALUES—cont'd

Test	Conventional Units	SI Units
Blood, Plasma, Serum—cont'd		
Iron	50-170 μg/dL	9-30 μmol/L
Lactate dehydrogenase, serum (LDH)	45-90 U/L	45-90 U/L
Luteinizing hormone, serum/plasma (LH)	Male: 6-23 mIU/mL	6-23 U/L
	Female: follicular phase 5-30 mIU/mL	5-30 U/L
	midcycle 75-150 mIU/mL	75-150 U/L
	postmenopause 30-200 mIU/mL	30-200 U/L
Osmolality, serum	275-295 mOsm/kg	275-295 mOsm/kg
Parathyroid hormone, serum, N-terminal	230-630 pg/mL	230-630 ng/L
Phosphatase (alkaline), serum (p-NPP at 30° C)	20-70 U/L	20-70 U/L
Phosphorus (inorganic), serum	3.0-4.5 mg/dL	1.0-1.5 mmol/L
Prolactin, serum (hPRL)	< 20 ng/mL	< 20 μg/L
Proteins, serum		
Total (recumbent)	6.0-8.0 g/dL	60-80 g/L
Albumin	3.5-5.5 g/dL	35-55 g/L
Globulin	2.3-3.5 g/dL	23-35 g/L
Thyroid-stimulating hormone, serum or plasma (TSH)	0.5-5.0 μU/mL	0.5-5.0 mU/L
Thyroidal iodine (^{123}I) uptake	8%-30% of administered dose/24 hr	0.08-0.30/24 hr
Thyroxine (T_4), serum	4.5-12 μg/dL	58-154 nmol/L
Triglycerides, serum	35-160 mg/dL	0.4-1.81 mmol/L
Triiodothyronine (T_3), serum (RIA)	115-190 ng/dL	1.8-2.9 nmol/L
Triiodothyronine (T_3) resin uptake	25%-38%	0.25-0.38
Urea nitrogen, serum (BUN)	7-18 mg/dL	1.2-3.0 mmol urea/L
Uric acid, serum	3.0-8.2 mg/dL	0.18-0.48 mmol/L
Cerebrospinal (CSF) Fluid		
Cell count	0-5 cells/mm^3	0-5 × 10^6/L
Chloride	118-132 mEq/L	118-132 mmol/L
Gamma globulin	3%-12% total proteins	0.03-0.12
Glucose	50-75 mg/dL	2.8-4.2 mmol/L
Pressure	70-180 mm H_2O	70-180 mm H_2O
Proteins, total	< 40 mg/dL	< 0.40 g/L
Hematology		
Bleeding time (template)	2-7 min	2-7 min
Erythrocyte count	Male: 4.3-5.9 million/mm^3	4.3-5.9 × 10^{12}/L
	Female: 3.5-5.5 million/mm^3	3.5-5.5 × 10^{12}/L
Erythrocyte sedimentation rate (Westergren)	Male: 0-15 mm/hr	0-15 mm/hr
	Female: 0-20 mm/hr	0-20 mm/hr

Continued

COMMON LABORATORY VALUES—cont'd

Test	Conventional Units	SI Units
Hematology—cont'd		
Hematocrit (Hct)	Male: 40%-54%	0.40-0.54
	Female: 37%-47%	0.37-0.47
Hemoglobin A_{IC}	≤ 6%	≤ 0.06%
Hemoglobin, blood (Hb)	Male: 13.5-17.5 g/dL	2.09-2.71 mmol/L
	Female: 12.0-16.0 g/dL	1.86-2.48 mmol/L
Hemoglobin, plasma	1-4 mg/dL	0.16-0.62 mmol/L
Leukocyte count and differential		
Leukocyte count	4500-11,000/mm^3	4.5-11.0 × 10^9/L
Segmented neutrophils	54%-62%	0.54-0.62
Bands	3%-5%	0.03-0.05
Eosinophils	1%-3%	0.01-0.03
Basophils	0%-0.75%	0-0.0075
Lymphocytes	25%-33%	0.25-0.33
Monocytes	3%-7%	0.03-0.07
Mean corpuscular hemoglobin (MCH)	25.4-34.6 pg/cell	0.39-0.54 fmol/cell
Mean corpuscular hemoglobin concentration (MCHC)	31%-37% Hb/cell	4.81-5.74 mmol Hb/L
Mean corpuscular volume (MCV)	80-100 μm^3	80-100 fl
Partial thromboplastin time (activated) (aPTT)	25-40 sec	25-40 sec
Platelet count	150,000-400,000/mm^3	150-400 × 10^9/L
Prothrombin time (PT)	12-14 sec	12-14 sec
Reticulocyte count	0.5%-1.5% of red cells	0.005-0.015
Thrombin time	< 2 sec deviation from control	< 2 sec deviation from control
Volume		
Plasma	Male: 25-43 mL/kg	0.025-0.043 L/kg
	Female: 28-45 mL/kg	0.028-0.045 L/kg
Red cell	Male: 20-36 mL/kg	0.020-0.036 L/kg
	Female: 19-31 mL/kg	0.019-0.031 L/kg
Sweat		
Chloride	0-35 mmol/L	0-35 mmol/L
Urine		
Calcium	100-300 mg/24 hr	2.5-7.5 mmol/24 hr
Creatinine clearance	Male: 97-137 mL/min	
	Female: 88-128 mL/min	
Estriol, total (in pregnancy)		
30 wk	6-18 mg/24 hr	21-62 μmol/24 hr
35 wk	9-28 mg/24 hr	31-97 μmol/24 hr
40 wk	13-42 mg/24 hr	45-146 μmol/24 hr
17-Hydroxycorticosteroids	Male: 3.0-9.0 mg/24 hr	8.2-25.0 μmol/24 hr
	Female: 2.0-8.0 mg/24 hr	5.5-22.0 μmol/24 hr
17-Ketosteroids, total	Male: 8-22 mg/24 hr	28-76 μmol/24 hr
	Female: 6-15 mg/24 hr	21-52 μmol/24 hr
Osmolality	50-1400 mOsm/kg	
Oxalate	8-40 μg/mL	90-445 μmol/L
Proteins, total	< 150 mg/24 hr	< 0.15 g/24 hr

TEST 1

DIRECTIONS: Each numbered item or incomplete statement is followed by options arranged in alphabetical or logical order. Select the best answer to each question. Some options may be partially correct, but there is only **ONE BEST** answer.

1. Three days after a 58-year-old man undergoes bowel resection, he begins hyperventilating and is found to have respiratory alkalosis. The following day, his condition has worsened. Findings include temperature that exceeds 40°C (> 104°F); profound hypotension; tachycardia; elevated blood urea nitrogen (BUN) and serum creatinine levels; low urinary output; and white blood cell count of 17,000/mm^3 with a shift to the left. The patient's sputum is purulent, and a Gram's stain shows the presence of gram-negative rods. Which of the following agents should be given for hemodynamic support?

❍ A. Aspirin
❍ B. Dopamine
❍ C. Furosemide
❍ D. Isoproterenol
❍ E. Nitroprusside

2. A 35-year-old man has taken an overdose of a drug whose metabolites are hepatotoxic but whose immediate symptoms of toxicity consist of nausea and vomiting. About 36 hours after ingesting the drug, he is taken to the hospital and found to have elevated levels of prothrombin and transaminase. To prevent hepatic failure and encephalopathy, he is treated with metoclopramide and acetylcysteine. The patient most likely took an overdose of which of the following drugs?

❍ A. Acetaminophen
❍ B. Diazepam
❍ C. Isoniazid
❍ D. Lithium
❍ E. Salicylate

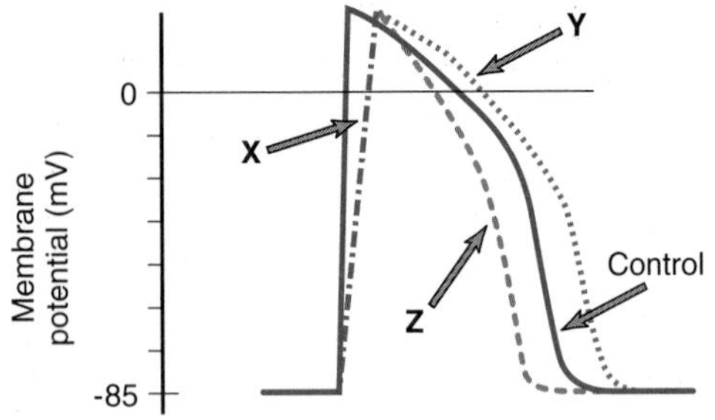

3. Curves X, Y, and Z in the figure above represent changes in the action potential of the cardiac muscle in response to the administration of various antiarrhythmic agents. Which of the following agents would be most likely to produce the changes depicted in curve Z?

- ❍ A. Amiodarone
- ❍ B. Bretylium
- ❍ C. Diltiazem
- ❍ D. Mexiletine
- ❍ E. Quinidine

4. A 56-year-old man has constant blood pressure values of about 150/98 mm Hg. Laboratory studies show that his plasma renin activity is elevated. Treatment with which of the following drugs would be most likely to reduce blood pressure and suppress renin release?

- ❍ A. Captopril
- ❍ B. Hydralazine
- ❍ C. Losartan
- ❍ D. Prazosin
- ❍ E. Propranolol

5. A previously healthy 49-year-old woman complains that she has been suffering from morning stiffness that persists for several hours after awakening. During the past 3 months, she has also had anorexia, fatigue, and generalized joint and muscle pain. A good first-line drug to treat this patient is

- ❍ A. allopurinol
- ❍ B. auranofin
- ❍ C. colchicine
- ❍ D. ibuprofen
- ❍ E. indomethacin

6. A 57-year-old man has been treated for hypertension for the past 7 years. Lately, he has gained about 7 kg (15 lb) and has begun to complain that his feet are swollen and that he is short of breath. When he is admitted to the hospital, clinical findings include blood pressure of 165/105 mm Hg, pulse of 105/min, and significant ankle edema, dyspnea, cyanosis, and tachycardia. His medical records show that he is currently taking hydrochlorothiazide, propranolol, and ibuprofen. Which of the following drugs would be the most appropriate treatment for this patient?

- ❍ A. Diazoxide
- ❍ B. Digoxin plus quinidine
- ❍ C. Furosemide plus lisinopril
- ❍ D. Hydralazine plus spironolactone
- ❍ E. Prazosin plus verapamil

7. A 54-year-old man with chronic renal failure has become increasingly fatigued over the past 3 months. Blood studies confirm the presence of normochromic anemia. Which of the following agents would most likely reverse his anemia?

- ❍ A. Epoetin alfa
- ❍ B. Folic acid
- ❍ C. Iron
- ❍ D. Sargramostim
- ❍ E. Vitamin B_{12}

8. A 12-year-old girl is diagnosed with acute lymphocytic leukemia. She has thrombocytopenia and anemia, and her white blood cell count is 150,000/mm^3. The patient begins treatment with vincristine and prednisone. Which of the following is the mechanism of action of vincristine?

- ❍ A. Alkylation of DNA
- ❍ B. Generation of free radicals
- ❍ C. Inhibition of dihydrofolate reductase
- ❍ D. Inhibition of mitotic spindle formation
- ❍ E. Inhibition of topoisomerase

9. A 57-year-old woman with a lengthy history of type 1 diabetes mellitus develops significant water retention and symptoms suggestive of pulmonary congestion. Laboratory studies show:

Serum creatinine	7 mg/dL
Blood urea nitrogen (BUN)	75 mg/dL
Serum sodium	145 mEq/L
Serum potassium	7.2 mEq/L
Serum chloride	100 mEq/L

Other laboratory data support a diagnosis of advanced renal disease, possibly as a result of long-standing diabetes. Shortly after the patient begins treatment with a diuretic, she exhibits cardiac conduction changes that progress to heart block and then to cardiac arrest. Which diuretic is most likely responsible for the cardiac effects in this patient?

❍ A. Chlorthalidone
❍ B. Ethacrynic acid
❍ C. Furosemide
❍ D. Hydrochlorothiazide
❍ E. Triamterene

10. A 45-year-old woman has a syndrome characterized by severe gastric hyperacidity, peptic ulcer disease, and gastrinomas. The most effective drug for treating this syndrome is

❍ A. famotidine
❍ B. mesalamine
❍ C. misoprostol
❍ D. omeprazole
❍ E. sucralfate

11. A 72-year-old man undergoes hip replacement surgery. Postoperative heparin treatment is begun, and the patient suddenly shows signs of gastrointestinal bleeding. Which of the following agents would immediately antagonize the effects of heparin?

❍ A. Aminocaproic acid
❍ B. Folic acid
❍ C. Protamine
❍ D. Vitamin B_{12}
❍ E. Vitamin K

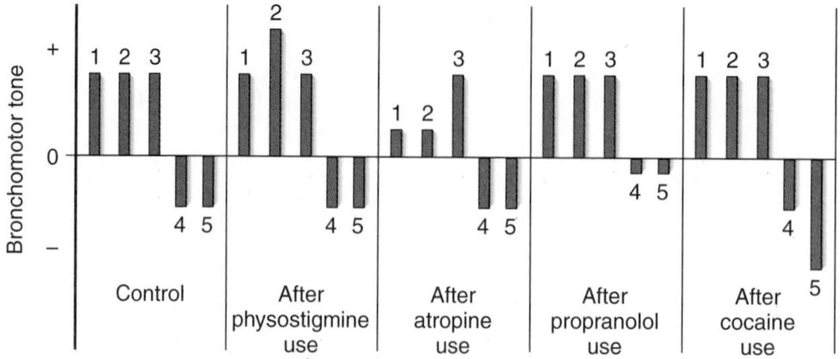

12. In the figure above, changes in bronchomotor tone are depicted in terms of constriction (+) or relaxation (–). The first panel of the figure (control) shows changes that were elicited by five different procedures (numbered 1 through 5), each of which was performed alone. The remaining panels show changes that were elicited by the same five procedures, each of which was performed after pretreatment with a different drug. Based on the results, procedure 5 is most likely the administration of

- ❍ A. ephedrine
- ❍ B. epinephrine
- ❍ C. histamine
- ❍ D. phenylephrine
- ❍ E. terbutaline

13. A 39-year-old woman who has been using albuterol for several years to treat her asthma complains of irregular heart beats. Holter monitoring confirms the presence of episodic premature ventricular contractions (PVCs), and she begins metoprolol therapy to suppress PVCs. The therapy worsens her asthmatic symptoms and does not completely diminish the PVCs, and therapy is stopped. Which of the following would be most appropriate for use in the management of her PVCs?

- ❍ A. Treatment with flecainide
- ❍ B. Treatment with nifedipine
- ❍ C. Treatment with procainamide
- ❍ D. Treatment with quinidine
- ❍ E. No drug treatment

14. Resistance to antibacterial agents is less likely to occur when patients are treated with a drug combination that inhibits sequential steps of intermediate metabolism in bacteria. Which of the following combinations acts in this manner?

- ❍ A. Amoxicillin plus clavulanate
- ❍ B. Ampicillin plus sulbactam
- ❍ C. Imipenem plus cilastatin
- ❍ D. Piperacillin plus tazobactam
- ❍ E. Trimethoprim plus sulfamethoxazole

15. A 41-year-old man is diagnosed with testicular cancer. Physical examination and pulmonary function studies and x-rays suggest that he also has a preexisting pulmonary disease. Which of the following antineoplastic drugs would be most likely to exacerbate the patient's pulmonary problems?

- ❍ A. Bleomycin
- ❍ B. Cisplatin
- ❍ C. Doxorubicin
- ❍ D. Methotrexate
- ❍ E. Vincristine

16. A 17-year-old boy who is being treated for leukemia develops a fever. He begins treatment with antibacterial, antiviral, and antifungal agents and 2 days later develops acute renal failure. Which of the following drugs is most likely responsible for this adverse effect?

❍ A. Acyclovir
❍ B. Amphotericin B
❍ C. Ampicillin
❍ D. Ceftazidime
❍ E. Vancomycin

17. A 55-year-old man who has been receiving anticoagulant treatment for many years is diagnosed with tuberculosis. Which of the following antimycobacterial agents would most likely induce cytochrome P450 enzymes in the patient's liver and thereby modify the effects of his anticoagulant treatment?

❍ A. Ethambutol
❍ B. Isoniazid
❍ C. Pyrazinamide
❍ D. Pyridoxine
❍ E. Rifampin

18. A 48-year-old man undergoes kidney transplantation. Because he is receiving a graft from an autologous donor, he must take immunosuppressive medications for life. Which of the following drugs is preferred to prevent rejection of the allografted kidney?

❍ A. Azathioprine
❍ B. Cyclophosphamide
❍ C. Cyclosporine
❍ D. Fluorouracil
❍ E. Vincristine

19. A 53-year-old man with a family history of hypercholesterolemia is found to have elevated cholesterol levels. The physician prescribes a drug that acts by inhibiting HMG-CoA reductase. This drug is

❍ A. cholestyramine
❍ B. colestipol
❍ C. gemfibrozil
❍ D. lovastatin
❍ E. niacin

20. A 71-year-old man is being treated with levodopa to alleviate the symptoms of Parkinson's disease. To potentiate the effects of levodopa, the physician begins concurrent treatment with a drug that decreases the metabolism of dopamine without producing life-threatening side effects. Which of the following drugs is most likely prescribed for this patient?

❍ A. Amantadine
❍ B. Bromocriptine
❍ C. Carbidopa
❍ D. Phenelzine
❍ E. Selegiline

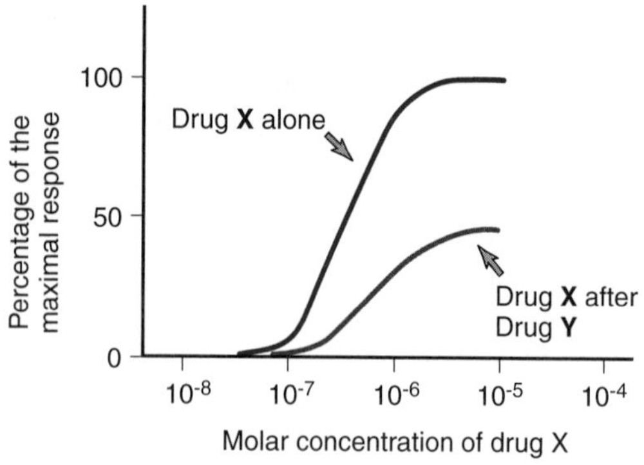

21. The figure above depicts the dose-response curve when drug X is given alone and when the drug is given in the presence of a fixed dose of drug Y. Drug Y elicits no response when it is given alone. The experimental system is an organ bath that contains a piece of vascular smooth muscle. Drug Y in this figure is a

- ❍ A. competitive antagonist
- ❍ B. full agonist
- ❍ C. noncompetitive antagonist
- ❍ D. partial agonist

22. A 9-year-old boy suffers from severe asthma. The wheezing and other symptoms have been inadequately controlled by his current treatment measures. Combination therapy with drugs chosen to target different mechanisms of action is recommended. Which of the following drugs would inhibit the bronchoconstrictor effect of increased parasympathetic tone?

- ❍ A. Cromolyn
- ❍ B. Ipratropium
- ❍ C. Theophylline
- ❍ D. Zafirlukast
- ❍ E. Zileuton

23. A 72-year-old man complains of blurred vision and red, painful eyes. His medical records show that he has ankylosing spondylitis and benign prostatic hyperplasia (BPH) but has no history of glaucoma. Slit-lamp examination confirms the diagnosis of iridocyclitis. A topical glucocorticoid is prescribed, along with ocular drops to dilate the pupils and thereby reduce the pain and prevent synechiae. A few days after he begins treatment, the patient complains that he cannot urinate. Which of the following drugs is most likely responsible for this side effect?

- ❍ A. Atropine
- ❍ B. Ephedrine
- ❍ C. Epinephrine
- ❍ D. Phenylephrine
- ❍ E. Prednisone

24. A 26-year-old woman is being treated with tranylcypromine for a major depressive disorder. She is injured in an automobile accident and is taken to the hospital and kept overnight for observation. The patient is given a pain medication, and later that night she becomes delirious, hyperpyretic, and comatose. Which of the following pain medications is most likely responsible for these adverse effects?

- ❍ A. Acetaminophen
- ❍ B. Codeine
- ❍ C. Ibuprofen
- ❍ D. Meperidine
- ❍ E. Morphine

25. A 29-year-old woman is recovering from a pulmonary embolism and is being treated with warfarin when she learns that she is pregnant. Which of the following is the most appropriate next step in the management of this patient?

❍ A. Continue warfarin therapy
❍ B. Stop warfarin and begin abciximab therapy
❍ C. Stop warfarin and begin aspirin therapy
❍ D. Stop warfarin and begin heparin therapy
❍ E. Stop warfarin and begin ticlopidine therapy

26. A 70-year-old man with gout is prescribed probenecid. He later develops a severe rash and stops taking the drug. Several days later, he begins monotherapy with allopurinol and experiences an acute attack of gouty arthritis. The allopurinol-induced attack could have been avoided by concurrent treatment with allopurinol and which of the following drugs?

❍ A. Aspirin
❍ B. Chloroquine
❍ C. Colchicine
❍ D. Ibuprofen
❍ E. Sulfinpyrazone

27. An 18-year-old woman with a history of depression is found unresponsive in her apartment with an empty bottle of amitriptyline lying nearby. Upon arrival in the emergency department, the patient is tachycardic, with an irregular pulse of 160/min. Her blood pressure is 86/54 mm Hg, and her temperature is 37.8°C (100°F). Physical examination shows dry mucous membranes, dilated pupils, absent bowel sounds, a distended urinary bladder, and persistent tonic-clonic seizures. The patient's tachycardia, fever, dry mucous membranes, dilated pupils, absent bowel sounds, and distended bladder are caused by the blockade of

❍ A. α-adrenergic receptors
❍ B. catecholamine reuptake
❍ C. dopamine receptors
❍ D. muscarinic receptors
❍ E. serotonin reuptake

28. A 25-year-old African-American man who is working as a Peace Corps volunteer in Africa receives a blood transfusion after a surgical procedure. He subsequently develops symptoms of malaria, and laboratory studies show that he is infected with *Plasmodium vivax*. His symptoms are controlled with chloroquine. Which of the following drugs would be the most effective against the exoerythrocytic form of *P. vivax*?

❍ A. Chloroquine
❍ B. Mefloquine
❍ C. Primaquine
❍ D. Pyrimethamine-sulfadoxine
❍ E. Quinine

29. One of the following drugs produces acute toxic effects by competing with pyridoxal 5-phosphate (the active form of vitamin B_6) for the enzyme glutamic acid decarboxylase. An overdose causes slurred speech and ataxia, with rapid development of seizures. Which of the following drugs produces these effects?

❍ A. Acetaminophen
❍ B. Amitriptyline
❍ C. Isoniazid
❍ D. Lithium
❍ E. Salicylate

30. A 37-year-old man is taken to the emergency department because he has a fever and is experiencing night sweats and increased fatigue. Laboratory studies show a white blood cell count of 140,000/mm^3 with a differential of > 90% leukemic blasts; a hematocrit of 29%; and a platelet count of 40,000/mm^3. A bone marrow aspirate confirms the diagnosis of acute nonlymphocytic leukemia. Which drug is most appropriate for induction therapy for this patient?

❍ A. Cisplatin
❍ B. Cytarabine
❍ C. Flutamide
❍ D. Streptozocin
❍ E. Vincristine

31. A 39-year-old woman with a history of pulmonary and extrapulmonary tuberculosis collapses while shopping and is taken to the emergency department. She complains that she has recently lost weight and now suffers from increasing fatigue and muscle weakness. She is also concerned about dark spots that have appeared over her knuckles and in her mouth. Laboratory findings include hyponatremia, hyperkalemia, a low plasma aldosterone level, and a high plasma renin level. The adrenocorticotropic hormone (ACTH) test is administered, and the patient's cortisol levels fail to rise in response to cosyntropin. Which of the following is the therapy of choice for long-term management of the patient's condition?

❍ A. ACTH replacement
❍ B. Albuterol
❍ C. Aldosterone
❍ D. Hydrocortisone plus fludrocortisone
❍ E. Insulin plus glucose infusion

32. A 55-year-old man has benign prostatic hyperplasia (BPH) and male pattern baldness. Which of the following agents would be most likely to alleviate both conditions?

❍ A. Cortisone
❍ B. Estradiol
❍ C. Finasteride
❍ D. Gonadotropins
❍ E. Testosterone

33. A 57-year-old postmenopausal woman with a small bone structure is diagnosed with osteoporosis. The patient does not want to take estrogen therapy but is willing to take calcium and vitamin D supplements. Which other drug could the physician prescribe to stop the progression of osteoporosis?

❍ A. Alendronate
❍ B. Finasteride
❍ C. Hydrochlorothiazide
❍ D. Leuprolide
❍ E. Rosiglitazone

34. A 26-year-old woman is infected simultaneously with *Treponema pallidum, Neisseria gonorrhoeae,* and *Chlamydia trachomatis.* Which of the following drugs would be most effective against these three sexually transmitted disease agents?

❍ A. Ampicillin
❍ B. Cephalexin
❍ C. Doxycycline
❍ D. Penicillin G
❍ E. Streptomycin

35. A 14-year-old girl with epilepsy is brought to the emergency department because she shows signs of increasing drowsiness and inattentiveness. Her father thinks that she might have taken an extra dose of her antiepileptic medication a few hours before he noticed her symptoms. Physical examination of the patient shows an ataxic gait, nystagmus, and gingival hyperplasia. Which of the following medications is the patient most likely taking?

❍ A. Carbamazepine
❍ B. Diazepam
❍ C. Ethosuximide
❍ D. Phenytoin
❍ E. Valproic acid

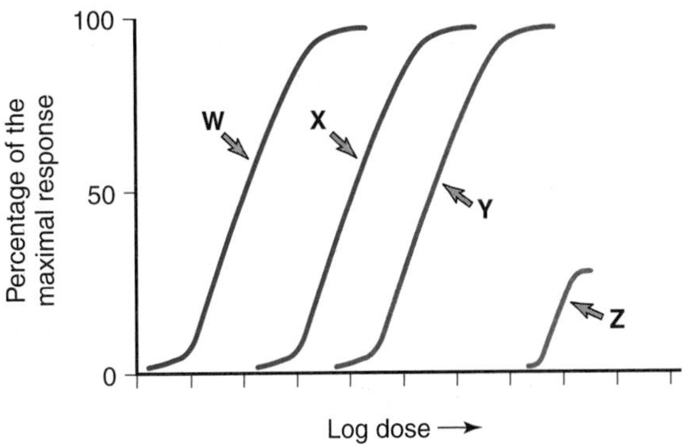

36. The figure above depicts dose-response curves for drugs W, X, Y, and Z after the addition of an appropriate dose of each drug to an isolated tissue in an organ bath. A comparison of the curves shows that drug W

❍ A. has a greater affinity for the receptor than drug X
❍ B. has greater intrinsic activity than drug X
❍ C. is an antagonist of drug X
❍ D. is an antagonist of drug Z
❍ E. is less potent than drug X

37. A 59-year-old woman with a *Pseudomonas aeruginosa* infection is prescribed cefepime. Concurrent treatment with which of the following drugs would be most likely to alter the serum concentration of cefepime?

❍ A. Amifostine
❍ B. Dexrazoxane
❍ C. Ketoconazole
❍ D. Phenytoin
❍ E. Probenecid

38. An 80-year-old man suffers a major depressive episode 2 years after his wife has died and his children have moved out of town. The medical records show that the patient has had two myocardial infarctions over the past 10 years and has a history of intermittent second-degree heart block. Which of the following drugs would be the most appropriate for treating his depression?

❍ A. Amitriptyline
❍ B. Desipramine
❍ C. Fluoxetine
❍ D. Imipramine
❍ E. Phenelzine

39. Which of the following drugs is a parenterally administered beta-lactam antibiotic that can be given in a single daily dose to treat bacterial meningitis in a child?

❍ A. Azithromycin
❍ B. Ceftriaxone
❍ C. Ciprofloxacin
❍ D. Fosfomycin
❍ E. Meropenem

40. A 40-year-old man is taken to the emergency department because his heart is beating irregularly. Examination and electrocardiographic studies show a respiratory rate of 26/min and the presence of paroxysmal supraventricular tachycardia (PSVT). The patient is treated with an intravenous bolus of an antiarrhythmic agent, and his sinus rhythm returns, but his respiratory rate increases to 45/min and he experiences a burning sensation in his chest. The antiarrhythmic agent most likely to cause these effects is

❍ A. adenosine
❍ B. esmolol
❍ C. lidocaine
❍ D. magnesium
❍ E. propranolol

41. A 44-year-old moderately obese woman is diagnosed with type 2 diabetes mellitus. Dietary modifications and sulfonylurea therapy fail to control the patient's glucose levels. Which oral antidiabetic agent with a minimal risk of causing hypoglycemia should be prescribed for this patient?

❍ A. Chlorpropamide
❍ B. Glipizide
❍ C. Glyburide
❍ D. Metformin
❍ E. Tolbutamide

42. A 65-year-old man receives a kidney transplant. He begins immunosuppressive therapy and is told that he must continue this therapy for the rest of his life. Which of the following drugs is used almost exclusively for immunosuppressive therapy?

❍ A. Cyclophosphamide
❍ B. Cyclosporine
❍ C. Methotrexate
❍ D. Prednisone
❍ E. Vincristine

43. A 39-year-old woman has been taking oral contraceptives for 13 years. She smokes two packs of cigarettes a day. Which of the following is the most serious adverse reaction that could occur with oral contraceptive use in this patient?

❍ A. Breakthrough bleeding
❍ B. Cerebral thrombosis
❍ C. Depression
❍ D. Hypotension
❍ E. Increase in the serum triglyceride level

44. A 47-year-old obese man with a blood pressure of 151/98 mm Hg begins antihypertensive therapy with a nonselective β-adrenergic receptor antagonist that can be taken once a day. Six months later, his blood pressure is under better control, but he complains of sexual dysfunction and is found to have an increase in his plasma triglyceride level and a decrease in his high-density lipoprotein (HDL) level. His physician stops his current treatment and begins treatment with a selective β_1-adrenergic receptor antagonist that has intrinsic sympathomimetic activity (ISA). Treatment with which of the following drugs is most likely to be initiated?

❍ A. Acebutolol
❍ B. Betaxolol
❍ C. Carvedilol
❍ D. Labetalol
❍ E. Pindolol

45. A 30-year-old woman complains that she has been having left-sided pulsatile headaches for the past 6 months. The headaches are preceded by bilateral flashes of light and a sensation of light-headedness. Ergotamine is prescribed. When this proves ineffective, the physician stops ergotamine treatment and begins treatment with a serotonin 5-HT_{1D} receptor agonist. Which of the following drugs is most likely to be given at this time?

❍ A. Buspirone
❍ B. Dihydroergotamine
❍ C. Metoclopramide
❍ D. Ondansetron
❍ E. Sumatriptan

46. When anticancer drugs are used, it is often difficult to achieve maximal beneficial effects with minimal adverse effects. This is also true with drugs that must be bioactivated before they become cytotoxic. Which of the following is an example of a prodrug that requires bioactivation?

❍ A. Busulfan
❍ B. Carmustine
❍ C. Cyclophosphamide
❍ D. Mechlorethamine
❍ E. Methotrexate

47. A 42-year-old man is currently taking drugs for hypertension and gastric pain and discomfort. When he visits his physician, he complains about breast enlargement and an unexpectedly abrupt decline of sexual potency. Which of the following drugs is most likely to cause these adverse effects?

❍ A. Aluminum hydroxide
❍ B. Cimetidine
❍ C. Hydrochlorothiazide
❍ D. Misoprostol
❍ E. Ranitidine

48. While undergoing a routine eye examination, a 55-year-old woman is found to have 20/70 visual acuity without correction in the right eye and 20/50 in the left eye. Tonometry shows an intraocular pressure of 38 mm Hg in both eyes; ophthalmoscopy shows physiologic cupping of the optic discs of both eyes; and a visual field examination shows a nerve fiber bundle defect. Treatment with echothiophate is prescribed. This drug exerts its beneficial effects by inhibiting which of the following enzymes?

❍ A. Acetylcholinesterase (AChE)
❍ B. Carbonic anhydrase (CA)
❍ C. Catechol-*O*-methyltransferase (COMT)
❍ D. Choline acetyltransferase (CAT)
❍ E. Tyrosine hydroxylase

49. A 23-year-old man develops excessive thirst after sustaining a severe head injury with a fracture at the base of the skull. His daily water intake is 5–6 L, and because of the ensuing polyuria, he has to get up several times during the night to void. Laboratory findings include serum osmolality > 300 mOsmol/kg, urine osmolarity < 300 mOsmol/kg, and serum sodium of 147 mEq/L. Which of the following is the treatment of choice for this patient?

- ❍ A. Administration of a thiazide diuretic
- ❍ B. Administration of anterior pituitary gland extract
- ❍ C. Administration of desmopressin
- ❍ D. Reduction of water intake
- ❍ E. Restriction of salt and protein intake

50. A 25-year-old man goes to the emergency department of a nearby hospital four times during a 4-week period suffering from chest pain, difficulty in breathing, dizziness, and sweating. Each time, physical examination shows no signs of cardiovascular or other problems. The patient is referred to a psychiatrist and is found to have no suicidal ideation. He is diagnosed with panic disorder. Which of the following anxiolytics is the most useful in the treatment of this disorder?

- ❍ A. Alprazolam
- ❍ B. Buspirone
- ❍ C. Diazepam
- ❍ D. Flurazepam
- ❍ E. Triazolam

ANSWERS AND DISCUSSIONS

1. *B* (dopamine) is correct. The patient's clinical and laboratory findings are consistent with the diagnosis of fulminant bacteremia with septic shock. For hemodynamic support, a pressor drug such as dopamine may be used. The effects of dopamine vary, depending on the rate of infusion. At low doses (0.5–2 μg/kg/min), the drug mainly acts on specific dopamine receptors in the renal, mesenteric, coronary, and intracerebral vasculature to cause vasodilation and thereby increase the renal blood flow and improve the glomerular filtration rate. These effects can be critical in patients with diminished renal perfusion. At moderate doses (2–10 μg/kg/min), dopamine also stimulates β_1-adrenergic receptors. This causes an increase in cardiac output while maintaining the dopamine-induced vasodilative effects. At high doses (> 10 μg/kg/min), dopamine stimulation of α_1-adrenergic receptors predominates to increase peripheral vascular resistance. In the case described, the patient's poor renal status may be secondary to greatly diminished vascular resistance and functional hypovolemia. Hypovolemia occurs because increased capillary permeability results in movement of fluid to extravascular spaces. In one third of patients with septic shock, aggressive replacement of fluids causes a significant improvement in blood pressure.

   A (aspirin) is incorrect. Nonsteroidal anti-inflammatory drugs may lower the patient's temperature, but they would not correct the hemodynamics.
   C (furosemide) is incorrect. Furosemide is a loop diuretic and would therefore be inappropriate. The patient requires fluid replacement.
   D (isoproterenol) is incorrect. Because isoproterenol activates β_2-adrenergic receptors in the vascular beds, it would cause a further drop in blood pressure and would therefore be inappropriate.
   E (nitroprusside) is incorrect. Nitroprusside would cause a much further drop in blood pressure and would therefore be inappropriate.

2. *A* (acetaminophen) is correct. The initial symptoms and signs of acetaminophen overdose are limited to nausea and vomiting. Signs of hepatotoxicity can be noted within 24–48 hours; liver failure may result in death. Liver toxicity is markedly enhanced by alcohol consumption. Metoclopramide is used to treat the patient's nausea and vomiting. Acetylcysteine inactivates the reactive metabolite that is responsible for hepatotoxicity. Ideally, acetylcysteine should be administered within 10 hours after exposure to the acetaminophen overdose.

B (diazepam) is incorrect. Diazepam causes central nervous system depression and is not associated with liver damage.
C (isoniazid) is incorrect. Although long-term use of isoniazid causes liver damage, short-term use does not. Acute isoniazid toxicity is due to the drug's competition with pyridoxal phosphate for the enzyme glutamate decarboxylase. This lowers the levels of GABA and leads to seizures. Acute isoniazid toxicity can be treated with pyridoxine.
D (lithium) and E (salicylate) are incorrect. Acute lithium toxicity and acute salicylate toxicity do not cause liver damage.

3. ***D*** (mexiletine) is correct. Mexiletine and other class IB antiarrhythmic drugs produce the changes depicted in curve Z. Mexiletine inhibits the fast sodium channels of the myocardial cell membrane and thereby decreases the rate of rise of the action potential. It decreases both the effective refractory period and the action potential duration.

A (amiodarone) is incorrect. Amiodarone is an antiarrhythmic drug that has some class IA effects and some class III effects. It increases the action potential duration and the effective refractory period.
B (bretylium) is incorrect. Bretylium is a class III antiarrhythmic drug. It does not decrease the action potential duration. It blocks potassium channels and delays repolarization.
C (diltiazem) is incorrect. Diltiazem is a class IV antiarrhythmic drug. It blocks calcium channels and increases the action potential duration.
E (quinidine) is incorrect. Quinidine and other class IA antiarrhythmic drugs produce the changes depicted in curve Y. Quinidine increases the action potential duration.

4. ***E*** (propranolol) is correct. Propranolol is used to treat hypertension and the subsequent decline of renal function in patients with scleroderma renal crisis (SRC). SRC is associated with elevated peripheral renin concentrations. Propranolol acts by blocking β-adrenergic receptors located on the surface of the juxtaglomerular cells and thereby decreases the release of renin. This affects the renin-angiotensin-aldosterone system and causes a reduction in blood pressure.

A (captopril) is incorrect. Captopril is an angiotensin-converting enzyme (ACE) inhibitor that is used in the treatment of hypertension, congestive heart failure, and various renal syndromes, including diabetic nephropathy and scleroderma. ACE is the enzyme responsible for converting angiotensin I to angiotensin II. Angiotensin II causes negative feedback inhibition of renin release in juxtaglomerular cells. By blocking ACE, captopril reduces the formation of angiotensin II and thereby reduces the feedback inhibition. As a result, renin release is enhanced, rather than suppressed, by captopril.

B (hydralazine) is incorrect. Hydralazine is an antihypertensive agent. It is a peripheral vasodilator that causes relaxation of arteriolar smooth muscle via a direct effect. The decrease in vascular resistance results in an increase in renin release.
C (losartan) is incorrect. Losartan was the first of a class of antihypertensive agents called angiotensin II receptor antagonists. Angiotensin II causes negative feedback inhibition of renin release in the juxtaglomerular cells. Losartan blocks this feedback inhibition. As a result, renin release is enhanced, rather than suppressed.
D (prazosin) is incorrect. Prazosin is a selective competitive inhibitor of vascular postsynaptic α_1-adrenergic receptors. Inhibition of these receptors causes a decrease in peripheral vascular resistance and blood pressure. The decrease in vascular resistance results in an increase in renin release.

5. ***D*** (ibuprofen) is correct. The patient's clinical manifestations are consistent with the diagnosis of rheumatoid arthritis. This disorder is frequently treated with ibuprofen, a nonsteroidal anti-inflammatory drug (NSAID) that is administered orally and has analgesic and antipyretic properties. Other indications for ibuprofen use include osteoarthritis, dysmenorrhea, ankylosing spondylitis, gout, psoriatic arthritis, and mild to moderate pain.

A (allopurinol) is incorrect. Allopurinol is not used to treat rheumatoid arthritis. It is used to prevent gout attacks or renal calculi and to prevent or treat uric acid nephropathy. The drug acts by inhibiting xanthine oxidase, thereby blocking the metabolism of hypoxanthine and xanthine (oxypurines) to uric acid.
B (auranofin) is incorrect. Auranofin is an oral antirheumatic drug that is used to treat early active cases of both adult and juvenile types of rheumatoid arthritis. The drug is less effective against chronic rheumatoid arthritis, and it is typically used only when salicylates or other NSAIDs do not provide satisfactory relief.
C (colchicine) is incorrect. Colchicine is not used to treat rheumatoid arthritis. It is used to treat acute gout attacks and is the preferred drug for use in the treatment of acute gouty arthritis. Colchicine has also been used in the management of amyloidosis, Behçet's syndrome, dermatitis herpetiformis, familial Mediterranean fever, Paget's disease, pericarditis, pseudogout, and biliary and hepatic cirrhosis.
E (indomethacin) is incorrect. Indomethacin is an NSAID that is used primarily in the treatment of rheumatoid arthritis and osteoarthritis. However, patients with rheumatoid arthritis initially would not be treated with indomethacin, because the drug is more toxic than ibuprofen.

6. *C* (furosemide plus lisinopril) is correct. Furosemide is a drug of choice for the treatment of peripheral edema or edema associated with congestive heart failure (CHF) or nephrotic syndrome. Lisinopril, an angiotensin-converting enzyme (ACE) inhibitor, can be used alone to treat hypertension or it can be used in combination with other drugs to treat patients with CHF.

A (diazoxide) is incorrect. Diazoxide would not be used to treat the patient described. Diazoxide is given parenterally to control hypertensive emergencies. It is given orally for use in the management of hypoglycemia associated with hyperinsulinemia. Because of its hypoglycemic and salt-retaining activities, the oral preparation is not appropriate in the treatment of chronic hypertension.
B (digoxin plus quinidine) is incorrect. There would be no reason to give digoxin plus quinidine to the patient described. Although digoxin has been used for decades in the management of patients with heart failure, ACE inhibitors have replaced digoxin as first-line therapy for CHF due to systolic dysfunction. Quinidine should be used cautiously in patients with CHF, because the direct negative inotropic effects of the drug can exacerbate this condition.
D (hydralazine plus spironolactone) is incorrect. Hydralazine is sometimes used in the treatment of CHF in patients with systolic dysfunction. Spironolactone is a potassium-sparing diuretic. Its diuretic action is too weak to be of value in the treatment of the patient described.
E (prazosin plus verapamil) is incorrect. Prazosin is sometimes useful in the management of heart failure. Verapamil should be used cautiously in patients with CHF or in patients taking β-adrenergic receptor antagonists, because verapamil can precipitate or exacerbate heart failure in these patients.

7. *A* (epoetin alfa) is correct. In healthy individuals, erythropoietin is synthesized in cells adjacent to the proximal renal tubule in response to low tissue oxygen levels. In patients with chronic renal failure, impairment of erythropoietin production leads to normochromic anemia. This form of anemia can be treated with epoetin alfa, a glycoprotein that stimulates red cell production. The glycoprotein is a recombinant analogue of naturally occurring erythropoietin and is derived from genetically modified cells of the Chinese hamster ovary. Epoetin alfa is also used to treat chemotherapy-induced anemia in patients with cancer and to treat zidovudine-induced anemia in patients with HIV infection.

B (folic acid) is incorrect. Folic acid is not used in the treatment of normochromic anemia. It is used in the diagnosis of folate deficiency and in the treatment of megaloblastic anemia, macrocytic anemia, and tropical sprue. Folic acid supplements are also given to pregnant women to decrease the risk of neural tube defects in their offspring.

C (iron) is incorrect. Iron is not used in the treatment of normochromic anemia. An iron preparation (usually ferrous sulfate) is used to treat microcytic hypochromic anemia associated with iron deficiency in patients who have cancer or who have lost a considerable amount of blood.
D (sargramostim) is incorrect. Sargramostim is not used in the treatment of normochromic anemia. Sargramostim is a recombinant DNA product that is similar to human granulocyte-macrophage colony-stimulating factor (GM-CSF). It stimulates the proliferation and differentiation of macrophage and granulocyte progenitor cells. Sargramostim is used to promote myeloid cell recovery in patients who have non-Hodgkin's lymphoma, acute lymphoblastic leukemia, or Hodgkin's disease and are undergoing bone marrow transplantation; to prolong survival in patients with delayed myeloid recovery following bone marrow transplantation; to promote myeloid recovery after standard-dose chemotherapy; and to treat drug-induced bone marrow toxicity or neutropenia associated with AIDS.
E (vitamin B_{12}) is incorrect. Cyanocobalamin (vitamin B_{12}) is not used in the treatment of normochromic anemia. It is used to treat pernicious anemia and vitamin B_{12} deficiency, as well as to determine vitamin B_{12} absorption in the Schilling test.

8. ***D*** (inhibition of mitotic spindle formation) is correct. Vincristine exerts its effects on the cell by binding to the crucial microtubule proteins of the mitotic spindle and causing a termination of mitotic spindle formation. The drug arrests cells in the metaphase of mitosis and is therefore said to be cell cycle–specific for the M phase.

A (alkylation of DNA), C (inhibition of dihydrofolate reductase), and E (inhibition of topoisomerase) are incorrect. Based on its mechanisms of action, vincristine is classified as a mitotic inhibitor. Cyclophosphamide is an example of a DNA alkylating drug; methotrexate is an example of a dihydrofolate reductase inhibitor; and etoposide is an example of a topoisomerase inhibitor.
B (generation of free radicals) is incorrect. Vincristine does not generate free radicals, but doxorubicin does. Free radicals can damage various elements of the cell, including the cell membranes, and eventually cause cell death. This is the mechanism responsible for doxorubicin-induced cardiac toxicity.

9. ***E*** (triamterene) is correct. In the case described, the administration of triamterene increased the level of potassium, and the high level of circulating potassium induced the cardiac conduction changes that cause cardiac arrest. Triamterene is a potassium-sparing diuretic that acts at the distal tubule to inhibit sodium-potassium exchange and cause hyperkalemia. Other agents that would induce similar effects and that would also be contraindicated in cases such as this include spironolactone and amiloride.

A (chlorthalidone) and D (hydrochlorothiazide) are incorrect. Treatment with chlorthalidone or hydrochlorothiazide is not appropriate in a diabetic patient, and these drugs are not effective in patients whose glomerular filtration rate is < 30 mL/min (serum creatinine > 3).
B (ethacrynic acid) and C (furosemide) are incorrect. Furosemide and ethacrynic acid are loop diuretics that would reduce sodium and water retention and would promote potassium loss.

10. *D* (omeprazole) is correct. The patient's manifestations are consistent with the diagnosis of Zollinger-Ellison syndrome. This syndrome is usually a fatal disorder in which hypersecretion of gastric acid is caused by gastrin-secreting tumors (gastrinomas). The most effective drug for treating Zollinger-Ellison syndrome is omeprazole, an orally administered agent that suppresses gastric acid secretion by inhibiting the proton pump (H^+,K^+-ATPase) in parietal cells. Omeprazole is also used in the short-term treatment of gastroesophageal reflux disease and gastric and duodenal ulcers.

A (famotidine) is incorrect. Famotidine, cimetidine, and ranitidine are orally or parenterally administered agents that reduce basal and nocturnal gastric acid secretions by competitively inhibiting the binding of histamine to H_2 receptors on the gastric basolateral membrane of parietal cells. Although these H_2 receptor antagonists can be used to treat Zollinger-Ellison syndrome, they are not as effective as omeprazole.
B (mesalamine) is incorrect. Sulfasalazine is a prodrug used in the treatment of ulcerative colitis. Sulfasalazine is cleaved by intestinal bacteria to yield sulfapyridine and mesalamine (5-aminosalicylic acid, or 5-ASA). Mesalamine has anti-inflammatory effects. Although its exact mechanisms of action are unknown, it is believed to act at least in part by blocking cyclooxygenase and thereby inhibiting prostaglandin production in the bowel mucosa.
C (misoprostol) is incorrect. Misoprostol is an orally administered synthetic prostaglandin E_1 analogue. It is primarily used to prevent gastric ulcers in patients who are taking nonsteroidal anti-inflammatory drugs (NSAIDs) on a long-term basis.
E (sucralfate) is incorrect. Sucralfate is an orally administered drug that is effective for use in the treatment of active duodenal ulcers and for maintenance therapy following the resolution of these ulcers. The efficacy of sucralfate in the treatment of gastric ulcers is comparable to the efficacy of cimetidine. Sucralfate reacts with hydrochloric acid in the stomach to form an adherent, paste-like substance capable of acting as an acid buffer.

11. *C* (protamine) is correct. When protamine comes into contact with heparin, it forms a salt, neutralizing the anticoagulant effect of heparin. Protamine, a strongly basic compound, forms complexes with heparin sodium and heparin calcium, which are acidic compounds. Formation of this complex can result in disruption of the heparin–antithrombin III complex that is responsible for the anticoagulant activity of heparin.

A (aminocaproic acid) is incorrect. Aminocaproic acid does not antagonize the effects of heparin. Aminocaproic acid is an inhibitor of fibrinolysis. It is indicated for use in the treatment of hyperfibrinolysis in patients who have undergone cardiac surgery and in patients with aplastic anemia; abruptio placentae; hepatic cirrhosis; or neoplastic diseases such as carcinoma of the prostate, lung, stomach, or cervix.
B (folic acid) is incorrect. Folic acid does not antagonize the effects of heparin. Folic acid is used to diagnose folate deficiency and to treat megaloblastic and macrocytic anemias and tropical sprue.
D (vitamin B_{12}) and E (vitamin K) are incorrect. Vitamin B_{12} and vitamin K do not antagonize the effects of heparin. Vitamin B_{12} is used to treat pernicious anemia and vitamin B_{12} deficiency. It is also used to assess vitamin B_{12} absorption in the Schilling test. Vitamin K is an antidote for warfarin overdose.

12. ***B*** (epinephrine) is correct. Epinephrine causes bronchorelaxation by stimulating β_2-adrenergic receptors. This response is blocked by propranolol and potentiated by cocaine. Cocaine blocks the uptake of epinephrine into the nerve terminal (uptake 1) and thereby prolongs the effects of epinephrine. Sympathetic nerve stimulation would produce a similar effect.

A (ephedrine) is incorrect. The effects of ephedrine would be attenuated by cocaine, since ephedrine is taken up into the nerve terminal and then causes the release of norepinephrine. Ephedrine also has some direct effects on β-adrenergic receptors.
C (histamine) is incorrect. The results of procedure 3 are consistent with the administration of histamine. When given alone, histamine causes bronchoconstriction. This effect is not blocked by atropine.
D (phenylephrine) is incorrect. Phenylephrine is an α_1-adrenergic receptor agonist and would therefore have no effects on the lung.
E (terbutaline) is incorrect. The results of procedure 4 are consistent with the administration of terbutaline, a selective β_2-adrenergic receptor agonist.

13. ***E*** (no drug treatment) is correct. The patient's PVCs are likely produced by albuterol. Therefore, every effort should be made to minimize the use of albuterol. PVCs in individuals who do not have heart disease carry little or no risk, so therapy with an anti-

arrhythmic drug is unnecessary. Although a selective β_1-blocker, such as metoprolol, is preferable to a nonselective β-blocker for patients with asthma, emphysema, chronic obstructive pulmonary disease (COPD), or other pulmonary conditions in which acute bronchospasm would put them at risk, therapy with any β-blocker should be avoided or used with extreme caution in these patients.

A (treatment with flecainide) is incorrect. As discussed in Option E, PVCs in individuals who do not have heart disease carry little or no risk, so therapy with an antiarrhythmic drug is unnecessary. Flecainide is a class IC antiarrhythmic agent that is administered orally and is indicated for the treatment of documented life-threatening arrhythmias. Flecainide was approved for the suppression of paroxysmal supraventricular tachycardia (PSVT) caused by both reentrant and nonreentrant mechanisms; however, the Cardiac Arrhythmia Suppression Trial (CAST) demonstrated that the drug had the propensity to cause proarrhythmic effects, so it is no longer considered a first-line agent for this use.
B (treatment with nifedipine) is incorrect. Nifedipine is a dihydropyridine-type calcium channel blocker. This type of calcium channel blocker has more prominent effects on vasodilation and coronary flow than do diltiazem and verapamil. Thus, it is not used to treat arrhythmias. It is used instead to treat Prinzmetal's angina, hypertension (slow-release formulation), and other vascular disorders, such as Raynaud's phenomenon.
C (treatment with procainamide) and D (treatment with quinidine) are incorrect. Procainamide and quinidine are class IA antiarrhythmic agents. These drugs are able to suppress supraventricular and ventricular arrhythmias, but their use places patients at risk for numerous side effects. About 80% of patients treated on a long-term basis with procainamide suffer from a lupus-like disorder, characterized by symptoms such as fever, chills, arthralgia, pericarditis, pleuritis, and skin rash. Adverse effects of quinidine therapy include cinchonism, diarrhea, hypotension, torsades de pointes, hepatitis, thrombocytopenia, and hemolytic anemia.

14. *E* (trimethoprim plus sulfamethoxazole) is correct. It is significantly more difficult for bacteria to develop resistance to two drugs that act on different steps in the same pathway. Trimethoprim plus sulfamethoxazole is a combination that is used extensively. It is generally bactericidal and acts by inhibiting sequential enzymes involved in the bacterial synthesis of folic acid. Sulfamethoxazole is a structural analogue of *p*-aminobenzoic acid (PABA), and it competitively inhibits the formation of dihydrofolic acid from PABA. Trimethoprim binds to and reversibly inhibits dihydrofolate reductase, preventing the formation of tetrahydrofolic acid from dihydrofolic acid.

A (amoxicillin plus clavulanate), B (ampicillin plus sulbactam), and D (piperacillin plus tazobactam) are incorrect. Amoxicillin, ampicillin, and piperacillin are beta-lactam antibiotics. Clavulanate, sulbactam, and tazobactam are irreversible inhibitors of bacterial beta-lactamases. When a beta-lactam antibiotic is used in combination with an appropriate beta-lactamase inhibitor, it will be effective against beta-lactamase–producing bacteria. The amoxicillin-clavulanate combination is effective against *Haemophilus influenzae* and penicillinase-producing anaerobes and is used to treat acute infections such as otitis media, sinusitis, and bacterial cystitis; uncomplicated gonorrhea; and chancroid caused by susceptible organisms. The ampicillin-sulbactam combination is effective against many beta-lactamase–producing bacteria and is used to treat infections such as moderate to severe intra-abdominal infections, gynecologic infections, and skin and soft tissue infections. The piperacillin-tazobactam combination is effective against gram-negative and anaerobic bacteria and is used to treat moderate to severe polymicrobial infections, including intra-abdominal, skin, soft tissue, and lower respiratory tract infections. In the treatment of *Pseudomonas aeruginosa* infections, piperacillin monotherapy is as effective as piperacillin-tazobactam combination therapy.

C (imipenem plus cilastatin) is incorrect. Imipenem is a carbapenem that is classified as a beta-lactam antibiotic. Imipenem is metabolized by dehydropeptidase, an enzyme found in the renal tubule border. Cilastatin is a drug that inhibits dehydropeptidase in the host. When used in combination with cilastatin, imipenem has a broader spectrum of activity than does any other currently available beta-lactam antibiotic. It has several traits that make it a superior antibiotic: it is extremely efficient in penetrating the bacterial cell wall; it is resistant to bacterial enzymes; and it has a high affinity for all bacterial penicillin-binding proteins. The combination is used to treat polymicrobial infections, especially those that are nosocomial or resistant to other antibiotics.

15. *A* (bleomycin) is correct. Bleomycin is a cell cycle–specific drug that acts during the G_2 phase of the cycle and exerts its chemotherapeutic effects by causing scission of single- and double-stranded DNA. Some degree of pulmonary toxicity occurs in up to 11% of patients treated with bleomycin. The most serious adverse effect is interstitial pneumonitis, which in rare cases progresses to pulmonary fibrosis and death.

B (cisplatin), C (doxorubicin), D (methotrexate), and E (vincristine) are incorrect. Treatment with cisplatin, doxorubicin, methotrexate, or vincristine is not associated with pulmonary toxicity. Cisplatin treatment is associated with nephrotoxicity. Doxorubicin treatment is associated with signs of cardiotoxicity, such as transient abnormal electrocardiographic rhythms and cumulative, dose-dependent cardiomyopathy. Methotrexate treatment is associated with signs of hepatotoxicity, including elevated levels of hepatic enzymes with short-term use and cirrhosis and fibrosis with long-term use. Vincristine treatment is associated with signs of neurotoxicity, including peripheral neuropathy, peripheral paresthesia, loss of deep tendon reflexes, numbness and tingling, and pain.

16. ***B*** (amphotericin B) is correct. Nephrotoxicity occurs in more than 80% of patients treated with large cumulative doses of amphotericin B. Patients with nephrotoxicity may suffer from azotemia, hypokalemia, hyposthenuria, nephrocalcinosis, renal tubular acidosis, or frank renal failure. Renal tubular acidosis may be present without concurrent systemic acidosis and is attributable in part to renal tubular necrosis following the lysis of cholesterol-rich lysosomal membranes of renal tubular cells.

A (acyclovir) and E (vancomycin) are incorrect. Acyclovir and vancomycin can cause nephrotoxicity, but they are less likely than amphotericin B to do so. In addition, acute renal failure does not usually develop so rapidly with these agents. Acyclovir-induced nephrotoxicity appears to result from crystallization of the drug within the nephron.
C (ampicillin) and D (ceftazidime) are incorrect. Adverse effects on the kidney are very rare with ampicillin use and are not associated with ceftazidime use.

17. ***E*** (rifampin) is correct. Rifampin induces cytochrome P450 enzymes. This causes a significant increase in the metabolism of many drugs, such as coumarin derivatives, oral contraceptives, cyclosporine, and chloramphenicol.

A (ethambutol) is incorrect. Ethambutol does not induce cytochrome P450 enzymes. Aluminum salts can reduce the rate or extent of ethambutol absorption.
B (isoniazid) is incorrect. Isoniazid inhibits, rather than induces, the hepatic metabolism of drugs that undergo oxidation, including warfarin.
C (pyrazinamide) is incorrect. Pyrazinamide does not induce cytochrome P450 enzymes. Pyrazinamide can increase serum uric acid levels and precipitate attacks of gout. Therefore, the doses of antigout agents, including allopurinol, colchicine, probenecid, and sulfinpyrazone, may need to be altered in patients treated with pyrazinamide. This is a pharmacodynamic interaction, rather than a pharmacokinetic interaction.
D (pyridoxine) is incorrect. Pyridoxine (vitamin B_6) does not induce cytochrome P450 enzymes. Pyridoxine is used to prevent or treat vitamin B_6 deficiency; to prevent or treat toxicity caused by isoniazid, cycloserine, or hydralazine; and to treat sideroblastic anemia associated with elevated serum iron levels.

18. *C* (cyclosporine) is correct. Cyclosporine is the preferred immunosuppressive agent for renal allografts. All of the other agents are considerably more cytotoxic. Nephrotoxicity is a common adverse effect of cyclosporine therapy and occurs in virtually all patients receiving this therapy. In renal transplant patients, it is difficult to differentiate cyclosporine-induced nephrotoxicity from allograft rejection or from hypertension-induced nephrosclerosis (also related to cyclosporine administration).

A (azathioprine) and B (cyclophosphamide) are incorrect. Azathioprine or cyclophosphamide can be used to prevent rejection of kidney allografts, but neither drug is the drug of choice, because both are more cytotoxic than cyclosporine. As an immunosuppressant, azathioprine is also useful in the treatment of rheumatoid arthritis, lupus nephritis, and psoriatic arthritis.
D (fluorouracil) and E (vincristine) are incorrect. Fluorouracil or vincristine is not typically used as an immunosuppressive agent to prevent rejection of kidney allografts.

19. *D* (lovastatin) is correct. Lovastatin is a prodrug with several active metabolites. After lovastatin is hydrolyzed to mevinolinic acid, it competes with HMG-CoA for HMG-CoA reductase, a hepatic microsomal enzyme. Interference with the activity of this enzyme reduces the quantity of mevalonic acid, a precursor of cholesterol. This process occurs within the hepatocyte and is one of two mechanisms responsible for reducing plasma cholesterol levels. Cholesterol also can be taken up from low-density lipoprotein (LDL) by endocytosis. Since de novo synthesis of cholesterol is impaired by lovastatin, the second mechanism is augmented. Thus, lovastatin also enhances clearance of LDL. Lovastatin exerts its effects mainly on total cholesterol and LDL levels, with minor effects seen on high-density lipoprotein (HDL) and triglyceride levels.

A (cholestyramine) and B (colestipol) are incorrect. Cholestyramine and colestipol are bile acid–binding resins. The drugs release chloride and combine with bile acids in the intestine to form insoluble, nonabsorbable complexes that are excreted in the feces, along with unchanged resin. Plasma cholesterol levels do not rise, because the newly formed cholesterol is now shunted into the bile acid synthesis pathway.
C (gemfibrozil) is incorrect. Gemfibrozil inhibits peripheral lipolysis and decreases hepatic extraction of free fatty acids. This in turn decreases hepatic triglyceride production. It also inhibits the synthesis and increases the clearance of apolipoprotein B, a carrier molecule for very low density lipoprotein (VLDL). In addition, it may accelerate the turnover and removal of cholesterol from the liver and increase the excretion of cholesterol into the feces.
E (niacin) is incorrect. The exact mechanism by which niacin (nicotinic acid) reduces lipid levels is unknown. Among the mechanisms that have been proposed are a decrease in hepatic synthesis of LDL and VLDL, the inhibition of free fatty acid

release from adipose tissue, and the inhibition of lipolysis. The inhibition of lipolysis may be due to the inhibitory action of niacin on lipolytic hormones.

20. *E* (selegiline) is correct. Selegiline decreases the metabolism of dopamine by inhibiting monoamine oxidase type B (MAO-B) but not type A (MAO-A). In the treatment of idiopathic Parkinson's disease, selegiline is used in combination with levodopa or in combination with both levodopa and carbidopa. Because of its selectivity for MAO-B, selegiline is purported to increase dopamine levels while causing fewer drug interactions and having a decreased risk of hypertension than do nonselective MAO inhibitors, such as phenelzine.

A (amantadine), B (bromocriptine), and C (carbidopa) are incorrect. Amantadine, bromocriptine, and carbidopa are drugs that are useful in the treatment of Parkinson's disease. All three drugs increase dopamine levels, but they do so by different mechanisms. Amantadine potentiates dopaminergic responses in the central nervous system (CNS) by causing the release of dopamine and norepinephrine from storage sites and inhibiting the reuptake of dopamine and norepinephrine. Bromocriptine, a synthetic dopamine agonist, acts by stimulating dopamine D_2 receptors and antagonizing D_1 receptors in the hypothalamus and the neostriatum of the CNS. Carbidopa inhibits the decarboxylation of peripheral levodopa, which then allows lower doses of levodopa to be used in the treatment of Parkinson's disease.
D (phenelzine) is incorrect. Unlike selegiline (discussed in Option E), phenelzine inhibits MAO-A. Phenelzine is used to treat depression.

21. *C* (noncompetitive antagonist) is correct. In this figure, drug X is a full agonist because it elicits a 100% response when given alone. Drug Y is a noncompetitive antagonist. A noncompetitive antagonist is a drug that shifts the dose-response curve for a full agonist downward and to the right. It prevents the full agonist from reaching a maximal response because it permanently alters a fraction of the receptors, usually by covalently binding to the receptors.

A (competitive antagonist) is incorrect. If drug Y were a competitive antagonist, it would cause a parallel shift to the right in the dose-response curve for drug X. A maximal response could still be achieved with drug X, but it would require a larger dose.
B (full agonist) and D (partial agonist) are incorrect. Drug Y is not an agonist, because it elicits no response when added to the organ bath alone.

22. ***B*** (ipratropium) is correct. Ipratropium antagonizes the action of acetylcholine by blocking muscarinic cholinergic receptors. It is often used as a bronchodilator in the management of bronchospasm associated with chronic obstructive pulmonary disease.

A (cromolyn), D (zafirlukast), and E (zileuton) are incorrect. Although cromolyn, zafirlukast, and zileuton are useful in the treatment of asthma, they do not act by inhibiting the bronchoconstrictor effect of increased parasympathetic tone. Cromolyn acts by inhibiting mast cell degranulation. This prevents the release of histamine and slow-reacting substance of anaphylaxis (SRS-A), which are mediators of type I allergic reactions. Cromolyn may also reduce the release of inflammatory leukotrienes. Zafirlukast acts by blocking leukotriene receptors, and zileuton acts by inhibiting 5-lipoxygenase, the first enzyme in the lipoxygenase pathway.
C (theophylline) is incorrect. Theophylline relaxes the smooth muscle of the bronchial airways and pulmonary blood vessels. In patients with asthma, theophylline reduces airway responsiveness to histamine, methacholine, adenosine, and allergens. The ability of theophylline to control chronic asthma, however, is greater than the relatively weak bronchodilator action of the drug. Theophylline may possess anti-inflammatory properties, as evidenced by its ability to attenuate late-phase reactions in asthma.

23. ***A*** (atropine) is correct. Ophthalmic preparations (drops or ointments) of atropine are used for the treatment of iridocyclitis and other forms of iritis and uveitis. Atropine, the prototypical antimuscarinic agent, produces mydriasis (dilation of pupils) and reduces ocular pain and inflammation. Urinary retention is a common side effect of antimuscarinic agents, even when they are used in an ophthalmic form. Urinary retention results from a decrease in the muscle tone and amplitude of contractions of the ureters and bladder. This side effect is especially likely to occur in patients with BPH.

B (ephedrine) is incorrect. Ephedrine is not available in an ophthalmic form and is not used in the treatment of ocular disorders.
C (epinephrine) and D (phenylephrine) are incorrect. Epinephrine and phenylephrine are direct-acting adrenergic receptor agonists that are available in ophthalmic forms. Although they both produce mydriasis, neither causes urinary retention. In patients with open-angle glaucoma, epinephrine decreases the intraocular pressure, produces short-term (brief) mydriasis, and may improve aqueous outflow. In patients with allergic conjunctivitis, phenylephrine stimulates α_1-adrenergic receptors on the dilator muscles and arterioles of the conjunctivas and thereby causes profound mydriasis and vasoconstriction.
E (prednisone) is incorrect. Although prednisone can be used to treat iridocyclitis, it must be given orally because it is not available in an ophthalmic form. Other corticosteroids are available for

topical ophthalmic use and are as effective as orally administered corticosteroids for use in the treatment of anterior ocular inflammation.

24. *D* (meperidine) is correct. Meperidine is an opioid agonist that can produce delirium, hyperpyrexia, convulsions, coma, and death in patients treated with a monoamine oxidase (MAO) inhibitor, such as tranylcypromine. These adverse effects may be due to inhibition of meperidine degradation or to the accumulation of serotonin, because meperidine blocks the neuronal reuptake of serotonin.

A (acetaminophen) and C (ibuprofen) are incorrect. Acetaminophen and ibuprofen would not produce these effects, because they do not interact with tranylcypromine.
B (codeine) and E (morphine) are incorrect. Meperidine (discussed in Option D) is most likely responsible for the adverse effects described, because in patients taking MAO inhibitors, meperidine is not as safe as the other opioid agonists, including codeine and morphine.

25. *D* (stop warfarin and begin heparin therapy) is correct. Warfarin and heparin are anticoagulants that are useful in the treatment of pulmonary embolism. Warfarin is contraindicated during pregnancy, because it crosses the placenta and is known to cause abnormalities in the fetus, particularly when taken during the first trimester. Warfarin is also contraindicated during and immediately after delivery, because it may cause maternal hemorrhaging. Because heparin does not cross the placenta, it can be used instead of warfarin, especially during the first trimester of pregnancy.

A (continue warfarin therapy) is incorrect. Refer to the explanation for Option D.
B (stop warfarin and begin abciximab therapy), C (stop warfarin and begin aspirin therapy), and E (stop warfarin and begin ticlopidine therapy) are incorrect. Abciximab, aspirin, and ticlopidine are antiplatelet drugs that are not useful in the management of a pulmonary embolism. According to the pregnancy categories established by the Food and Drug Administration, ticlopidine is a category B drug, and abciximab is a category C drug. Controlled human studies of abciximab during pregnancy have not been completed; thus, risks to the fetus have not been clearly delineated. Aspirin is classified as a category C drug during the first and second trimesters. Aspirin increases the risk of perinatal mortality, intrauterine growth retardation, and postmaturity syndrome (with fetal damage or death due to decreased placental function in prolonged pregnancy). Moreover, the regular use of aspirin late in pregnancy may result in constriction or premature closure of the ductus arteriosus in the fetus.

26. ***C*** (colchicine) is correct. When allopurinol treatment is initiated, an acute attack of gouty arthritis sometimes occurs. The attack is due to the resorption of uric acid from tissues. To avoid this effect, colchicine can be given early in the course of allopurinol treatment.

A (aspirin) and B (chloroquine) are incorrect. Neither aspirin nor chloroquine is used to treat gout. In fact, low doses of aspirin increase the plasma levels of uric acid.
D (ibuprofen) is incorrect. Nonsteroidal anti-inflammatory drugs (NSAIDs) can be used on a short-term basis to control acute gouty arthritis. Indomethacin is the NSAID most frequently used for this purpose, but ibuprofen is sometimes used. An allopurinol-induced attack cannot be avoided by concurrent treatment with allopurinol and ibuprofen.
E (sulfinpyrazone) is incorrect. Sulfinpyrazone is not the drug of choice to treat an acute attack of gouty arthritis. Furthermore, the use of sulfinpyrazone during the early course of allopurinol treatment increases the risk of forming renal calculi.

27. ***D*** (muscarinic receptors) is correct. Amitriptyline and other tricyclic antidepressants (TCAs) block α-adrenergic and muscarinic receptors and also block the reuptake of catecholamines and serotonin. The symptoms listed in the question are caused by the blockade of muscarinic receptors.

A (α-adrenergic receptors), B (catecholamine reuptake), and E (serotonin reuptake) are incorrect. Refer to the explanation for Option D. The blockade of α-adrenergic receptors is responsible for the hypotensive actions of TCAs, including orthostatic hypotension, which can occur even with therapeutic doses. The blockade of catecholamine and serotonin reuptake contributes to the antidepressant effects of TCAs and also contributes to the cardiotoxicity of these drugs.
C (dopamine receptors) is incorrect. TCAs do not block dopamine receptors. Chlorpromazine and other antipsychotic agents are examples of drugs that block dopamine receptors.

28. ***C*** (primaquine) is correct. *P. vivax* and *P. ovale* are *Plasmodium* species that have a persistent exoerythrocytic (hepatic) form. If this form is not eradicated, relapses will occur. Primaquine is the only antimalarial drug that blocks exoerythrocytic schizogony; other antimalarial agents block erythrocytic schizogony. In patients infected with *P. vivax* or *P. ovale,* primaquine is given in combination with a blood schizonticidal agent, such as chloroquine. Patients with reduced glucose-6-phosphate dehydrogenase levels are at increased risk for acute hemolytic anemia when they are treated with primaquine. The degree of hemolysis in these patients is dependent on ethnic origin and dosage level. In patients of African descent, the degree of hemolysis is often mild and possibly self-limiting. In those of Asian or Mediterranean descent, hemolysis can be severe. Primaquine use should be discontinued at the first signs of hemolytic anemia.

A (chloroquine) is incorrect. As discussed in Option C, chloroquine is not effective against the exoerythrocytic form of *P. vivax* or *P. ovale;* therefore, it must be given in combination with primaquine to treat patients infected with these forms of malaria. Chloroquine can be used alone to treat patients with malaria that is caused by *P. malariae* or a chloroquine-sensitive strain of *P. falciparum.*

B (mefloquine) and E (quinine) are incorrect. Mefloquine and quinine act as blood schizonticides. They are not effective against the exoerythrocytic form of *P. vivax* or *P. ovale.* Mefloquine is given orally for the prevention or treatment of malaria caused by chloroquine-resistant strains of *P. falciparum* or by other *Plasmodium* species. Quinine can be given orally or parenterally to treat chloroquine-resistant malaria.

D (pyrimethamine-sulfadoxine) is incorrect. Pyrimethamine-sulfadoxine is not effective against the exoerythrocytic form of *P. vivax* or *P. ovale.* Pyrimethamine and sulfadoxine have been used together in an oral preparation to treat or prevent malaria; however, the combination is no longer recommended for malaria prophylaxis, because it places individuals at risk for fatal toxic epidermal necrolysis. Pyrimethamine inhibits parasitic dihydrofolate reductase, whereas sulfadoxine antagonizes parasitic *p*-aminobenzoic acid (PABA). When given together, the drugs have a synergistic effect on folic acid–dependent biochemical pathways.

29. *C* (isoniazid) is correct. The drug described in the question is isoniazid. Pyridoxine is a specific antidote for isoniazid toxicity and is usually effective in terminating diazepam-resistant seizures that occur in patients who have taken an isoniazid overdose.

A (acetaminophen) is incorrect. An acetaminophen overdose may cause hepatic necrosis, a dose-dependent adverse effect that is potentially fatal. Renal tubular necrosis, hypoglycemic coma, and thrombocytopenia may also occur.

B (amitriptyline) is incorrect. An amitriptyline overdose may cause drowsiness; hypothermia; tachycardia and other arrhythmic abnormalities, such as bundle branch block; electrocardiographic evidence of impaired conduction; congestive heart failure; polyradiculoneuropathy; dilated pupils; disorders of ocular motility; convulsions; severe hypotension; stupor; and coma.

D (lithium) is incorrect. A toxic dose of lithium is very close to the therapeutic doses. Serum lithium concentrations should not be allowed to rise above 2.0 mEq/L during the early treatment phase. Serum concentrations above 3.0 mEq/L can produce adverse effects involving multiple organ systems. Adverse effects

that suggest lithium toxicity include anorexia, visual impairment or disturbance, drowsiness, muscular weakness, fasciculations, myoclonia, ataxia, slurred speech, tremor, confusion, seizures, arrhythmias, stupor, and coma.
E (salicylate) is incorrect. A salicylate overdose causes central nervous system stimulation, with early symptoms including vomiting, hyperpnea, hyperactivity, and convulsions. Subsequent symptoms include depression, coma, respiratory failure, and collapse. These symptoms are accompanied by severe electrolyte disturbances.

30. *B* (cytarabine) is correct. Cytarabine is the cornerstone of induction therapy for acute nonlymphocytic leukemia.

A (cisplatin) is incorrect. Cisplatin is a cell cycle–nonspecific (CCNS) anticancer agent that is used in the treatment of various tumors. It is particularly valuable when used in the treatment of testicular carcinoma, making a previously deadly disease potentially curable.
C (flutamide) is incorrect. Flutamide is a nonsteroidal antiandrogen that is used to treat metastatic prostate cancer. It is most effective when used simultaneously with a luteinizing hormone–releasing hormone (LHRH) agonist, such as leuprolide acetate.
D (streptozocin) is incorrect. Streptozocin is a CCNS anticancer agent. Like carmustine and lomustine, it is a member of the nitrosourea family. Streptozocin is used to treat pancreatic islet cell carcinoma, carcinoid tumor, colorectal cancer, and pancreatic adenocarcinoma. It has specific activity only in pancreatic cancers and some gastrointestinal tumors.
E (vincristine) is incorrect. Vincristine is a cell cycle–specific (CCS) anticancer agent that is used to treat breast carcinoma, colorectal cancer, squamous cell carcinoma of the head and neck, Hodgkin's disease, non-Hodgkin's lymphoma, small cell lung cancer, multiple myeloma, soft tissue sarcomas, osteogenic sarcoma, brain tumors, and acute lymphoblastic leukemia. Its actions are similar to those of vinblastine, but its toxicities differ significantly.

31. *D* (hydrocortisone plus fludrocortisone) is correct. If the tuberculous process destroys more than 90% of both adrenal cortices, symptoms of Addison's disease become apparent. The patient's history, clinical and laboratory findings, and results in the ACTH test are consistent with the diagnosis of primary adrenal insufficiency. Hydrocortisone and fludrocortisone each have glucocorticoid (anti-inflammatory) properties and mineralocorticoid (salt-retaining) properties. Hydrocortisone is the pharmaceutical preparation of cortisol (the hormone secreted by the adrenal cortex). Fludrocortisone is a fluorinated form of hydrocortisone that has much stronger salt-retaining properties, similar to those of aldosterone.

A (ACTH replacement) is incorrect. ACTH replacement would not improve the patient's condition, because the destroyed adrenal cortices cannot produce more cortisol.
B (albuterol) and E (insulin plus glucose infusion) are incorrect. Severe hyperkalemia can lead to cardiac arrest and therefore requires rapid therapeutic intervention. In patients with adrenocortical insufficiency, a β_2-adrenergic agonist (e.g., albuterol) or insulin can be used to induce rapid cellular potassium uptake and thereby effectively combat life-threatening hyperkalemia. If insulin is used for this purpose, it is usually given concomitantly with bicarbonate. Glucose infusion can be given to prevent hypoglycemia. Although the drugs listed in Options B and E may help in the emergency care of adrenal insufficiency, they are not used in the long-term management of the disease.
C (aldosterone) is incorrect. Aldosterone is an adrenal steroid that has strong mineralocorticoid properties. It is not available in pharmaceutical preparations.

32. *C* (finasteride) is correct. Finasteride is a specific inhibitor of 5α-reductase, an intracellular enzyme that converts testosterone to dihydrotestosterone (DHT). DHT normally stimulates the growth of prostate tissue, and increased amounts of DHT are found in atrophic hair follicles. By blocking the synthesis of DHT, finasteride reduces serum DHT concentrations by as much as 70%, which helps reverse BPH and baldness.

A (cortisone) is incorrect. Cortisone is a corticosteroid hormone secreted by the adrenal cortex. In addition to having glucocorticoid properties, cortisone has significant mineralocorticoid properties and is used clinically as replacement therapy in patients with adrenocortical insufficiency. Cortisone treatment would not improve the conditions of the patient described.
B (estradiol) is incorrect. Theoretically, estrogens would be effective in alleviating the patient's symptoms. However, their use would result in the chemical castration of an otherwise healthy man.
D (gonadotropins) and E (testosterone) are incorrect. Gonadotropins increase DHT levels. The use of gonadotropins or testosterone would exacerbate the patient's symptoms.

33. *A* (alendronate) is correct. Alendronate is a bisphosphonate that is used to treat osteoporosis in postmenopausal women and to treat Paget's disease of bone. Unlike other bisphosphonates, alendronate is able to strengthen bone rather than simply prevent bone loss. Alendronate binds to hydroxyapatite in bone, thereby inhibiting osteoclast activity. It does not interfere with the recruitment and attachment of osteoclasts.

B (finasteride) and D (leuprolide) are incorrect. Finasteride and leuprolide are not used to treat osteoporosis. Finasteride is a synthetic analogue of testosterone. It acts as a competitive inhibitor of type II 5α-reductase and is used in the treatment of symp-

tomatic benign prostatic hyperplasia (BPH). Leuprolide is a synthetic analogue of naturally occurring gonadotropin-releasing hormone (GnRH). It is used as a hormonal antagonist in the treatment of advanced prostatic cancer or breast cancer, and it is also used as hormonal therapy in the treatment of endometriosis.
C (hydrochlorothiazide) is incorrect. Hydrochlorothiazide is not used to treat osteoporosis. Hydrochlorothiazide is a thiazide diuretic that is indicated in the treatment of edema and hypertension. It has also been used to treat diabetes insipidus and hypercalciuria, although these uses have not been approved by the Food and Drug Administration.
E (rosiglitazone) is incorrect. Rosiglitazone is a member of the thiazolidinedione class of drugs, which are also called insulin sensitizers and are used to improve glycemic control in patients with type 2 diabetes mellitus. Rosiglitazone is used as an adjunct to diet and exercise in these patients and is sometimes given in combination with metformin.

34. ***C*** (doxycycline) is correct. Doxycycline is effective against *T. pallidum* (the agent of syphilis), *N. gonorrhoeae* (the agent of gonorrhea), and *C. trachomatis* (an agent of urethritis, cervicitis, and lymphogranuloma venereum). A second drug, such as ceftriaxone or a fluoroquinolone, may be added to treat the patient's gonorrhea infection.

A (ampicillin) is incorrect. Ampicillin would be the drug of choice for the treatment of uncomplicated gonorrhea, but it is ineffective in the treatment of syphilis and *Chlamydia* infections.
B (cephalexin) is incorrect. Cephalexin is not effective against *T. pallidum* and *C. trachomatis*. Cephalexin is a first-generation cephalosporin that has excellent activity against most gram-positive bacteria. It is used mainly to treat otitis media and to treat respiratory tract infections caused by susceptible staphylococci, *Streptococcus pneumoniae,* and group A β-hemolytic streptococci.
D (penicillin G) is incorrect. Penicillin G would be the drug of choice for the treatment of syphilis. It is also effective in the treatment of gonorrhea, but it is ineffective in the treatment of *Chlamydia* infections.
E (streptomycin) is incorrect. Streptomycin should not be used in the treatment of infections caused by any of the three pathogens.

35. ***D*** (phenytoin) is correct. The patient's clinical manifestations (especially the gingival hyperplasia) are typical of the side effect profile of phenytoin.

A (carbamazepine) and B (diazepam) are incorrect. Carbamazepine and diazepam do not cause gingival hyperplasia. Most of the adverse effects of these drugs are central nervous system (CNS) effects. In patients treated with carbamazepine, these effects include ataxia, blurred vision, diplopia, dizziness, drowsiness, fatigue, and hallucinations. In patients treated with diazepam,

these effects include ataxia, confusion, depression, dizziness, drowsiness, fatigue, headache, syncope, tremor, and vertigo.
C (ethosuximide) is incorrect. Ethosuximide does not cause gingival hyperplasia. Gastrointestinal effects are the most commonly reported side effects of ethosuximide. These effects include abdominal pain, anorexia, diarrhea, epigastric distress, nausea, vomiting, and weight loss. The most common CNS effects of ethosuximide include ataxia, dizziness, drowsiness, fatigue, headache, and an increase in libido.
E (valproic acid) is incorrect. Valproic acid does not cause gingival hyperplasia. Valproic acid can cause CNS depression, especially if the patient is concomitantly taking another anticonvulsant drug. The most serious problem with valproic acid use is hepatic failure.

36. *A* (has a greater affinity for the receptor than drug X) is correct. In comparison with drug X, drug W has a greater affinity for the receptor, is more potent, and has the same intrinsic activity.

B (has greater intrinsic activity than drug X) and E (is less potent than drug X) are incorrect. Refer to the explanation for Option A.
C (is an antagonist of drug X) and D (is an antagonist of drug Z) are incorrect. Drug W is not an antagonist of drug X or drug Z. Drugs W, X, and Y are full agonists, and drug Z is a partial antagonist.

37. *E* (probenecid) is correct. Cefepime is a fourth-generation cephalosporin. When high tissue concentrations of a cephalosporin or a penicillin are needed, probenecid can be administered concurrently. Probenecid delays the renal clearance of cephalosporins and penicillins, thereby elevating their serum concentrations and prolonging their half-lives.

A (amifostine) is incorrect. Amifostine is not known to interact with cefepime. Amifostine is a phosphorylated sulfhydryl-containing prodrug that protects healthy tissues from the cytotoxic actions of radiation therapy or chemotherapy. Amifostine is used to prevent cisplatin-induced nephrotoxicity in patients with ovarian cancer and non–small cell lung cancer.
B (dexrazoxane) is incorrect. Dexrazoxane is not known to interact with cefepime. Dexrazoxane is a cyclic derivative of a heavy metal chelator called EDTA (ethylenediaminetetraacetic acid). Dexrazoxane is used to reduce the incidence and severity of doxorubicin-induced cardiomyopathy in women with breast cancer. Dexrazoxane rapidly enters cardiac cells and is hydrolyzed to a compound that chelates with intracellular iron. By limiting the ability of the iron to react with superoxide anions and H_2O_2 (formed from the redox cycling of doxorubicin), dexrazoxane prevents the formation of the highly toxic hydroxyl radical.
C (ketoconazole) is incorrect. Ketoconazole is not known to interact with cefepime. However, ketoconazole inhibits the metabolism of many other drugs by inhibiting CYP3A4, an isozyme of the cytochrome P450 microsomal enzyme system.

D (phenytoin) is incorrect. Phenytoin is not known to interact with cefepime. However, phenytoin induces hepatic microsomal enzymes and thereby enhances the clearance of other drugs metabolized by these enzymes. Drugs that may be affected by phenytoin include cardiac glycosides, corticosteroids, cyclosporine, doxycycline, estrogens, levodopa, lidocaine, methadone, oral contraceptives, tacrolimus, theophylline, vitamin D, and some anticonvulsants.

38. *C* (fluoxetine) is correct. Fluoxetine is the prototype of the selective serotonin reuptake inhibitors (SSRIs) and has a longer half-life than other SSRIs. The SSRIs are structurally distinct from other classes of antidepressants, including monoamine oxidase inhibitors (MAO inhibitors) and tricyclic antidepressants (TCAs). Fluoxetine is effective in the treatment of major depressive disorders and causes far fewer significant side effects than do TCAs.

A (amitriptyline), B (desipramine), and D (imipramine) are incorrect. Amitriptyline, desipramine, and imipramine are TCAs. These drugs have a quinidine-like effect on the heart and can precipitate conduction disturbances in patients who have a preexisting cardiac disease. TCAs sometimes cause orthostatic hypotension, an adverse effect that occurs secondary to α-adrenergic receptor blockade. They also cause dry mouth, urinary hesitancy, and blurred vision, all of which are anticholinergic effects.
E (phenelzine) is incorrect. Phenelzine is an MAO inhibitor. MAO inhibitors have many side effects and interact with numerous drugs. They are used to treat major depressive disorders when other agents fail.

39. *B* (ceftriaxone) is correct. The beta-lactam antibiotics include penicillins, cephalosporins, monobactams, and carbapenems. Because most beta-lactam antibiotics are rapidly excreted via tubular secretion, they have short half-lives and must be administered three or four times a day. Ceftriaxone is a parenterally administered third-generation cephalosporin. It has significant activity against gram-negative organisms and also penetrates the cerebrospinal fluid in concentrations that make it useful for the treatment of meningitis. Because ceftriaxone has the longest half-life of all cephalosporins, it can be administered once a day and is a useful antibiotic for both inpatient and outpatient therapy.

A (azithromycin) is incorrect. Azithromycin is not a beta-lactam antibiotic. It is a semisynthetic macrolide whose structure is similar to that of erythromycin. Azithromycin can be given once a day and causes less gastrointestinal intolerance than does erythromycin.
C (ciprofloxacin) is incorrect. Ciprofloxacin is not a beta-lactam antibiotic. It is a broad-spectrum fluoroquinolone. Ciprofloxacin is used to treat many serious infections caused by gram-negative bacteria, but resistance has developed in strains of

Pseudomonas aeruginosa and *Serratia marcescens*. It is generally active against aerobic gram-positive bacteria, but resistance has been noted in strains of *Staphylococcus aureus* and *Streptococcus pneumoniae*.
D (fosfomycin) is incorrect. Fosfomycin is not a beta-lactam antibiotic. It is a drug whose structure is similar to that of phospho-*enol*pyruvate, one of the precursors involved in the synthesis of peptidoglycan. Unlike beta-lactam antibiotics, fosfomycin disrupts the building of bacterial cell walls by inhibiting the formation of cell wall precursors, rather than inhibiting peptide cross-linking. Fosfomycin is given as a single dose in the treatment of uncomplicated urinary tract infections that are caused by *Escherichia coli* or *Enterococcus faecalis*.
E (meropenem) is incorrect. Meropenem is a beta-lactam antibiotic, and it must be given three times a day. Like imipenem, meropenem is a carbapenem antibiotic. Unlike imipenem, meropenem does not require concomitant administration of a renal enzyme inhibitor (such as cilastatin). Meropenem is used to treat complicated intra-abdominal infections in adults and children and to treat bacterial meningitis in children. Meropenem and imipenem have similar spectrums of action, although meropenem is more active against *Haemophilus influenzae, Neisseria gonorrhoeae, P. aeruginosa,* and members of the family Enterobacteriaceae.

40. *A* (adenosine) is correct. Adenosine is a purine nucleotide that has an extremely short half-life (about 10 seconds) and is used for the emergency treatment of acute PSVT, including the type associated with Wolff-Parkinson-White syndrome. Flushing, bronchospasm, and dyspnea are common side effects of adenosine treatment. Cardiac arrhythmias (such as premature ventricular contractions, premature atrial contractions, sinus bradycardia, sinus tachycardia, atrioventricular block, and skipped beats) also occur with adenosine treatment, but they usually last only a few seconds because of the drug's short half-life. Other adverse effects include dizziness, headache, chest pressure, nausea, vomiting, light-headedness, and paresthesia.

B (esmolol) is incorrect. Esmolol is used to control supraventricular tachyarrhythmias (including sinus tachycardia and PSVT) or to control the ventricular rate in patients with atrial fibrillation or atrial flutter. Unlike adenosine (which is used in the emergency department setting), esmolol is primarily used in the perioperative setting. The most common side effects of esmolol are hypotensive symptoms, such as dizziness, diaphoresis, and headache.
C (lidocaine) and D (magnesium) are incorrect. Lidocaine and magnesium are not used in the treatment of PSVT. Lidocaine is used to treat ventricular fibrillation or ventricular tachycardia during cardiopulmonary resuscitation and to treat ventricular arrhythmias resulting from digitalis toxicity, myocardial infarction, or cardiac manipulation during surgery. Magnesium is used in the management of sustained ventricular arrhythmias or torsades de pointes associated with magnesium depletion, cardiac

disease, or cardiotoxicity induced by antiarrhythmic agents or cardiac glycosides.
E (propranolol) is incorrect. Propranolol is not used in the emergency treatment of PSVT, but it is often used to prevent PSVT.

41. ***D*** (metformin) is correct. Insulin resistance is a common pathophysiologic problem in obese patients with type 2 diabetes mellitus. Metformin acts by increasing insulin sensitivity in these patients. Unlike the sulfonylurea drugs, it rarely causes hypoglycemia, because it does not significantly change insulin concentrations. Chlorpropamide, glipizide, glyburide, and tolbutamide are all oral sulfonylurea drugs. These drugs increase insulin secretion and are useful in the treatment of nonobese patients with type 2 diabetes mellitus.

A (chlorpropamide), B (glipizide), C (glyburide), and E (tolbutamide) are incorrect. Chlorpropamide and tolbutamide are first-generation sulfonylureas and are not as potent as glipizide and glyburide, which are second-generation sulfonylureas. Chlorpropamide is more likely than the other sulfonylureas to produce a disulfiram-like reaction after ingestion of ethanol. Tolbutamide is the shortest-acting and least potent of the group. The sulfonylureas are administered orally to lower blood glucose in patients with type 2 diabetes mellitus. When a sulfonylurea is administered, it binds to adenosine triphosphate (ATP)–sensitive potassium channels on the surface of pancreatic islet cells and thereby reduces potassium conductance and causes membrane depolarization. Depolarization stimulates calcium ion influx through voltage-sensitive calcium channels and increases the intracellular concentration of calcium ions. This in turn induces the secretion, or exocytosis, of insulin. During sulfonylurea therapy, hypoglycemia sometimes occurs and can be severe. Manifestations include hunger, pallor, nausea, fatigue, perspiration, headache, palpitations, numbness of the mouth, tingling in the fingers, tremors, muscle weakness, blurred vision, hypothermia, uncontrolled yawning, irritability, mental confusion, tachycardia, shallow breathing, and loss of consciousness.

42. ***B*** (cyclosporine) is correct. Cyclosporine is used almost exclusively for immunosuppressive therapy. It is used primarily to prevent allograft rejection, but it is also given to treat autoimmune conditions such as uveitis, psoriasis, rheumatoid arthritis, inflammatory bowel disease, and certain nephropathies. Cyclosporine acts by inhibiting the production or release of various lymphokines, including interleukin-1 and interleukin-2.

A (cyclophosphamide) is incorrect. Cyclophosphamide is a cell cycle–nonspecific antineoplastic agent. It is also an immunosuppressant agent that is used in the management of various immunologic disorders, including nephrotic syndrome, Wegener's granulomatosis, rheumatoid arthritis, graft-versus-host disease, and graft rejection.

C (methotrexate) is incorrect. Methotrexate is used to treat a broad array of neoplasms and numerous immunologic disorders, including rheumatoid arthritis.
D (prednisone) is incorrect. Prednisone is used to prevent allograft rejection and to treat asthma, systemic lupus erythematosus, and many other inflammatory disorders. It is also used in induction therapy for acute lymphoblastic leukemia.
E (vincristine) is incorrect. Vincristine is a cell cycle–specific antineoplastic agent that is used in the management of breast cancer, colorectal cancer, squamous cell carcinoma of the head and neck, Hodgkin's disease, non-Hodgkin's lymphoma, acute lymphoblastic leukemia, small cell lung cancer, multiple myeloma, soft tissue and osteogenic sarcomas, and brain tumors.

43. *B* (cerebral thrombosis) is correct. The following warning, issued by the Food and Drug Administration in 1982, pertains to all birth control pills: "Cigarette smoking increases the risk of serious cardiovascular side effects from oral contraceptive use." This risk increases with age and with heavy smoking (15 or more cigarettes per day) and is quite marked in women over 35 years of age. Women who use oral contraceptives should be strongly advised not to smoke. Oral contraceptives have been shown to increase both the relative and attributable risks of cerebrovascular events (thrombotic and hemorrhagic strokes), although in general the risk is greatest among hypertensive women over 35 years of age who smoke.

A (breakthrough bleeding) is incorrect. Breakthrough bleeding and spotting may occur in patients taking oral contraceptives, especially during the first 3 months of use. Nonhormonal causes should be considered and adequate diagnostic measures taken to rule out pregnancy and cancer. If these causes of breakthrough bleeding have been excluded, a change to another contraceptive formulation may solve the problem, or the problem may resolve with time.
C (depression) is incorrect. The use of oral contraceptives in women with a history of depression should be carefully monitored, and contraceptive use should be discontinued if moderate or severe depression occurs.
D (hypotension) is incorrect. Hypertension, rather than hypotension, is associated with the use of oral contraceptives.
E (increase in the serum triglyceride level) is incorrect. A small proportion of women will have persistent hypertriglyceridemia while taking oral contraceptives. However, this risk is not as serious as the risk of cerebral thrombosis.

44. ***A*** (acebutolol) is correct. Acebutolol is a cardioselective β_1-adrenergic receptor antagonist that has mild ISA (similar to the ISA of pindolol). Nonselective β-blockers increase plasma triglyceride levels and decrease HDL levels. However, agents with ISA have no clinically important adverse effects on plasma lipid levels. In fact, studies suggest that agents with both cardioselectivity and ISA may decrease total cholesterol and low-density lipoprotein (LDL) levels.

B (betaxolol) is incorrect. Betaxolol is a selective β_1-blocker. It has no ISA and no significant membrane-stabilizing activity (MSA), so it differs from pindolol (which has ISA) and propranolol (which has significant MSA). Betaxolol is relatively lipid-soluble but is less lipid-soluble than propranolol. Betaxolol is one of the most potent and selective of the β-blockers available. Its selectivity for the β_1 receptor makes it a preferred drug for the treatment of patients with bronchospastic pulmonary disease.
C (carvedilol) and D (labetalol) are incorrect. Carvedilol and labetalol are agents that block α_1, β_1, and β_2 receptors and thereby cause vasodilation and a decrease in the total peripheral resistance. These actions decrease the blood pressure without causing a substantial decrease in the resting heart rate, cardiac output, or stroke volume. Carvedilol also has antioxidant properties. Labetalol has some ISA, but carvedilol does not. Carvedilol is appropriate for treating hypertension in patients with renal disease or diabetes mellitus.
E (pindolol) is incorrect. Pindolol is a nonselective β-blocker that has ISA and is given orally.

45. ***E*** (sumatriptan) is correct. The patient's complaints are consistent with the diagnosis of a migraine headache disorder, with migraine attacks preceded by an aura. Sumatriptan is approved for the treatment of migraine headaches with or without aura, but it is not indicated for the prevention of migraine attacks. Sumatriptan is a drug that is structurally similar to serotonin (5-hydroxytryptamine, or 5-HT) and acts by stimulating 5-HT_{1D} receptors. These receptors have been identified on basal arteries and in the vasculature of the dura mater. The drug's therapeutic effect is a result of selective vasoconstriction of inflamed and dilated cranial blood vessels in the carotid circulation.

A (buspirone) is incorrect. Buspirone exhibits the highest affinity for 5-HT_{1A} receptors. It is used to treat anxiety.
B (dihydroergotamine) is incorrect. Dihydroergotamine (DHE) is a semisynthetic ergot alkaloid that is administered parenterally or intranasally to terminate migraine headaches. Because less toxic agents are available, DHE is considered most appropriate for treating patients who have severe migraine disorder. DHE binds with high affinity to all known 5-HT_1 receptors and to a number of other biogenic amine receptors, including $5\text{-HT}_{2A/2C}$ receptors, α_1- and α_2-adrenergic receptors, and dopamine D_2 receptors. However, the drug's therapeutic effect in the treatment of

migraine headaches is thought to be due primarily to its agonist activity at 5-HT_{1D} receptors.
C (metoclopramide) is incorrect. Metoclopramide is a drug that enhances gastrointestinal motility and is an effective antiemetic. Its mechanism of action is complex. Unlike bethanechol, metoclopramide enhances motility without stimulating gastric secretions. Peripherally, metoclopramide augments cholinergic activity either by causing release of acetylcholine from postganglionic nerve endings or by sensitizing muscarinic receptors on smooth muscle. The net effect of the drug's activities is a remarkable coordination of gastric and duodenal motility. Metoclopramide is used to terminate severe migraine attacks. In patients who are responsive to DHE, metoclopramide is given prior to administration of DHE to offset DHE-induced nausea. In patients who are not responsive to DHE, metoclopramide is used as an alternative treatment.
D (ondansetron) is incorrect. Ondansetron selectively blocks serotonin 5-HT_3 receptors. It is used to control vomiting.

46. *C* (cyclophosphamide) is correct. Cyclophosphamide is a prodrug that must be activated by the cytochrome P450 system in order to become cytotoxic. The hepatic microsomal system converts cyclophosphamide to aldophosphamide and 4-hydroxycyclophosphamide. These are further converted to acrolein and phosphoramide mustard. The mustard compound is a potent alkylator of DNA. When DNA-DNA interstrand cross-links form, DNA processing stops, causing cell death.

A (busulfan) and D (mechlorethamine) are incorrect. Busulfan and mechlorethamine do not require bioactivation. These drugs are bifunctional alkylating agents that exert their chemotherapeutic effects by substituting alkyl groups for hydrogen ions in a number of organic compounds. Busulfan reacts readily with thiol groups on amino acids. Mechlorethamine reacts readily with phosphate, amino, hydroxyl, sulfhydryl, carboxyl, and imidazole groups on amino acids. When these reactions occur, DNA-DNA interstrand cross-linking and DNA-protein cross-linking take place. This leads to DNA strand breakage and interferes with DNA replication, RNA transcription, and nucleic acid function.
B (carmustine) is incorrect. Carmustine does not require bioactivation. Carmustine has two chloroethyl groups that alkylate nucleic acids and cell proteins and form DNA-DNA or DNA-protein cross-links. During carmustine decomposition, isocyanates are also formed and can react by carbamoylating the lysine residues of proteins.
E (methotrexate) is incorrect. Methotrexate does not require bioactivation. It acts by inhibiting dihydrofolate reductase.

47. ***B*** (cimetidine) is correct. Cimetidine is a histamine H_2 receptor antagonist that is effective in the treatment of dyspepsia, peptic ulcer disease, and other gastrointestinal conditions associated with gastric acidity. Cimetidine use can cause endocrinologic dysfunction. Adverse effects include gynecomastia, galactorrhea, elevated prolactin levels, impotence, and decreased libido. Gynecomastia is due to the weak antiandrogenic action of cimetidine. Impotence and decreased libido are reversible upon discontinuation of cimetidine treatment.

A (aluminum hydroxide) is incorrect. Aluminum hydroxide does not cause gynecomastia or sexual dysfunction. Aluminum hydroxide is an antacid that has no effect on gastric acid secretion. The drug acts by partially neutralizing gastric secretions and thereby increasing the pH of gastric contents. This increase in pH inhibits the proteolytic activity of pepsin and promotes the healing of peptic ulcers. Antacids are no longer considered the primary therapy for peptic ulcer disease, and aluminum salts are considered the least potent of the antacids.

C (hydrochlorothiazide) is incorrect. Adverse effects of hydrochlorothiazide therapy include impotence but not breast enlargement.

D (misoprostol) is incorrect. Misoprostol does not cause gynecomastia or sexual dysfunction. Misoprostol is a synthetic prostaglandin E_1 analogue that is used to prevent gastric and duodenal ulcers in patients who are taking nonsteroidal anti-inflammatory drugs (NSAIDs) on a long-term basis.

E (ranitidine) is incorrect. Like cimetidine (discussed in Option B), ranitidine is a histamine H_2 receptor antagonist that is effective in the treatment of dyspepsia, peptic ulcer disease, and other gastrointestinal conditions associated with gastric acidity. Although ranitidine can cause gynecomastia, decreased libido, and impotence, the incidence of these adverse effects is considerably lower with ranitidine treatment than with cimetidine treatment.

48. ***A*** (acetylcholinesterase) is correct. The patient's ophthalmologic findings are consistent with the diagnosis of open-angle glaucoma. Echothiophate is an indirect-acting cholinergic receptor agonist that inhibits AChE and thereby potentiates the action of acetylcholine on the parasympathomimetic receptors. The drug is used as a miotic in diagnostic tests, to decrease intraocular pressure in patients with glaucoma, and to treat strabismus.

B (carbonic anhydrase) and C (catechol-*O*-methyltransferase) are incorrect. Echothiophate does not inhibit CA or COMT. An example of a CA inhibitor is acetazolamide, a drug that is used to prevent and treat altitude sickness and is also used as an adjunct in the treatment of glaucoma and epilepsy. An example of a COMT inhibitor is tolcapone, a drug that is given orally and is

used as an adjunct to levodopa-carbidopa in the treatment of Parkinson's disease.
D (choline acetyltransferase) and E (tyrosine hydroxylase) are incorrect. Echothiophate does not inhibit CAT or tyrosine hydroxylase. There is no known selective and specific inhibitor of CAT. Tyrosine hydroxylase is the rate-limiting step in catecholamine synthesis. Methyltyrosine inhibits tyrosine hydroxylase, but its use is limited to the treatment of pheochromocytoma.

49. *C* (administration of desmopressin) is correct. The patient's clinical and laboratory findings are consistent with the diagnosis of diabetes insipidus due to damage of the hypothalamus. This condition occurs rather frequently after head trauma and responds promptly to treatment with desmopressin, which is a synthetic analogue of vasopressin (antidiuretic hormone, or ADH). Desmopressin acts to maintain serum and urine osmolality within a physiologically acceptable range. It increases the reabsorption of water at the level of the renal collecting duct, thereby reducing urinary flow and increasing urine osmolality.

A (administration of a thiazide diuretic) and E (restriction of salt and protein intake) are incorrect. The findings in this case are consistent with the diagnosis of diabetes insipidus due to damage of the hypothalamus. This condition is not treated with thiazide diuretics or restriction of salt and protein intake. However, nephrogenic diabetes insipidus is treated with these measures. In patients with nephrogenic diabetes insipidus, volume depletion increases proximal tubular reabsorption and decreases the delivery of fluid to the distal nephron. Protein restriction is beneficial because it reduces daily solute excretion, thereby attenuating polyuria. Thiazide diuretics are also beneficial because they increase the excretion of sodium, chloride, and water by inhibiting sodium ion transport across the renal tubular epithelium. As a result, hypernatremia is prevented in patients with nephrogenic diabetes insipidus.
B (administration of anterior pituitary gland extract) is incorrect. Vasopressin is produced in the supraoptic and paraventricular nuclei of the hypothalamus as a prohormone. After cleavage to the mature form, it is transported down long axons to the posterior part of the pituitary gland for storage. The anterior part of the pituitary gland has no role in the pathogenesis of diabetes insipidus. Therefore, anterior pituitary gland extract would not be indicated.
D (reduction of water intake) is incorrect. The reduction of water intake is contraindicated. Patients who are not able or not permitted to respond to their need for water may develop severe, even life-threatening, hypernatremia as a result of osmotic brain shrinkage.

50. *A* (alprazolam) is correct. Alprazolam is an orally administered benzodiazepine that is used in the management of symptoms associated with panic disorder and other anxiety disorders.

B (buspirone) is incorrect. Buspirone is an orally administered anxiolytic that is structurally and pharmacologically distinct from all other anxiolytics, including benzodiazepines and barbiturates. Buspirone is used in the management of generalized anxiety disorder.

C (diazepam) is incorrect. Diazepam is a long-acting benzodiazepine. It is similar to chlordiazepoxide and clorazepate in that all three generate the same active metabolite. Diazepam is used orally in the short-term management of anxiety disorders. It can be used either orally or parenterally as a skeletal muscle relaxant or in the treatment of alcohol withdrawal. It is used parenterally as an antianxiety agent, sedative, amnestic, anticonvulsant, and anesthetic adjunct.

D (flurazepam) and E (triazolam) are incorrect. Flurazepam and triazolam are orally administered benzodiazepines that are used as hypnotic agents in the short-term management of insomnia.

TEST 2

DIRECTIONS: Each numbered item or incomplete statement is followed by options arranged in alphabetical or logical order. Select the best answer to each question. Some options may be partially correct, but there is only **ONE BEST** answer.

1. A 17-year-old girl at 30 weeks' gestation is in preterm labor. She has a history of mitral valve insufficiency and is admitted to the obstetrical unit of the hospital because she is experiencing back pain, cramps, and contractions. The contractions vary in intensity, last about 30 seconds, and are approximately 15 minutes apart. A vaginal examination indicates 2 cm of cervical dilation. The obstetrician decides to administer ritodrine. The patient should be monitored carefully for which of the following side effects of this tocolytic agent?

❍ A. Change in urinary output
❍ B. Gastrointestinal symptoms
❍ C. Increase in blood glucose level
❍ D. Increase in intraocular pressure
❍ E. Pulmonary edema

2. A 51-year-old obese man complains of recurrent pain in the right upper quadrant of his abdomen. Ultrasonography confirms the presence of radiolucent cholesterol gallstones. The patient is a poor candidate for surgery. Which of the following could be used to treat his cholelithiasis?

❍ A. Chenodiol
❍ B. Cholestyramine
❍ C. Gemfibrozil
❍ D. Lovastatin
❍ E. Niacin

3. A 45-year-old man has severe persistent asthma with bronchial hyperreactivity due to airway inflammation. His responsiveness to treatment with a variety of β_2-adrenergic receptor agonists has been decreasing. Therapy with which of the following immunosuppressive agents would most likely be recommended?

❍ A. Azathioprine
❍ B. Cyclophosphamide
❍ C. Cyclosporine
❍ D. Flunisolide
❍ E. Methotrexate

4. A 75-year-old woman has stable angina pectoris, ischemia, and stenosis of an artery that perfuses a large segment of the myocardium that lacks collateral vessels. She is scheduled to undergo percutaneous transluminal coronary angioplasty (PTCA) to revascularize the myocardium. Which of the following agents would most likely be given to prevent platelet aggregation during PTCA and acts by binding to glycoprotein receptors on platelet cells?

❍ A. Abciximab
❍ B. Aminocaproic acid
❍ C. Aprotinin
❍ D. Aspirin
❍ E. Ticlopidine

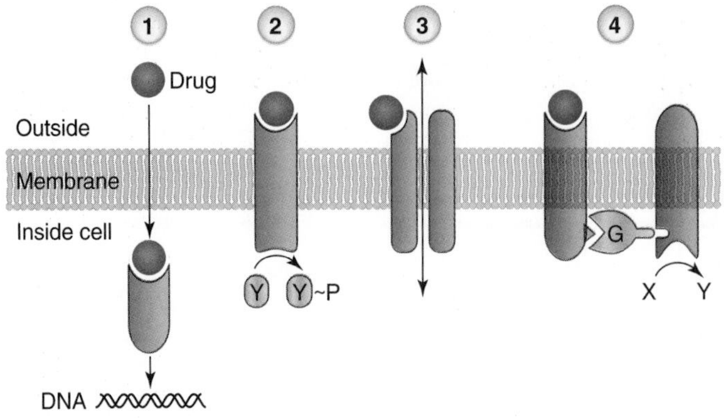

5. The figure above depicts four different transmembrane signaling mechanisms for drugs and hormones. Which agent will act via mechanism 3 to produce a beneficial effect?

- ❍ A. α-Adrenergic receptor agonist
- ❍ B. Histamine
- ❍ C. Insulin
- ❍ D. Nicotinic receptor agonist
- ❍ E. Serotonin 5-HT_1 receptor agonist

6. For the past 2 years, a 36-year-old woman has been taking 1000 mg of acetaminophen every 4–6 hours for back pain. Each day, she has also been consuming an average of five drinks containing gin and tonic. One morning, after partying the night before, she takes 2000 mg of acetaminophen as soon as she gets out of bed. She suffers from nausea and vomiting for about 2 hours and then begins to experience severe abdominal pain. She goes to the emergency department and is found to have hypoprothrombinemia and elevated hepatic enzyme levels. Which of the following agents would be an appropriate antidote?

- ❍ A. Acetylcysteine
- ❍ B. Ammonium chloride
- ❍ C. Meperidine
- ❍ D. Ondansetron
- ❍ E. Sodium bicarbonate

7. A 62-year-old man with a history of diabetes mellitus and moderate hypertension suffers from erectile dysfunction. Which of the following drugs would be most appropriate in the treatment of impotence in this patient?

- ❍ A. Nitroglycerin
- ❍ B. Pioglitazone
- ❍ C. Sildenafil
- ❍ D. Testosterone
- ❍ E. Zafirlukast

8. A 68-year-old man who recently suffered a myocardial infarction (MI) is injured in an automobile accident and develops cerebral edema and increased intracranial pressure. Mannitol infusion is started to decrease the cerebral edema. Which of the following is the most serious adverse effect of mannitol?

- ❍ A. Hyperkalemia
- ❍ B. Hypernatremia
- ❍ C. Hypertension
- ❍ D. Premature ventricular contractions
- ❍ E. Pulmonary edema

9. For the past 10 months, a 27-year-old woman has had episodes of watery diarrhea and abdominal pain. She says that the pain is relieved by defecation, and she now has as many as 10 stools a day. She has anorexia and has lost about 7 kg (15 lb) during the past 3 months. Laboratory and sigmoidoscopy results are consistent with the diagnosis of severe acute ulcerative colitis. Which of the following drugs is most likely to induce disease remission?

❍ A. Azathioprine
❍ B. Fludrocortisone
❍ C. Hydrocortisone
❍ D. Sulfasalazine
❍ E. Thalidomide

10. A 55-year-old man has hypercholesterolemia and hypertension. After he begins treatment, he develops muscle weakness and pain and is found to have an increased serum creatine kinase level. Which of the following drugs is most likely responsible for these adverse effects?

❍ A. Enalapril
❍ B. Gemfibrozil
❍ C. Hydrochlorothiazide
❍ D. Lovastatin
❍ E. Metoprolol

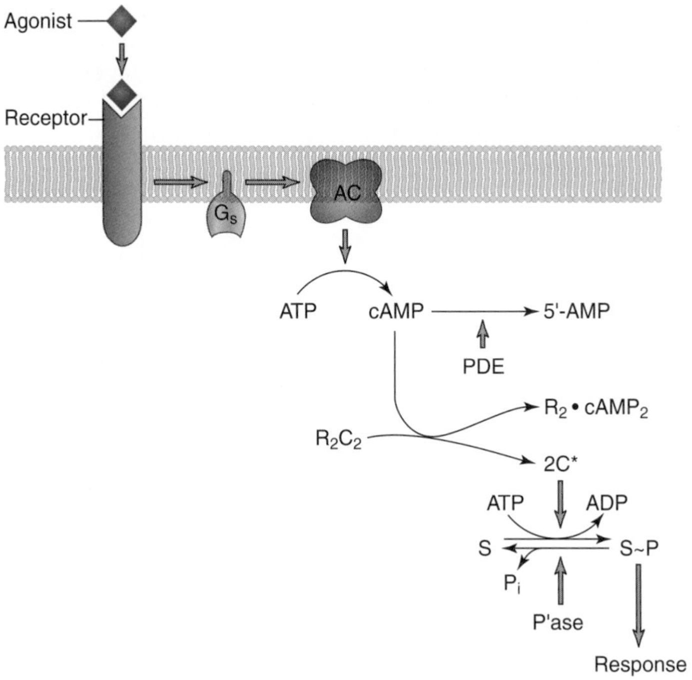

Abbreviations: G_s, stimulatory G protein; AC, adenylyl cyclase; ATP, adenosine triphosphate; cAMP, cyclic adenosine monophosphate; PDE, phosphodiesterases; R, regulatory subunit; C, catalytic subunit; S~P, phosphorylated substrate; P_i, inorganic phosphate; and P'ase, phosphatases.

11. The figure above depicts a signaling pathway in which a cell surface receptor couples with adenylyl cyclase via a G_s protein. Which of the following agonists increases cAMP via this pathway?

❍ A. Clonidine
❍ B. Isoproterenol
❍ C. Nicotine
❍ D. Phenylephrine
❍ E. Prednisone

12. A 66-year-old man with Parkinson's disease has been successfully treated for 3 years with a combination of levodopa and carbidopa. Lately, he has begun to experience rigidity, bradykinesia, and postural control problems associated with the "wearing off" effects of the drug combination. His physician decides to add a catechol-*O*-methyltransferase (COMT) inhibitor to the treatment regimen. Which of the following drugs would most likely be added?

❍ A. Amantadine
❍ B. Pergolide
❍ C. Selegiline
❍ D. Tolcapone
❍ E. Trihexyphenidyl

13. A 70-year-old man with acute angle-closure glaucoma is brought to the emergency department because he is experiencing extreme pain in his left eye and is seeing halos around lights. He has an intensely red left eye and a steamy-appearing cornea. Which of the following drugs would be considered appropriate medical treatment for this disorder?

❍ A. Atropine
❍ B. Edrophonium
❍ C. Furosemide
❍ D. Pilocarpine
❍ E. Timolol

14. A 30-year-old woman attempts suicide by swallowing seventy-five 325-mg tablets of ferrous sulfate. She is admitted to the hospital 6 hours later, diaphoretic and lethargic, and is experiencing abdominal pain, nausea, and vomiting. Her vomitus is guaiac-positive. Other findings include blood pressure of 83/58 mm Hg, pulse of 140/min, respirations of 35/min, temperature of 37.2°C (99°F), and serum iron concentration of 700 mg/dL. In addition to providing supportive care, it would be most appropriate to treat this patient with

❍ A. ammonium chloride
❍ B. hemodialysis
❍ C. intramuscular deferoxamine
❍ D. oral deferoxamine
❍ E. penicillamine

15. A 76-year-old woman suffers from postprandial heartburn, difficulty in swallowing food, and difficulty in sleeping because of gastrointestinal reflux. She has been taking antacids plus an over-the-counter preparation of famotidine, but these drugs fail to control her symptoms. Which of the following is the most appropriate therapy for this patient?

❍ A. Bethanechol
❍ B. Cetirizine
❍ C. Cisapride
❍ D. Lansoprazole
❍ E. Metoclopramide

16. A 25-year-old woman experiences urinary frequency and a burning sensation when she urinates. Two days later, she comes to the physician's office. A urine sample is sent for culture. Before the results of culture are completed, treatment with which of the following drugs should be started?

❍ A. Metronidazole
❍ B. Nitrofurantoin
❍ C. Penicillin G
❍ D. Tetracycline
❍ E. Trimethoprim-sulfamethoxazole

17. The teacher of a 13-year-old student notices that the student has episodes of staring and inattention that last from 5 to 10 seconds. Routine physical examination and laboratory studies show normal results, but an EEG shows a 3-Hz spike-and-wave pattern. The drug of choice for treating the patient is

❍ A. carbamazepine
❍ B. diazepam
❍ C. ethosuximide
❍ D. phenobarbital
❍ E. phenytoin

18. A 15-year-old girl has severe cramping pain that begins a few hours before the start of her menstrual flow. She says that the pain has occurred monthly for the past 9 months. She also complains of headaches and of being very tired during her menstrual period. Which of the following is the most appropriate therapy?

❍ A. Acetaminophen
❍ B. Celecoxib
❍ C. Dexamethasone
❍ D. Ibuprofen
❍ E. Indomethacin

19. A 53-year-old man suffers from watery diarrhea, hypokalemia, renal failure, and a VIPoma that arose in the pancreas and metastasized to other sites. After the pancreatic tumor is removed, which of the following drugs is most likely to be given to inhibit the release of vasoactive intestinal polypeptide (VIP) from the sites of metastasis?

❍ A. Leuprolide
❍ B. Nafarelin
❍ C. Octreotide
❍ D. Protirelin
❍ E. Sermorelin

20. A 68-year-old man suffers a heart attack and is treated prophylactically with warfarin. Later, his physician decides to add an antihyperlipoproteinemic agent to the treatment regimen. Which of the following agents is most likely to potentiate the anticoagulant effect of warfarin?

❍ A. Cholestyramine
❍ B. Colestipol
❍ C. Gemfibrozil
❍ D. Niacin
❍ E. Pravastatin

21. A farmer sprays his fruit orchard with parathion. Later in the day, he notes an increase in salivation, lacrimation, and urination, and has diarrhea. Which of the following drugs would be the drug of choice for treating these symptoms of poisoning?

❍ A. Amyl nitrite
❍ B. Atropine
❍ C. Dimercaprol
❍ D. Disulfiram
❍ E. Edetate calcium disodium

22. Estrogen receptor–positive tumor cells are detected in a 54-year-old postmenopausal woman with breast cancer. Which of the following drugs would act by blocking the estrogen receptors in her breast tissue?

❍ A. Levonorgestrel
❍ B. Nafarelin
❍ C. Octreotide
❍ D. Sermorelin
❍ E. Tamoxifen

23. A 28-year-old woman with chronic disseminated intravascular coagulation (DIC) develops thrombotic problems that require immediate treatment. Which of the following agents would be most appropriate for use in the management of the patient's DIC?

❍ A. Aspirin
❍ B. Celecoxib
❍ C. Heparin
❍ D. Ticlopidine
❍ E. Warfarin

24. A 58-year-old man weighs 90 kg (198 lb), and his blood pressure is 140/96 mm Hg. He has pitting edema in both legs. His physician prescribes exercise, restricted sodium intake, and a diuretic agent. Taking inappropriately high doses of which of the following diuretics would be most likely to produce profound diuresis and vascular collapse?

❍ A. Acetazolamide
❍ B. Furosemide
❍ C. Hydrochlorothiazide
❍ D. Spironolactone
❍ E. Triamterene

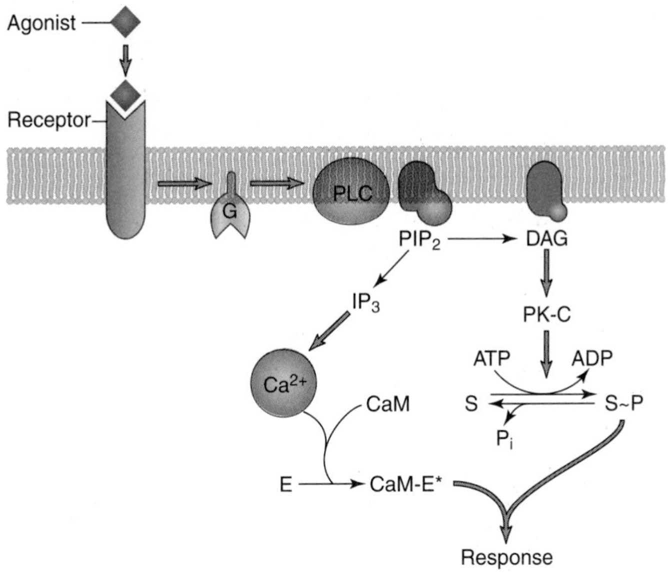

Abbreviations: G, G protein; PLC, phospholipase C; PIP_2, phosphatidylinositol 4,5-bisphosphate; DAG, diacylglycerol; IP_3, inositol triphosphate; CaM, calmodulin; E, calmodulin-binding enzyme; CaM-E*, activated state; PK-C, protein kinase C; ATP, adenosine triphosphate; ADP, adenosine diphosphate; S, substrate for protein kinase C; S~P, phosphorylated substrate; and P_i, inorganic phosphate.

25. A 37-year-old woman who has partial seizures with secondary generalized tonic-clonic seizures has been treated with carbamazepine for 3 years. The therapy has been only minimally successful, and the physician plans to add another drug to the treatment regimen. Which of the following drugs is most likely to be added?

❍ A. Clonazepam
❍ B. Cyclobenzaprine
❍ C. Ethosuximide
❍ D. Lamotrigine
❍ E. Lorazepam

26. The figure above depicts a signaling pathway for some types of drugs and hormones. Which of the following agonists exerts its effects via this pathway?

❍ A. Acetylcholine acting on a muscarinic receptor
❍ B. Acetylcholine acting on a nicotinic receptor
❍ C. Diazepam acting on a benzodiazepine receptor
❍ D. Insulin acting on an insulin receptor
❍ E. Isoproterenol acting on a β_1-adrenergic receptor

27. A 13-month-old girl who has an earache is taken to a pediatric clinic, and ampicillin is prescribed. Five days after she begins taking the drug, her condition worsens, and she has a temperature as high as 39.4°C (103°F). The pediatrician reexamines the child and notes that meningeal irritation is present. The child is hospitalized and diagnosed with meningitis caused by a beta-lactamase–positive strain of *Haemophilus influenzae*. Which of the following drugs is most likely to provide effective treatment?

❍ A. Benzathine penicillin G
❍ B. Ceftriaxone
❍ C. Erythromycin
❍ D. Penicillin V
❍ E. Procaine penicillin G

28. A 57-year-old woman is brought to the emergency department because the left side of her face and arm feel weak. Arteriography shows a thrombotic cerebral arterial occlusion. Which of the following drug combinations is most likely to cause this complication?

❍ A. Albuterol plus prednisone
❍ B. Codeine plus acetaminophen
❍ C. Estrogen plus progestin
❍ D. Imipenem plus cilastatin
❍ E. Propranolol plus hydrochlorothiazide

29. A 47-year-old semiconscious woman is receiving mechanical ventilatory support in the intensive care unit. Administration of which of the following drugs would be most likely to prevent her random, spontaneous thoracic movements from interfering with the efficiency of this support?

❍ A. Baclofen
❍ B. Dantrolene
❍ C. Neostigmine
❍ D. Pancuronium
❍ E. Succinylcholine

30. A 34-year-old man returns to the United States after an extended stay in rural Africa. Within a few months of his return, he develops a cough, fever, chills, and muscle aches and is diagnosed with schistosomiasis. Which of the following drugs is most likely to be effective in the treatment of this disease?

❍ A. Mebendazole
❍ B. Metronidazole
❍ C. Niclosamide
❍ D. Praziquantel
❍ E. Pyrantel pamoate

31. The cytoplasmic domain of the insulin receptor is the site of activation of which of the following enzymes?

❍ A. Adenylyl cyclase
❍ B. Phosphodiesterase
❍ C. Phospholipase C
❍ D. Phosphoprotein phosphatase
❍ E. Tyrosine kinase

32. A 20-year-old man has polymorphic, erythematous, and well-circumscribed edematous papules (wheals) over his entire body. The patient says that the lesions cause intense itching, appeared overnight, and have been present for 2 days. He has driven his automobile to the appointment and needs to drive himself home. Which of the following is the first-line treatment for this patient?

❍ A. Chlorpheniramine
❍ B. Famotidine
❍ C. Fexofenadine
❍ D. Prednisone
❍ E. Triamcinolone cream

33. A 42-year-old man who collapsed at work in a metal-plating factory is taken to the emergency department by ambulance. The patient is unresponsive to external stimuli, has impaired respiration, and exudes a bitter almond odor. Intravenous treatment with sodium nitrite is begun immediately. The therapeutic efficacy of nitrite in the treatment of poisoning of this type is due to which of the following actions?

❍ A. Decrease in intracranial pressure
❍ B. Formation of methemoglobin
❍ C. Increase in coronary arterial blood flow
❍ D. Increase in oxidative phosphorylation
❍ E. Relaxation of the nonvascular smooth muscle

34. A 56-year-old postmenopausal woman has metastatic breast cancer, with cancer cells that are positive for both estrogen and progesterone receptors. The physician plans to treat her with a drug that inhibits the conversion of androgens to estrogens in peripheral tissues. Which of the following is the most appropriate treatment for this patient?

❍ A. Aminoglutethimide
❍ B. Goserelin
❍ C. Octreotide
❍ D. Procarbazine
❍ E. Tamoxifen

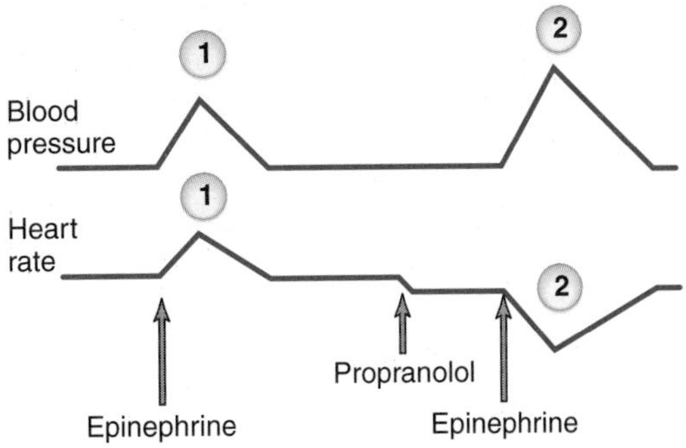

35. The figure above shows the blood pressure and heart rate response to epinephrine before (1) and after (2) the administration of propranolol. The heart rate is reduced when epinephrine is given in the presence of propranolol because

❍ A. propranolol directly stimulates the vagus nerve
❍ B. propranolol inhibits the central effects of epinephrine
❍ C. propranolol inhibits the effects of circulating norepinephrine
❍ D. propranolol is a quinidine-like agent that decreases the heart rate
❍ E. the increasing blood pressure activates the baroreceptor reflex

36. A 4-year-old boy is brought to his pediatrician's office because he has been behaving strangely. He shows increasing irritability and has experienced several episodes of vigorous vomiting, although he has not complained of nausea. The boy's mother mentions that the family has recently moved into an old house, and they have just finished remodeling it. The patient's laboratory studies show hypochromic microcytic anemia with basophilic stippling. An x-ray of the long bones shows broad bands of increased density at the metaphyses. Which of the following is the most likely cause of these findings?

❍ A. Benzene poisoning
❍ B. Dioxin poisoning
❍ C. Ipecac ingestion
❍ D. Iron poisoning
❍ E. Lead poisoning

37. A 28-year-old man with kyphosis, limited neck motion and chest expansion, low back pain, and radiographic evidence of sclerosis of the sacroiliac joints is diagnosed with ankylosing spondylitis. Which of the following is the most appropriate treatment for this patient?

❍ A. Corticosteroids
❍ B. Gold salts
❍ C. Indomethacin
❍ D. Penicillamine
❍ E. Salicylates

38. A 42-year-old man has mild hypertension. For the past 3 years, he has been able to control his blood pressure by modifying his diet and exercising, but he now requires drug therapy. A few weeks after he begins taking an antihypertensive agent, he complains of a nonproductive cough and is found to have hyperkalemia. Which of the following medications is most likely responsible for these adverse effects?

❍ A. Hydrochlorothiazide
❍ B. Lisinopril
❍ C. Metoprolol
❍ D. Nifedipine
❍ E. Valsartan

39. A 51-year-old man complains that he has attacks of excruciating pain in his big toe. Examination of the foot shows that the first metatarsophalangeal joint is swollen, hot, red, and tender. Laboratory findings include a serum uric acid level of 15.7 mg/dL. Which of the following is the most appropriate treatment to prevent future attacks of pain?

❍ A. Allopurinol
❍ B. Corticosteroids
❍ C. Indomethacin
❍ D. Morphine
❍ E. Salicylates

40. A 28-year-old woman is hospitalized for intense epigastric pain and hematemesis. Endoscopic examination shows the presence of a large peptic ulcer on the bulbus of the duodenum. On visualization, the bleeding has already stopped. A mucosal biopsy yields positive results for *Helicobacter pylori*. After the patient's acute symptoms are treated, therapy with which of the following regimens would most likely prevent recurrence of the peptic ulcer?

❍ A. Aluminum hydroxide plus famotidine
❍ B. Bismuth, metronidazole, and tetracycline
❍ C. Lansoprazole plus cephalexin
❍ D. Omeprazole, cimetidine, and trimethoprim-sulfamethoxazole (TMP-SMX)
❍ E. Sucralfate, ranitidine, and calcium carbonate

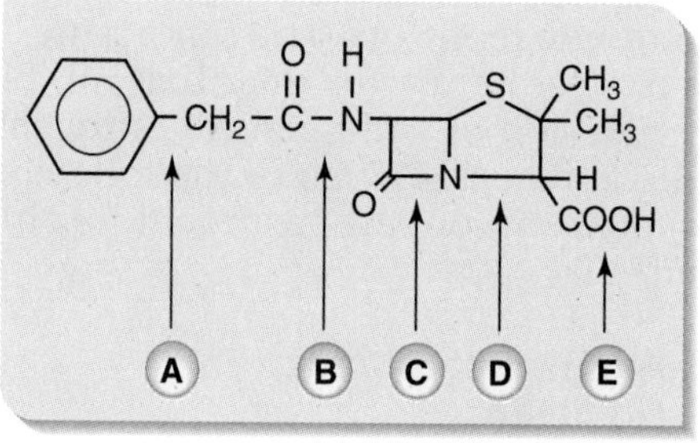

41. The figure above shows the structure of penicillin G. Five sites on the structure are labeled with the letters A through E. The site of action of penicillinase is

❍ A. site A
❍ B. site B
❍ C. site C
❍ D. site D
❍ E. site E

42. A 24-year-old woman in her 25th week of pregnancy is admitted to the hospital because of preeclampsia, with manifestations of visual disturbances, headache, increasing blood pressure, proteinuria, and rapid development of edema. To control the patient's blood pressure, the physician decides to use a drug that is a potent blocker of both α- and β-adrenergic receptors. Which of the following is most likely to be used?

❍ A. Atenolol
❍ B. Labetalol
❍ C. Minoxidil
❍ D. Pindolol
❍ E. Terazosin

43. A 49-year-old woman has small cell lung carcinoma. Radiotherapy and chemotherapy are effective in reducing the size of her primary tumor. However, ectopic tumor tissue continues to produce an excess of adrenocorticotropic hormone (ACTH). Which of the following drugs would substantially decrease the cortisol levels in this patient?

❍ A. Clomiphene
❍ B. Finasteride
❍ C. Mitotane
❍ D. Spironolactone
❍ E. Tamoxifen

44. A 72-year-old man is scheduled to have a tooth extraction. He has a history of mitral valve prolapse and is allergic to penicillin. Which of the following antibiotics should be prescribed prior to the extraction to prevent endocarditis in this patient?

❍ A. Amoxicillin
❍ B. Chloramphenicol
❍ C. Doxycycline
❍ D. Erythromycin
❍ E. Tetracycline

45. A 5-year-old girl suffers from itching and scaling of the skin and is constantly scratching. Physical examination of the girl shows dryness of the skin, localized hair loss, and hyperkeratosis on the medial side of the soles of her feet. The girl's mother says that she has been giving her daughter cod liver oil capsules for the past 7 months. The patient's clinical findings are most likely due to

❍ A. vitamin A deficiency
❍ B. vitamin D deficiency
❍ C. vitamin E deficiency
❍ D. vitamin A toxicity
❍ E. vitamin E toxicity

46. A 45-year-old woman is diagnosed with acute myelogenous leukemia (AML). Physical findings include chronic progressive fatigue, gingival hyperplasia, petechial bleeding of the skin, and enlarged spleen. Laboratory findings include extremely low granulocyte and platelet counts. Which of the following is the most appropriate treatment for this patient?

❍ A. Chlorambucil plus prednisone
❍ B. Cladribine plus interferon alfa
❍ C. Cytarabine plus idarubicin
❍ D. Hydroxyurea
❍ E. Prednisone

47. An 18-year-old woman complains of severe pain in her right eye, accompanied by a watery discharge. The eyelid shows swelling and vesicles, and the conjunctiva is red. Fluorescein staining of the cornea shows a typical picture of dendritic keratitis. Which of the following drugs should be applied topically before the results of the culture are known?

❍ A. Betamethasone
❍ B. Interferon alfa
❍ C. Ketoconazole
❍ D. Tetracycline
❍ E. Vidarabine

48. A 76-year-old man develops an intra-abdominal infection caused by a beta-lactamase–producing gram-negative organism. The patient has a history of renal problems and is allergic to penicillin. Which of the following drugs would be most useful for treating the infection?

❍ A. Aztreonam
❍ B. Cefepime
❍ C. Ceftazidime
❍ D. Metronidazole
❍ E. Nitrofurantoin

49. A 34-year-old woman with schizophrenia has been treated for several years with various drugs. She is now being treated with fluphenazine and complains of amenorrhea and galactorrhea. It would be most appropriate to switch her medication to

❍ A. chlorpromazine
❍ B. haloperidol
❍ C. olanzapine
❍ D. promethazine
❍ E. thioridazine

50. A 43-year-old woman undergoes nasopharyngeal surgery in an outpatient surgical facility. She will be given an antibiotic to prevent postsurgical infection. Her medical records indicate that 5 years ago she had an anaphylactic reaction to penicillin G. Which of the following antibiotics is most appropriate to prescribe for this patient?

❍ A. Amoxicillin
❍ B. Cefazolin
❍ C. Clindamycin
❍ D. Metronidazole
❍ E. Nafcillin

ANSWERS AND DISCUSSIONS

1. *E* (pulmonary edema) is correct. Women who are treated with ritodrine should be carefully monitored for pulmonary edema, which can occur even during the postpartum period. This life-threatening adverse effect occurs more frequently when corticosteroids are used concomitantly. Preexisting cardiovascular disease is a contributory factor and may be unmasked by the development of pulmonary edema.

   A (change in urinary output) and D (increase in intraocular pressure) are incorrect. Ritodrine use is not associated with marked changes in urinary flow or intraocular pressure.
   B (gastrointestinal symptoms) is incorrect. Gastrointestinal symptoms can occur in women treated with ritodrine, but these symptoms are usually mild.
   C (increase in blood glucose level) is incorrect. Women who are treated with ritodrine may experience increases in their insulin and blood glucose levels, but these increases are usually transient and stabilize within 48–72 hours, even during continued ritodrine infusion. The infants of women who have been treated with ritodrine may have hypoglycemia, hyperglycemia, or adynamic ileus.

2. *A* (chenodiol) is correct. Chenodiol, or chenodeoxycholic acid, is a bile acid produced in the liver. All bile acids increase the output of bile, but only chenodiol and ursodiol decrease the secretion of biliary cholesterol. When chenodiol is administered, the proportion of chenodiol in bile acids increases and the proportion of biliary cholesterol decreases. After long-term administration, chenodiol also reduces the hepatic production of cholesterol. This alteration in the ratio of bile acid to cholesterol desaturates the bile surrounding the gallstone, thereby allowing for the gradual dissolution of the stone.

   B (cholestyramine) is incorrect. Cholestyramine is a polymeric resin that is used to treat hypercholesterolemia with concomitant hypertriglyceridemia.
   C (gemfibrozil) is incorrect. Gemfibrozil is a fibric acid derivative. Although it effectively lowers serum triglyceride levels and also produces favorable changes in lipoprotein levels, it is not as effective as the HMG-CoA reductase inhibitors for use in the treatment of hyperlipoproteinemia.
   D (lovastatin) and E (niacin) are incorrect. Lovastatin is an HMG-CoA reductase inhibitor that is indicated for the treatment of primary hypercholesterolemia. Niacin is used as an adjunct in the

treatment of patients who have primary hyperlipoproteinemia type IIa, IIb, III, IV, or V and have an increased risk of coronary artery disease.

3. ***D*** (flunisolide) is correct. Flunisolide is administered via an oral metered-dose inhaler in the management of corticosteroid-dependent bronchial asthma or via a nasal spray to relieve symptoms associated with seasonal or perennial rhinitis, such as rhinorrhea, nasal congestion, postnasal drip, sneezing, and pharyngeal itching. Flunisolide is more effective for the management of allergic rhinitis than nonallergic rhinitis. The moisturizing effects of the vehicle in flunisolide nasal solutions may be partially responsible for the drug's beneficial effects.

A (azathioprine), B (cyclophosphamide), C (cyclosporine), and E (methotrexate) are incorrect. Azathioprine, cyclophosphamide, cyclosporine, and methotrexate are all immunosuppressive agents, but none is used to treat bronchial hyperreactivity due to airway inflammation. Azathioprine is used to treat rheumatoid arthritis, lupus nephritis, and psoriatic arthritis. Cyclophosphamide is a cell cycle–nonspecific antineoplastic agent that is used to treat many types of cancer, including lymphomas, leukemias, carcinomas, and sarcomas. Cyclosporine is used to prevent allograft rejection and to treat autoimmune disorders. Methotrexate is used to treat several types of cancer and immune-mediated disease.

4. ***A*** (abciximab) is correct. Abciximab is the Fab fragment of a chimeric human-murine monoclonal antibody. Abciximab is given in combination with aspirin and heparin to prevent myocardial infarctions and other cardiac complications in patients who are scheduled to undergo PTCA. Abciximab and aspirin both prevent platelet aggregation, but they do so by different means. Abciximab acts by binding to glycoprotein IIb/IIIa receptors on platelets, whereas aspirin acts by inhibiting the synthesis of thromboxane and other mediators of platelet aggregation.

B (aminocaproic acid) is incorrect. Aminocaproic acid is an inhibitor of fibrinolysis. It is indicated for use in the treatment of bleeding in patients who have undergone cardiac surgery or have disorders such as aplastic anemia; abruptio placentae; hepatic cirrhosis; or carcinoma of the prostate, lung, stomach, or cervix.
C (aprotinin) is incorrect. Aprotinin is a proteolytic enzyme inhibitor that is indicated for use during repeat coronary artery bypass surgery, when patients are likely to bleed excessively. It is useful during the initial surgery if there is an especially high risk of bleeding (e.g., in patients who have impaired hemostasis or patients who were pretreated with aspirin or other nonsteroidal anti-inflammatory drugs) or if transfusion is unacceptable or unavailable.
D (aspirin) is incorrect. Refer to the discussion for Option A.

E (ticlopidine) is incorrect. Ticlopidine inhibits platelet aggregation by blocking the ADP pathway. Ticlopidine may be a more efficacious inhibitor than aspirin, but because of rare cases of severe bone marrow toxicity, ticlopidine use is limited to patients who are intolerant of or unresponsive to aspirin.

5. ***D*** (nicotinic receptor agonist) is correct. Nicotinic receptor agonists signal via ligand-gated sodium channels (mechanism 3). They do not act via the three other signal mechanisms depicted in the figure: intracellular receptors that regulate gene expression (mechanism 1); ligand-regulated transmembrane enzymes, such as protein tyrosine kinases (mechanism 2); and G proteins and second messengers (mechanism 4).

A (α-adrenergic receptor agonist), B (histamine), and E (serotonin 5-HT_1 receptor agonist) are incorrect. Histamine, α-adrenergic receptor agonists, and 5-HT_1 agonists all signal via G proteins and second messengers (mechanism 4).
C (insulin) is incorrect. Insulin signals via ligand-regulated transmembrane enzymes (mechanism 2).

6. ***A*** (acetylcysteine) is correct. Acetaminophen and alcohol act synergistically to produce hepatotoxicity. Acetylcysteine is used as an antidote to treat acute acetaminophen overdose.

B (ammonium chloride) and E (sodium bicarbonate) are incorrect. Ammonium chloride or sodium bicarbonate would not be helpful in the treatment of an acute acetaminophen overdose. Ammonium chloride is used to correct metabolic alkalosis in patients suffering from chloride depletion secondary to diuretic therapy, gastric fistula drainage, nasogastric suction, or vomiting. Sodium bicarbonate is a systemic alkalinizing agent that is used in the management of metabolic and respiratory acidosis.
C (meperidine) is incorrect. Meperidine is an opioid analgesic; it would not be useful in the treatment of an acute acetaminophen overdose.
D (ondansetron) is incorrect. Ondansetron is a selective 5-HT_3 receptor antagonist that is used in the management of chemotherapy-induced nausea and vomiting.

7. ***C*** (sildenafil) is correct. A penile erection occurs when nitric oxide is released in the corpus cavernosum during sexual stimulation. The nitric oxide activates guanylyl cyclase and causes an increase in the level of cyclic guanosine monophosphate (cGMP). This increase leads to smooth muscle relaxation in the corpus cavernosum, thereby allowing the inflow of blood and resulting in an erection. In men with erectile dysfunction, sildenafil acts by inhibiting the breakdown of cGMP by type 5 phosphodiesterase. Sildenafil was originally developed as an antianginal agent, but was found to be more effective in the treatment of impotence.

A (nitroglycerin) is incorrect. Sublingual nitroglycerin is the drug of choice for relieving acute angina attacks, but it is not helpful for use in the treatment of erectile dysfunction. In patients who take nitroglycerin, the drug is converted to nitric oxide. Nitric oxide activates guanylyl cyclase and thereby stimulates the synthesis of cGMP. Then cGMP activates a series of protein kinase–dependent phosphorylations in the smooth muscle cells, eventually resulting in the dephosphorylation of the myosin light chain of the smooth muscle fiber. Dephosphorylation of the myosin light chain signals the cells to release calcium. This relaxes the smooth muscle cells, produces vasodilation, and relieves angina pectoris. To date, no commercial preparation of nitroglycerin is available to selectively release nitric oxide in the corpus cavernosum and thereby produce penile erection.

B (pioglitazone) and E (zafirlukast) are incorrect. Pioglitazone is a thiazolidinedione that acts as an insulin sensitizer and is used in the treatment of type 2 diabetes mellitus. Zafirlukast is a leukotriene receptor antagonist that is given orally in the treatment of asthma. Pioglitazone and zafirlukast are not helpful for use in the treatment of erectile dysfunction.

D (testosterone) is incorrect. Testosterone, the primary androgen in the body, is used in the management of congenital or acquired hypogonadism and is also used in the palliative treatment of breast cancer in postmenopausal women. It is not helpful in the treatment of erectile dysfunction.

8. *E* (pulmonary edema) is correct. Although all of the adverse effects listed can occur with mannitol use, acute pulmonary edema is the most serious. Inadequate urine output or rapid administration of large doses of mannitol can cause accumulation of the drug, overexpansion of the extracellular fluid, and circulatory overload. This in turn causes pulmonary edema and congestive heart failure. Accumulation of mannitol is more likely to occur in patients with acute or chronic renal failure than in other patients.

A (hyperkalemia), B (hypernatremia), C (hypertension), and D (premature ventricular contractions) are incorrect. Although all of the adverse effects listed can occur with mannitol use, acute pulmonary edema (discussed in Option E) is the most serious. During mannitol treatment, patients may exhibit electrolyte imbalances, such as hyperkalemia (caused by movement of intracellular potassium to the extracellular space); hypokalemia (caused by an increase in the excretion of potassium); hypernatremia (caused by a water loss that exceeds the sodium loss); and hyponatremia (caused by shifts in the relationship of sodium-free intracellular fluid to extracellular fluid and by an increase in the excretion of sodium). Mannitol-induced electrolyte imbalances can lead to hypertension and to premature ventricular contractions.

9. *C* (hydrocortisone) is correct. Immediate hospitalization and the parenteral administration of a corticosteroid are recommended to induce disease remission in patients with severe acute ulcerative colitis. Prednisone or hydrocortisone is initially given 2–4 times a day.

A (azathioprine) is incorrect. Immunosuppressive agents, such as azathioprine, have been used to treat ulcerative colitis. However, serious side effects occur in most patients and offset the limited value of azathioprine.
B (fludrocortisone) is incorrect. Fludrocortisone is a mineralocorticoid that is used in the treatment of patients with adrenocortical insufficiency and salt-losing adrenogenital syndrome. It is not used in the treatment of patients with ulcerative colitis.
D (sulfasalazine) is incorrect. Sulfasalazine is extensively used in the treatment of inflammatory bowel diseases. However, corticosteroids are more prompt than sulfasalazine in inducing disease remission in cases of severe acute ulcerative colitis.
E (thalidomide) is incorrect. Thalidomide attenuates symptoms associated with increased levels of tumor necrosis factor alpha (TNF-α). It is under investigation for use in the treatment of Crohn's disease but not for treating ulcerative colitis.

10. *D* (lovastatin) is correct. Lovastatin and other "statin" drugs (such as atorvastatin, fluvastatin, pravastatin, and simvastatin) are HMG-CoA reductase inhibitors that are used in the treatment of hypercholesterolemia. Asymptomatic elevations of creatine kinase levels occur in about 11% of patients treated with these drugs; however, more serious adverse effects, such as rhabdomyolysis, can also occur. Myalgia (muscle aches or cramps), fever, tiredness, or myasthenia occurs in up to 3% of patients, and myopathy occurs in about 1%. The risk is greater if a "statin" drug is administered with gemfibrozil, with lipid-lowering doses of nicotinic acid, or with cyclosporine or other immunosuppressive agents.

A (enalapril), C (hydrochlorothiazide), and E (metoprolol) are incorrect. Enalapril is an angiotensin-converting enzyme inhibitor; hydrochlorothiazide is a thiazide diuretic; and metoprolol is a selective β_1-adrenergic receptor antagonist. These drugs are used to treat hypertension. They do not produce muscle toxicity.
B (gemfibrozil) is incorrect. Gemfibrozil effectively lowers the serum triglyceride level and also produces favorable changes in lipoprotein levels. However, the HMG-CoA reductase inhibitors (see the explanation for Option D) are more effective than gemfibrozil in the treatment of hyperlipoproteinemia and would therefore be more likely to have been prescribed for this patient. The concomitant use of gemfibrozil and an HMG-CoA reductase inhibitor increases the risk of myopathy and rhabdomyolysis. Therapy should be discontinued if creatine kinase levels are elevated or myalgia occurs.

11. ***B*** (isoproterenol) is correct. Isoproterenol is a β_1-adrenergic receptor agonist. Both β_1- and β_2-adrenergic receptor agonists are linked to a G_s protein. They signal by increasing cAMP production.

A (clonidine) is incorrect. Clonidine and other α_2-adrenergic receptor agonists are linked to an inhibitory G protein (G_i protein). They signal by decreasing cAMP production.
C (nicotine) is incorrect. Nicotinic agonists signal by opening sodium channels.
D (phenylephrine) is incorrect. Phenylephrine and other α_1-adrenergic receptor agonists signal via the polyphosphoinositide pathway.
E (prednisone) is incorrect. Prednisone and other glucocorticoids signal by increasing gene expression.

12. ***D*** (tolcapone) is correct. All of the drugs listed are useful in the treatment of Parkinson's disease. However, tolcapone is the only one that acts as a COMT inhibitor.

A (amantadine) and C (selegiline) are incorrect. Tolcapone, amantadine, and selegiline all increase dopamine levels, but they do so by different mechanisms. Tolcapone inhibits COMT. Amantadine, an antiviral agent, releases dopamine and norepinephrine from storage sites and inhibits the reuptake of dopamine and norepinephrine. Selegiline selectively inhibits monoamine oxidase type B (MAO-B).
B (pergolide) and E (trihexyphenidyl) are incorrect. Pergolide is a potent dopamine receptor agonist that acts at both D_1 and D_2 receptors. Trihexyphenidyl is a muscarinic receptor antagonist.

13. ***D*** (pilocarpine) is correct. A topical ophthalmic preparation of pilocarpine is used in the treatment of acute angle-closure glaucoma, as well as in the treatment of chronic open-angle glaucoma.

A (atropine) is incorrect. In patients with acute angle-closure glaucoma, atropine is contraindicated because it can induce cycloplegia and mydriasis and thereby increase intraocular pressure.
B (edrophonium) and C (furosemide) are incorrect. Edrophonium and furosemide are not used in the treatment of glaucoma. Edrophonium is a rapid-acting, short-duration cholinesterase inhibitor that is used in the diagnosis of myasthenia gravis. Furosemide is a loop diuretic that is used in the treatment of hypertension and heart failure.
E (timolol) is incorrect. Timolol is not used in the treatment of acute angle-closure glaucoma. Topical preparations of timolol are used in the treatment of chronic open-angle glaucoma and ocular hypertension.

14. ***C*** (intramuscular deferoxamine) is correct. Deferoxamine can be administered intramuscularly, intravenously, or subcutaneously to treat an iron overdose.

A (ammonium chloride) and E (penicillamine) are incorrect. Ammonium chloride and penicillamine are not used in the treatment of an iron overdose. Ammonium chloride is used to correct metabolic alkalosis that results from chloride depletion following the use of diuretics or following vomiting, gastric fistula drainage, or nasogastric suction. Penicillamine is used in the treatment of Wilson's disease, cystinuria, and rheumatoid arthritis.
B (hemodialysis) is incorrect. Hemodialysis is not effective in cases of iron overdose, because iron is tightly bound to numerous proteins.
D (oral deferoxamine) is incorrect. Oral administration of deferoxamine to prevent absorption of iron from the gut is controversial. It certainly would not be indicated 6 hours after iron ingestion.

15. ***D*** (lansoprazole) is correct. Famotidine is a histamine H_2 receptor antagonist that is available in low-dose over-the-counter preparations and is frequently used in the treatment of gastrointestinal reflux disease (GERD). For the patient described here, it would be appropriate to prescribe high-dose therapy with a proton pump inhibitor (such as lansoprazole or omeprazole) or an H_2 receptor antagonist (such as cimetidine, famotidine, nizatidine, or ranitidine).

A (bethanechol) and E (metoclopramide) are incorrect. Because of the severity of the patient's disease, bethanechol or metoclopramide would not provide adequate therapy. Moreover, these drugs would increase the likelihood of adverse effects in an elderly patient. The use of bethanechol (a cholinergic agonist) is associated with urinary frequency, abdominal cramps, and blurred vision. The use of metoclopramide (a dopamine antagonist) is associated with drowsiness, restlessness, drug-induced parkinsonism, and tardive dyskinesia.
B (cetirizine) is incorrect. Cetirizine, an active metabolite of hydroxyzine, is an H_1 receptor antagonist (not an H_2 receptor antagonist); thus, it is not helpful in the management of GERD. Cetirizine is used in the treatment of allergic rhinitis and chronic urticaria.
C (cisapride) is incorrect. Cisapride used in combination with other drugs that inhibit its clearance is associated with serious side effects, such as QT prolongation and torsades de pointes. For this reason, cisapride is no longer routinely available. As of May 2000, cisapride is available only via investigational protocols for the treatment of GERD in patients who are unresponsive to other drugs.

16. *E* (trimethoprim-sulfamethoxazole) is correct. Acute uncomplicated cystitis in women usually responds well to treatment with trimethoprim-sulfamethoxazole (TMP-SMX). Treatment can be modified later if the responsible pathogen or pathogens are not sensitive to TMP-SMX.

A (metronidazole) is incorrect. Acute uncomplicated cystitis is usually not treated with metronidazole. Metronidazole is used to treat trichomoniasis in symptomatic patients and their asymptomatic sexual contacts.
B (nitrofurantoin) is incorrect. While TMP-SMX is a good choice in the treatment of acute uncomplicated cystitis in nonpregnant women, nitrofurantoin is a better choice in pregnant women who have creatinine clearance values greater than 40 mL/min and have not yet reached the 38th week of gestation. Nitrofurantoin is contraindicated in pregnant women who are in labor or have reached their 38th week of gestation.
C (penicillin G) is incorrect. Penicillin G is not a drug of choice for cystitis.
D (tetracycline) is incorrect. Tetracycline is used as an alternative drug for the treatment of urinary tract infections caused by susceptible organisms.

17. *C* (ethosuximide) is correct. The patient's EEG findings are consistent with the diagnosis of generalized absence seizures (petit mal seizures). Ethosuximide is the drug of choice for treating this type of generalized seizure in children. It is not effective for treating generalized tonic-clonic seizures or partial seizures. Therefore, if ethosuximide is used to manage absence seizures in a patient who suffers from these other types of seizures, concurrent administration of other antiepileptic drugs is required.

A (carbamazepine) is incorrect. The patient's seizures are generalized absence seizures. Carbamazepine is an antiepileptic drug that is used to treat generalized tonic-clonic seizures (grand mal seizures) and partial seizures. In children, carbamazepine use is preferable to phenobarbital use because carbamazepine has fewer adverse effects on behavior and alertness. Carbamazepine is also effective in the management of pain of neurologic origin (such as trigeminal neuralgia) and in the treatment of some psychiatric disorders (such as bipolar disorder and intermittent explosive disorder).
B (diazepam) is incorrect. The patient's seizures are generalized absence seizures. Diazepam is an antiepileptic drug that is used to treat status epilepticus and has been shown to be effective in preventing the recurrence of febrile seizures. In addition, diazepam is used as an anxiolytic, sedative, or amnestic agent; a skeletal muscle relaxant; an adjunct for anesthesia; and a treatment for alcohol withdrawal.
D (phenobarbital) is incorrect. The patient's seizures are generalized absence seizures. Phenobarbital is a barbiturate that has antiepileptic properties. Although it is not effective in the treat-

ment of absence seizures, it is generally effective in the treatment of the various other types of seizures.
E (phenytoin) is incorrect. The patient's seizures are generalized absence seizures. Phenytoin is an antiepileptic drug that can be used alone or in combination with other anticonvulsants to prevent tonic-clonic seizures and partial seizures with complex symptoms (psychomotor seizures). Phenytoin also can be used to prevent seizures from occurring during surgery.

18. *D* (ibuprofen) is correct. The patient's clinical manifestations are consistent with the diagnosis of primary dysmenorrhea. Ibuprofen is a nonsteroidal anti-inflammatory drug (NSAID) that is used to treat dysmenorrhea as well as rheumatoid arthritis and osteoarthritis.

A (acetaminophen) and E (indomethacin) are incorrect. Acetaminophen and indomethacin are nonselective cyclooxygenase (COX) inhibitors. Acetaminophen has only weak anti-inflammatory actions; thus, it would not be very effective in treating the symptoms of dysmenorrhea. Indomethacin has stronger anti-inflammatory actions and would be effective in treating the symptoms of dysmenorrhea; however, less toxic NSAIDs, such as ibuprofen, would be preferred.
B (celecoxib) is incorrect. Celecoxib is a selective COX-2 inhibitor. It is approved for the treatment of osteoarthritis and rheumatoid arthritis, but it is not currently indicated for the treatment of dysmenorrhea.
C (dexamethasone) is incorrect. Dexamethasone is a glucocorticoid that is used as an anti-inflammatory or immunosuppressive agent. It is not recommended in the treatment of dysmenorrhea.

19. *C* (octreotide) is correct. Octreotide is a synthetic analogue of somatostatin. In comparison with somatostatin, octreotide has a longer half-life; shows greater selectivity for inhibiting glucagon, growth hormone, and insulin release; and is associated with a lower incidence of rebound hypersecretion following discontinuation of its use. Somatostatin is approved for the control of watery diarrhea associated with VIPomas and for the control of flushing and diarrhea associated with metastatic carcinoid tumors. It has also been used to control diarrhea in patients with AIDS, as well as to treat esophageal varices, acromegaly, and pituitary tumors that secrete thyrotropin.

A (leuprolide) and B (nafarelin) are incorrect. Leuprolide and nafarelin are synthetic analogues of gonadotropin-releasing hormone (GnRH). Leuprolide is used in the treatment of advanced prostate cancer and breast cancer and is also used as hormonal therapy for patients with endometriosis. Nafarelin is used to treat precocious puberty and endometriosis.
D (protirelin) is incorrect. Protirelin, a synthetic thyrotropin-releasing hormone (TRH), is not used to inhibit the release of VIP.

It is used to assess thyroid function in patients with pituitary or hypothalamic dysfunction.
E (sermorelin) is incorrect. Sermorelin, a synthetic growth hormone–releasing hormone (GHRH), is not used to inhibit the release of VIP. It is used to treat growth hormone deficiency and to assess the ability of the pituitary gland to secrete growth hormone.

20. *C* (gemfibrozil) is correct. Gemfibrozil can potentiate the effects of warfarin. While warfarin may be added to the regimen of patients already receiving gemfibrozil, prothrombin times should be carefully monitored if gemfibrozil is added to the regimen of patients receiving warfarin.

A (cholestyramine) and B (colestipol) are incorrect. Cholestyramine and colestipol are bile acid–binding resins. When one of these resins is used concurrently with warfarin, it may either increase or decrease warfarin's hypoprothrombinemic effects. When the resin binds with vitamin K in the diet, it impairs vitamin K absorption, and this in turn can increase warfarin's hypoprothrombinemic effects. When the resin binds with warfarin directly, it impairs warfarin's bioavailability and decreases its hypoprothrombinemic effects. To avoid altering warfarin's pharmacokinetics, a bile acid–binding resin should be taken 4–6 hours before or after warfarin is taken.
D (niacin) is incorrect. Niacin does not alter the hypoprothrombinemic effects of warfarin.
E (pravastatin) is incorrect. Pravastatin and lovastatin are both drugs that act by inhibiting HMG-CoA reductase. When lovastatin is added to a stabilized regimen of warfarin therapy, hypoprothrombinemia and clinical bleeding sometimes occur. However, pravastatin does not appear to interact with warfarin; thus, it is the preferred HMG-CoA reductase inhibitor to be used during warfarin therapy.

21. *B* (atropine) is correct. Atropine is indicated in the treatment of a cholinergic crisis caused by poisoning with an organophosphate, such as parathion. The principal effects of atropine treatment are a reduction in salivary, bronchial, and sweat gland secretions; mydriasis; cycloplegia; changes in heart rate; contraction of sphincter muscles in the bladder and gastrointestinal tract; decreased gastric secretion; and decreased gastric motility.

A (amyl nitrite) is incorrect. Amyl nitrite is not used to treat organophosphate poisoning. It is used as an antidote to treat cyanide poisoning. Amyl nitrite oxidizes hemoglobin to form methemoglobin. The methemoglobin binds excess cyanide and forms cyanmethemoglobin, a nontoxic compound.
C (dimercaprol) and E (edetate calcium disodium) are incorrect. Dimercaprol and edetate calcium disodium are not used to treat organophosphate poisoning. Dimercaprol is a heavy metal chelator used in the treatment of acute arsenic, mercury, gold, or lead

poisoning. Edetate calcium disodium (calcium EDTA, or $CaNa_2$ EDTA) is a parenteral drug used in the treatment of lead toxicity; this agent should not be confused with the non–calcium-containing salt (edetate disodium) that is used in the treatment of hypercalcemia.

D (disulfiram) is incorrect. Disulfiram is not used to treat organophosphate poisoning. It is used in the management of ethanol abuse. Disulfiram competes with nicotinamide adenine dinucleotide (NAD) for binding sites on aldehyde dehydrogenase. This action interferes with the hepatic oxidation of acetaldehyde.

22. ***E*** (tamoxifen) is correct. Tamoxifen is used as an adjunct to breast surgery in the treatment of breast cancer. The activity of tamoxifen varies, depending on the type of tissue involved. In breast tissue, which requires estrogen for growth and development, the drug acts as an antagonist at estrogen receptors. In other tissue, the drug acts as a weak agonist at estrogen receptors. Thus, tamoxifen is often referred to as a partial agonist.

A (levonorgestrel), C (octreotide), and D (sermorelin) are incorrect. Levonorgestrel, octreotide, and sermorelin are not used to treat breast cancer. Levonorgestrel is a progestin that can be used alone or in combination with estrogen for contraception. Octreotide is a somatostatin analogue that inhibits the secretion of pituitary and gastrointestinal hormones (including serotonin, gastrin, vasoactive intestinal polypeptide, insulin, glucagon, secretin, motilin, pancreatic polypeptide, growth hormone, and thyrotropin) and is used in the treatment of carcinoid tumors, VIPomas, and acromegaly. Sermorelin is a growth hormone–releasing hormone (GHRH) analogue that is used in the diagnosis and treatment of growth hormone deficiency.

B (nafarelin) is incorrect. Although nafarelin has been used in clinical trials to treat breast cancer, it does not act by blocking estrogen receptors. Nafarelin is a gonadotropin-releasing hormone (GnRH) analogue that can be administered intranasally to treat endometriosis, precocious puberty, hirsutism, and benign prostatic hyperplasia (BPH) and to suppress ovulation in infertile women prior to in vitro fertilization.

23. ***C*** (heparin) is correct. Heparin is indicated for use in the management of DIC. In patients with this disorder, treatment should also be directed toward finding the underlying cause and removing the stimulus for continued clotting and bleeding episodes.

A (aspirin) and D (ticlopidine) are incorrect. Aspirin and ticlopidine are antiplatelet drugs, rather than anticoagulant drugs. Antiplatelet drugs are not used in the treatment of DIC.

B (celecoxib) is incorrect. Celecoxib is not used in the treatment of DIC. Celecoxib is a selective cyclooxygenase-2 (COX-2) inhibitor. Nonselective COX inhibitors act as antiplatelet drugs; celecoxib does not.

E (warfarin) is incorrect. Like heparin, warfarin is an anticoagulant drug. Unlike heparin, warfarin is administered orally. Warfarin must be taken for several days before it reaches its maximal effect; thus, it is not used in the immediate treatment of DIC.

24. ***B*** (furosemide) is correct. Furosemide is a loop diuretic that is used in the management of edema associated with congestive heart failure, cirrhosis, and renal diseases, including nephrotic syndrome. It is also used to treat mild to moderate hypertension and as adjunct therapy in patients with hypertensive crisis and acute pulmonary edema. Polyuria during furosemide treatment places patients at risk for excessive fluid loss and dehydration. The risk is increased when large doses of furosemide are used and sodium intake is restricted. Hypovolemia can lead to orthostatic hypotension and hemoconcentration. These adverse effects are more serious in elderly individuals and patients with chronic heart diseases.

A (acetazolamide) is incorrect. Acetazolamide acts by inhibiting carbonic anhydrase. Inhibition of this enzyme reduces the availability of hydrogen and bicarbonate ions for active transport and also reduces the hydrogen ion concentrations in the lumen of renal tubules. These actions alkalinize the urine and cause an increase in the excretion of bicarbonate, sodium, potassium, and water. A reduction in plasma bicarbonate results in metabolic acidosis, which rapidly reverses the diuretic effect. Because acetazolamide is such a weak diuretic, it is seldom prescribed as a diuretic agent.

C (hydrochlorothiazide) is incorrect. Hydrochlorothiazide is a thiazide diuretic that is used in the management of edema and hypertension. It increases the excretion of sodium, chloride, and water by inhibiting sodium ion transport across the renal tubular epithelium. It causes diuresis primarily by inhibiting active chloride reabsorption at the distal portion of the ascending limb or, more likely, the early part of the distal tubule (i.e., the cortical diluting segment). Hydrochlorothiazide would be less likely than furosemide to produce profound diuresis and vascular collapse.

D (spironolactone) and E (triamterene) are incorrect. Spironolactone, triamterene, and amiloride are potassium-sparing diuretics. Spironolactone is a competitive antagonist of aldosterone and has a slow-onset, moderate diuretic effect. Like amiloride, triamterene is an epithelial sodium channel blocker; however, unlike amiloride, triamterene increases the urinary excretion of magnesium. Triamterene is a relatively weak diuretic and antihypertensive agent and is most often used in the management of hypokalemia, especially in patients who are intolerant of or unresponsive to potassium supplements.

25. *D* (lamotrigine) is correct. Lamotrigine is an effective anticonvulsant when used as an adjunct in the treatment of refractory partial seizures with or without secondary generalized tonic-clonic seizures. Lamotrigine appears to stabilize neuronal membranes by acting at voltage-sensitive sodium channels. This decreases the presynaptic release of glutamate and aspartate and thereby decreases the frequency of seizures. The mechanism of action of lamotrigine is somewhat similar to that of carbamazepine and phenytoin.

A (clonazepam), C (ethosuximide), and E (lorazepam) are incorrect. Clonazepam, ethosuximide, and lorazepam are anticonvulsant drugs, but they are not used in the treatment of partial seizures. Clonazepam has been used to prevent generalized absence, atonic, and myoclonic seizures. However, because of the development of tolerance and a worsening of seizure activity when clonazepam is withdrawn, the drug is mainly reserved for the treatment of refractory myoclonic seizures. Ethosuximide is the drug of choice for managing absence seizures, and lorazepam is used in the treatment of status epilepticus.
B (cyclobenzaprine) is incorrect. Cyclobenzaprine is not an anticonvulsant drug. It is a skeletal muscle relaxant that is structurally related to amitriptyline. Cyclobenzaprine relieves muscle spasms via a central action, probably at the brain stem level, with no direct action on the neuromuscular junction or the muscle. It is not a peripheral neuromuscular blocker. Treatment with cyclobenzaprine reduces pain and tenderness and improves mobility.

26. *A* (acetylcholine acting on a muscarinic receptor) is correct. When acetylcholine binds to a muscarinic cholinergic receptor, it stimulates the IP_3-DAG cascade. It also enhances intracellular concentrations of cyclic guanosine monophosphate (cGMP), causes changes in K^+ conductance, and inhibits adenylyl cyclase activity.

B (acetylcholine acting on a nicotinic receptor) is incorrect. Nicotinic cholinergic receptors are ligand-gated membrane ion channels. When acetylcholine binds to these receptors, it increases the membrane conductance directly by altering the receptor conformation.
C (diazepam acting on a benzodiazepine receptor) is incorrect. Diazepam exerts its effects via the $GABA_A$ receptor complex, not via the IP_3-DAG cascade.
D (insulin acting on an insulin receptor) and E (isoproterenol acting on a β_1-adrenergic receptor) are incorrect. Insulin and isoproterenol do not exert their effects via the IP_3-DAG system. When insulin binds to an insulin receptor, it activates tyrosine kinase and causes changes in cellular phosphorylation patterns. When isoproterenol binds to a β receptor, it activates a G_s protein,

which then enhances adenylyl cyclase activity and causes an increase in the concentration of cyclic adenosine monophosphate (cAMP).

27. ***B*** (ceftriaxone) is correct. Like other third-generation cephalosporins, ceftriaxone has significant activity against gram-negative organisms and is able to penetrate the cerebrospinal fluid (CSF) in concentrations that make it useful in the treatment of beta-lactamase–negative and beta-lactamase–positive meningitis.

A (benzathine penicillin G) and E (procaine penicillin G) are incorrect. Benzathine and procaine penicillin G are only administered intramuscularly. Serum concentrations of penicillin can be detected for up to 30 days following the administration of benzathine penicillin G. The serum concentrations are lower but more prolonged with the benzathine form than with the procaine form, and they are lower but more prolonged with the procaine form than with either the potassium or the sodium forms. Penicillin penetrates inflamed meninges; however, only minimal CSF levels are attained after administration of benzathine or procaine penicillin G injections. Thus, these drugs are unacceptable in the treatment of *H. influenzae* meningitis. Procaine penicillin G is also unacceptable because procaine can cause adverse reactions independent of penicillin G. An immediate-onset, toxic reaction occurs in some individuals and lasts for 15–30 minutes. Manifestations include anxiety, agitation, confusion, combativeness, hallucinations, and seizures.
C (erythromycin) is incorrect. Because only small amounts of erythromycin penetrate the CSF, this drug would not be used to treat *H. influenzae* meningitis.
D (penicillin V) is incorrect. Although all of the antibiotics listed as options may be effective against *H. influenzae,* only ceftriaxone is able to penetrate the blood-brain barrier and reach CSF concentrations that are effective in the treatment of meningitis. Moreover, penicillin G and penicillin V are not effective against beta-lactamase–producing bacteria. Penicillin V is preferable to penicillin G when oral administration is desired, because penicillin V has better gastric acid stability and therefore reaches higher plasma levels.

28. ***C*** (estrogen plus progestin) is correct. The combination of estrogen and progestin effectively inhibits ovulation through selective inhibition of pituitary function. The most severe complications are vascular thrombotic events.

A (albuterol plus prednisone) is incorrect. The most common adverse reactions associated with albuterol use are related to the drug's sympathomimetic effects. The severity of the adverse effects associated with prednisone use increases as the length of treatment increases. Adverse effects do not include vascular thrombotic events.

B (codeine plus acetaminophen) is incorrect. The use of codeine and acetaminophen together produces a greater analgesic effect than does the use of acetaminophen alone or the use of higher doses of codeine. Moreover, the use of codeine and acetaminophen in combination causes fewer adverse reactions than does the use of equianalgesic doses of either drug alone. Adverse reactions do not include vascular thrombotic events.
D (imipenem plus cilastatin) is incorrect. Nausea, vomiting, and diarrhea are among the most frequent side effects reported during treatment with imipenem plus cilastatin. Because pseudomembranous colitis can also occur, it is important to consider this diagnosis in patients who develop diarrhea after they begin treatment with imipenem plus cilastatin. Adverse effects do not include vascular thrombotic events.
E (propranolol plus hydrochlorothiazide) is incorrect. Patients treated with hydrochlorothiazide should be monitored closely for signs of electrolyte imbalance, including hyponatremia, hypokalemia, hypomagnesemia, and hypochloremia. Most of the adverse effects of propranolol represent overextensions of the drug's therapeutic effect. Adverse effects do not include vascular thrombotic events.

29. ***D*** (pancuronium) is correct. Pancuronium is a nondepolarizing neuromuscular blocking agent that would be useful in preventing the patient's ineffective respiratory movements. In contrast to succinylcholine (which is a depolarizing neuromuscular blocking agent), pancuronium has little agonist activity and therefore has no depolarizing effect at the motor end plate. Pancuronium has a long duration of action, and its effects can be reversed by cholinesterase inhibitors, such as neostigmine.

A (baclofen) and B (dantrolene) are incorrect. Baclofen and dantrolene are spasmolytic drugs. Unlike neuromuscular blocking agents, these drugs are not used to cause muscle paralysis during surgical procedures or mechanical ventilation. By acting as a $GABA_B$ receptor agonist, baclofen decreases the number and severity of muscle spasms and relieves associated pain, clonus, and muscle rigidity in patients with multiple sclerosis and other neurodegenerative diseases. Dantrolene decreases muscle contraction by interfering with the release of calcium ion from the sarcoplasmic reticulum in skeletal muscle cells. This "uncouples" the excitation-contraction process. Dantrolene is useful in treating malignant hyperthermia.
C (neostigmine) is incorrect. Neostigmine use would not be appropriate in this case. Neostigmine is a drug that inhibits cholinesterase and thereby potentiates the action of acetylcholine on skeletal muscle and smooth muscle. Neostigmine is used for the reversal of nondepolarizing neuromuscular blockade (e.g., for the reversal of the effects of pancuronium).
E (succinylcholine) is incorrect. Unlike pancuronium (see the discussion for Option D), succinylcholine is a depolarizing neuromuscular blocking agent and has a short duration of action. Succinylcholine competes with acetylcholine for the cholinergic

receptors on the motor end plate. Succinylcholine causes a more prolonged depolarization than acetylcholine, because it has a high affinity for these receptors and a strong resistance to cholinesterase. Depolarization results in fasciculation of the skeletal muscles, followed by muscle paralysis. The effects of succinylcholine cannot be reversed by a cholinesterase inhibitor.

30. *D* (praziquantel) is correct. Praziquantel is an anthelmintic agent that is used to treat schistosomiasis, clonorchiasis, and opisthorchiasis. It acts by increasing the cell membrane permeability of trematodes, thereby causing their vacuolation and disintegration.

A (mebendazole) and E (pyrantel pamoate) are incorrect. Mebendazole and pyrantel pamoate are not indicated in the treatment of schistosomiasis. Mebendazole and pyrantel pamoate are broad-spectrum anthelmintic agents that are particularly effective against gastrointestinal nematodes, such as whipworms, pinworms, and hookworms, and are considered the drugs of choice in treating infections caused by these nematodes. Mebendazole selectively damages cytoplasmic microtubules in the absorptive and intestinal cells of nematodes but not of the host. Pyrantel pamoate causes a depolarizing neuromuscular blockade in helminths by stimulating the release of acetylcholine, inhibiting cholinesterase, and stimulating ganglionic neurons.

B (metronidazole) is incorrect. Metronidazole is not indicated for use in the treatment of schistosomiasis. Metronidazole is effective against several protozoa, including *Entamoeba histolytica, Giardia lamblia,* and *Trichomonas vaginalis*. It is also one of the most effective drugs available against anaerobic bacteria.

C (niclosamide) is incorrect. Niclosamide is not indicated in the treatment of schistosomiasis. Niclosamide is an anthelmintic agent that is used to treat infections with cestodes, such as beef, fish, and dwarf tapeworms. It acts by blocking mitochondrial oxidative phosphorylation and inhibiting glucose uptake in these parasites.

31. *E* (tyrosine kinase) is correct. Insulin and several growth factors have receptors with extracellular and cytoplasmic domains. Binding to the extracellular domain of the receptor activates a tyrosine kinase on the cytoplasmic domain. This causes the autophosphorylation of specific tyrosine residues and the phosphorylation of substrate proteins.

A (adenylyl cyclase) and C (phospholipase C) are incorrect. Isoproterenol and other β-adrenergic receptor agonists are examples of agents that signal via the adenylyl cyclase pathway. Phenylephrine and other α_1-adrenergic receptor agonists are examples of agents that signal via the phospholipase C pathway.

B (phosphodiesterase) is incorrect. Sildenafil is an example of an agent that exerts its activity by inhibiting a phosphodiesterase. The drug is a specific phosphodiesterase that inhibits the breakdown of cyclic guanosine monophosphate (cGMP) in the corpus cavernosum of the penis.

D (phosphoprotein phosphatase) is incorrect. As discussed in Option E, insulin is an agent that signals via activation of tyrosine kinase. This causes the autophosphorylation of specific tyrosine residues and the phosphorylation of substrate proteins. However, the cascade of effects initiated by a chemical signal often involves a series of phosphorylation and dephosphorylation reactions, with phosphorylation catalyzed by kinases and dephosphorylation catalyzed by phosphatases. Many transmitters are known to signal by activating different kinases. The effects of transmitter signals on phosphatases are not well understood.

32. *C* (fexofenadine) is correct. The patient's clinical manifestations are consistent with the diagnosis of acute urticaria. Fexofenadine, a second-generation H_1 receptor antagonist, is highly efficacious in the treatment of this condition. Fexofenadine does not cross the blood-brain barrier and is therefore not sedating. Although fexofenadine is an active metabolite of terfenadine (a drug withdrawn from the market in 1999), fexofenadine lacks the life-threatening cardiovascular side effects of terfenadine.

A (chlorpheniramine) is incorrect. Chlorpheniramine is a competitive H_1 receptor antagonist of the propylamine group of antihistamines. It is effective for use in the treatment of histamine-mediated conditions, such as urticaria and allergic rhinitis. However, like other first-generation H_1 receptor antagonists, it has sedative effects. These effects, which result from antagonism at central histamine receptors, would interfere with driving an automobile.

B (famotidine) is incorrect. In patients with urticaria, H_2 receptor antagonists such as famotidine have little effect if given alone. Doxepin, a tricyclic antidepressant that acts as a combined H_1 and H_2 antagonist, is effective in the treatment of chronic idiopathic urticaria.

D (prednisone) and E (triamcinolone cream) are incorrect. Systemic corticosteroids such as prednisone have no role in the treatment of relatively innocuous conditions, such as acute urticaria, because their potential side effects outweigh their potential benefits. In cases of urticaria in which the itching is severe and prevents the patient from sleeping, a topical corticosteroid, such as triamcinolone cream, may be given as adjunct therapy to achieve more rapid relief, but the topical drug should be used for only a short period of time.

33. *B* (formation of methemoglobin) is correct. The patient's history and clinical manifestations are consistent with the diagnosis of cyanide poisoning. In patients with this type of poisoning, sodium nitrite is an effective antidote because it is able to oxidize hemoglobin to form methemoglobin. The methemoglobin then binds to cyanide and forms cyanmethemoglobin, a nontoxic compound.

A (decrease in intracranial pressure), C (increase in coronary arterial blood flow), and E (relaxation of the nonvascular smooth muscle) are incorrect. Sodium nitrite and other nitrites have a wide range of effects. For example, they can cause headaches because of their effects on the cerebral vasculature. They will increase the total coronary blood flow in individuals with healthy hearts, although they will simply redistribute the blood to ischemic areas in patients who have ischemia. And, they will relax all types of smooth muscle, including bronchial, biliary, gastrointestinal, ureteral, and uterine smooth muscle. However, these effects are not related to the actions of nitrites in treating cyanide poisoning.
D (increase in oxidative phosphorylation) is incorrect. Sodium nitrite does not increase oxidative phosphorylation.

34. *A* (aminoglutethimide) is correct. Aminoglutethimide is an adrenal steroid inhibitor that is used to suppress adrenal function in patients with Cushing's syndrome, or in those with breast or prostate cancer. Aminoglutethimide blocks aromatase, thereby inhibiting the conversion of androgens to estrogens in peripheral tissues. The drug also inhibits the enzymatic conversion of cholesterol to pregnenolone, thereby reducing the synthesis of glucocorticoids, mineralocorticoids, estrogens, and androgens.

B (goserelin) and E (tamoxifen) are incorrect. Goserelin and tamoxifen are helpful for use in the management of breast cancer, but they do not inhibit the conversion of androgens to estrogens in peripheral tissues. Goserelin is an analogue of gonadotropin-releasing hormone (GnRH). In addition to being used as palliative treatment in advanced breast or prostate cancer, goserelin is used in the management of endometriosis and dysfunctional uterine bleeding. Tamoxifen is a nonsteroidal, antiestrogenic, antineoplastic agent. Tamoxifen is used as an adjunct to breast surgery in patients with breast cancer, and it is also used in the prevention of breast cancer in women at high risk.
C (octreotide) and D (procarbazine) are incorrect. Octreotide and procarbazine are not used to treat breast cancer. Octreotide, an analogue of somatostatin, is used to control symptoms associated with VIPomas (such as watery diarrhea) and symptoms associated with metastatic carcinoid tumors (such as flushing and diarrhea). Procarbazine is a cell cycle–specific antineoplastic agent that is used to treat Hodgkin's disease. Procarbazine is an atypical DNA

alkylating agent that is not cross-resistant to other alkylating agents.

35. ***E*** (the increasing blood pressure activates the baroreceptor reflex) is correct. Drugs that elevate blood pressure cause reflex bradycardia as long as other drugs are not present to block the reflex arc. Before propranolol is administered, epinephrine causes a direct stimulation of the heart that is only partially masked by the reflex vagal effect.

A (propranolol directly stimulates the vagus nerve) is incorrect. Propranolol does not directly stimulate the vagus nerve.
B (propranolol inhibits the central effects of epinephrine) is incorrect. Propranolol inhibits some of the central effects of epinephrine, but this action is unrelated to the decrease in heart rate associated with the administration of epinephrine.
C (propranolol inhibits the effects of circulating norepinephrine) is incorrect. Propranolol does not block all of the effects of circulating norepinephrine. It blocks only the stimulating effects that circulating norepinephrine has on the heart.
D (propranolol is a quinidine-like agent that decreases the heart rate) is incorrect. Propranolol has a negative inotropic effect on the heart rate, and additional negative inotropic effects occur if propranolol or other β-adrenergic receptor antagonists are used with diltiazem, disopyramide, quinidine, or verapamil. In the presence of propranolol, epinephrine causes a decrease in heart rate because of the reflex bradycardia mediated through vagal slowing of the heart in association with the pressor response.

36. ***E*** (lead poisoning) is correct. The paint used in old houses may contain lead. Lead poisoning should be suspected when a child has gastrointestinal or central nervous system (CNS) symptoms, microcytic anemia (with or without basophilic stippling), and lead lines in the distal long bones. The diagnosis of lead poisoning is confirmed by a finding of a high level of lead in the blood. Patients with lead poisoning are treated parenterally with edetate calcium disodium (EDTA) for 5 days and are then given oral succimer.

A (benzene poisoning) is incorrect. Benzene is used as a solvent. Acute benzene poisoning would cause CNS symptoms, whereas chronic benzene poisoning would cause hematologic changes. With long-term exposure to benzene, there may be an increase in the erythrocyte, leukocyte, and thrombocyte counts before the onset of aplastic anemia. Poisoning with benzene would not account for the x-ray findings described in the patient.
B (dioxin poisoning) is incorrect. Dioxin is a highly toxic compound that is formed in the combustion of polychlorinated hydrocarbons. Individuals exposed to high levels of dioxin may initially experience symptoms such as nausea, vomiting, myalgia, and irritation of the skin, eyes, and mucous membranes. After a latency period of several weeks, they may develop chloracne, por-

phyria cutanea tarda, hirsutism, or hyperpigmentation. Levels of hepatic transaminases and blood lipids may be elevated.
C (ipecac ingestion) is incorrect. Ipecac syrup is used to induce vomiting after poisoning with some types of substances. A child who accidentally ingested ipecac syrup would experience nausea and vomiting. If an individual who has anorexia and bulimia repeatedly ingested ipecac to induce vomiting, it could cause dehydration, an electrolyte imbalance, and myopathy. Ingestion of ipecac would not account for the other findings described in the patient.
D (iron poisoning) is incorrect. Symptoms of iron poisoning include nausea, vomiting, diarrhea, and hypotension. They do not include the laboratory and x-ray findings described in the patient.

37. *C* (indomethacin) is correct. Indomethacin is a nonsteroidal anti-inflammatory drug (NSAID) that also has antipyretic and analgesic properties. It is used primarily in the treatment of rheumatoid arthritis, osteoarthritis, and ankylosing spondylitis. By inhibiting cyclooxygenase and lipoxygenase, indomethacin reduces the formation of proinflammatory mediators (such as prostaglandins and leukotrienes) and also inhibits migration of leukocytes into the inflamed area. Indomethacin may also exert its immunomodulating effects by inhibiting phosphodiesterase.

A (corticosteroids) is incorrect. Corticosteroids are the most powerful drugs used for the prevention and suppression of inflammation. They inhibit the first step in the arachidonic acid cascade (i.e., they inhibit the action of phospholipase A_2), thereby preventing the production of prostaglandins and leukotrienes. In spite of this rather general anti-inflammatory activity, corticosteroids are not very efficacious in the treatment of ankylosing spondylitis.
B (gold salts) is incorrect. Gold salts are efficacious in the treatment of rheumatoid arthritis but not in the treatment of ankylosing spondylitis. Gold salts are thought to act either by preventing macrophages from processing antigens or by inhibiting the release of lysosomal enzymes.
D (penicillamine) is incorrect. Penicillamine has some antirheumatic effects but is not useful in the management of ankylosing spondylitis. Penicillamine appears to act by suppressing both the formation of collagen and the circulating levels of IgM rheumatoid factor and by depressing T-cell (but not B-cell) activity. Penicillamine is commonly used as a chelating compound for the removal of excess copper in Wilson's disease. It is also used to dissolve cysteine stones in the urinary tract.
E (salicylates) is incorrect. Salicylates are not efficacious in the treatment of ankylosing spondylitis. Unlike indomethacin, which inhibits both cyclooxygenase and lipoxygenase, salicylates inhibit only the cyclooxygenase branch of the arachidonic acid cascade. Salicylates also lack the immunomodulating properties of indomethacin.

38. *B* (lisinopril) is correct. Lisinopril is an angiotensin-converting enzyme (ACE) inhibitor that is given orally in the treatment of hypertension and congestive heart failure. ACE inhibitors can cause kinins to accumulate in the respiratory tract and thereby result in a persistent nonproductive cough. They also cause hyperkalemia.

A (hydrochlorothiazide) is incorrect. The adverse effects of hydrochlorothiazide include hyponatremia, hypokalemia, hypomagnesemia, and hypochloremia. They do not include a persistent cough.
C (metoprolol) is incorrect. The adverse effects of metoprolol are usually mild and temporary. They often occur at the onset of therapy and diminish over time. They do not include a persistent cough.
D (nifedipine) and E (valsartan) are incorrect. The adverse effects of nifedipine and valsartan do not include a persistent cough. Most of the adverse effects of nifedipine are related to vasodilative actions, which are greater with regular-release capsules than with the extended-release products. These adverse effects are usually not serious and respond well to dosage reduction. Valsartan is generally well tolerated.

39. *A* (allopurinol) is correct. The patient's clinical and laboratory findings are consistent with the diagnosis of gout. Allopurinol is used to prevent gout in patients who have experienced repeated attacks of the disorder. Allopurinol is also used to prevent hyperuricemia and uric acid nephropathy in cancer patients who are undergoing radiation therapy or chemotherapy. In these cancer patients, hyperuricemia is associated with rapid cell turnover and massive cell destruction. Allopurinol acts by inhibiting xanthine oxidase and thereby blocking the conversion of xanthine and hypoxanthine (oxypurines) to uric acid.

B (corticosteroids) is incorrect. Intra-articular corticosteroids may be used to terminate an acute attack of gout, but they would not be effective in preventing future attacks. Prolonged use of intra-articular corticosteroids is contraindicated because it would lead to cartilage atrophy and osteoporosis and would eventually destroy the affected joints.
C (indomethacin) is incorrect. Because of its anti-inflammatory and pain-relieving properties, indomethacin is sometimes effective in terminating an acute attack of gout. However, the drug is not effective in preventing repeated attacks of gout.
D (morphine) is incorrect. To terminate an acute attack of gout, it may be necessary to give a strong pain reliever for a brief period of time. If morphine is used, one dose is usually enough. Long-term use could lead to addiction and would not prevent repeated attacks of gout.
E (salicylates) is incorrect. Because salicylates interfere with the renal handling of uric acid, they should not be used in the management of gout.

40. ***B*** (bismuth, metronidazole, and tetracycline) is correct. *H. pylori* infection of the mucosa is found in association with most peptic ulcers of the duodenum and stomach. To prevent recurrence, this pathogen must be eradicated. Combination therapy with bismuth, metronidazole, and tetracycline achieves an eradication rate of 90% or more. The addition of omeprazole may further aid the healing process and reduce the length of treatment.

A (aluminum hydroxide plus famotidine) is incorrect. Aluminum hydroxide, an antacid, and famotidine, a histamine H_2 receptor antagonist, would not prevent the recurrence of peptic ulcers; they would bring about only temporary relief of symptoms.
C (lansoprazole plus cephalexin) is incorrect. Although proton pump inhibitors such as lansoprazole are used in the treatment of *H. pylori* infection, they do not eradicate the infection. *H. pylori* is resistant to cephalexin.
D (omeprazole, cimetidine, and trimethoprim-sulfamethoxazole) is incorrect. In patients with peptic ulcer disease, omeprazole inhibits the secretion of gastric acid and thereby supports the healing process. Omeprazole does not eradicate *H. pylori,* so it would not prevent recurrence. Cimetidine and TMP-SMX also do not eradicate *H. pylori.*
E (sucralfate, ranitidine, and calcium carbonate) is incorrect. Sucralfate is a sulfate disaccharide that has multiple mechanisms of action and is useful in the management of peptic ulcer disease. In clinical trials, it was found to be as effective as histamine H_2 receptor antagonists, such as ranitidine, and to cause few side effects. Calcium carbonate is a chemical buffer for acids. Because this combination does not eradicate *H. pylori,* it would not prevent recurrence.

41. ***C*** (site C) is correct. Penicillinase is a beta-lactamase. Beta-lactamases cleave the beta-lactam ring and thereby inactivate beta-lactam antibiotics.

A (site A), B (site B), D (site D), and E (site E) are incorrect. Site C is the site of action of penicillinase. Site A is the side chain that is altered in semisynthetic penicillins to change the bacterial spectrum, acid stability, or penicillinase resistance of the drug. Site B can be cleaved by amidases in the gastrointestinal tract. Site D is a five-membered ring in penicillins and a six-membered ring in cephalosporins. Site E shows the carboxylic acid group that is responsible for the active renal tubular secretion of penicillins.

42. ***B*** (labetalol) is correct. Labetalol is one of several antihypertensive agents that can be used in the management of moderate, pregnancy-induced hypertension. By inhibiting both α- and β-adrenergic receptors, labetalol causes vasodilation and a decrease in total peripheral resistance. This decreases the blood pressure without causing a substantial reduction in the resting heart rate, cardiac output, or stroke volume.

A (atenolol) and D (pindolol) are incorrect. Moderate, pregnancy-induced hypertension is sometimes treated with atenolol or pindolol. Unlike labetalol, however, these agents block only β-adrenergic receptors. Atenolol is a competitive β_1-blocker. Pindolol is a β_1- and β_2-blocker with intrinsic sympathomimetic activity (ISA).
C (minoxidil) and E (terazosin) are incorrect. Minoxidil and terazosin are usually not used to treat pregnancy-induced hypertension. Minoxidil is a direct vasodilator, and terazosin is an α_1-blocker.

43. ***C*** (mitotane) is correct. Either mitotane or ketoconazole can be used to inhibit adrenal steroidogenesis when ectopic tumors produce an excess of ACTH. Ketoconazole blocks many of the same steps as metyrapone and, in some sites, has been shown to be a more potent inhibitor.

A (clomiphene) is incorrect. Clomiphene does not decrease cortisol levels. Clomiphene stimulates the pituitary to release follicle-stimulating hormone (FSH) and luteinizing hormone (LH). It is a nonsteroidal drug that is used to induce ovulation in infertile women.
B (finasteride) is incorrect. Finasteride is a synthetic analogue of testosterone. It acts as a competitive inhibitor of type II 5α-reductase, an intracellular enzyme that converts testosterone to dihydrotestosterone (DHT). Finasteride is used in the treatment of benign prostatic hyperplasia.
D (spironolactone) is incorrect. Spironolactone is a potassium-sparing diuretic that is used in combination with a thiazide diuretic to treat hypertension. Spironolactone is also indicated for use in the management of severe heart failure and in the treatment of ascites associated with cirrhosis. Unapproved uses include the treatment of polycystic ovary syndrome and hirsutism in women.
E (tamoxifen) is incorrect. Tamoxifen is a nonsteroidal antiestrogen that is used as an adjunct to breast surgery in the treatment of breast cancer.

44. ***D*** (erythromycin) is correct. Antibiotics should be taken before dental procedures are performed in individuals who have a history of valvular heart disease. In those allergic to penicillin, erythromycin is the drug of choice. In those not allergic to penicillin, amoxicillin is frequently used.

A (amoxicillin) is incorrect. As discussed in Option D, amoxicillin is frequently used for antibiotic prophylaxis. However, it would be contraindicated in a patient allergic to penicillin.
B (chloramphenicol), C (doxycycline), and E (tetracycline) are incorrect. Chloramphenicol, doxycycline, or tetracycline would not be the drug of choice for antibiotic prophylaxis. Although chloramphenicol is active against a wide range of organisms, including gram-positive bacteria, gram-negative bacteria such as *Chlamydia* and *Rickettsia,* and many anaerobic bacteria, it is seldom used today because it is more toxic than other antibiotics that are also effective against these organisms. Doxycycline and other tetracyclines are broad-spectrum antibiotics that are mainly used to treat *Chlamydia, Rickettsia,* and *Mycoplasma pneumoniae* infections. Doxycycline can be given once a day to treat nongonococcal urethritis and cervicitis. Because of its minimal renal clearance, doxycycline is the tetracycline of choice in treating infections in patients with poor renal function.

45. ***D*** (vitamin A toxicity) is correct. The patient's skin disorder and hair loss are most likely due to vitamin A toxicity. A long-term excess of vitamin A can cause hypervitaminosis A, with manifestations including increased intracranial pressure, massive desquamation, xerosis, lip fissures, fatigue, malaise, irritability, psychiatric changes mimicking severe depression or schizophrenia, anorexia, abdominal discomfort, nausea and vomiting, mild fever, excessive sweating, slow growth, and arthralgia.

A (vitamin A deficiency) is incorrect. The patient's clinical manifestations are caused by an excess (not a deficiency) of vitamin A. Vitamin A is required for embryonic development, bone development, testicular and ovarian function, night vision, and the maintenance of mucosal and epithelial surfaces.
B (vitamin D deficiency) is incorrect. Skin disorders and hair loss are not symptoms of vitamin D deficiency. A deficiency of vitamin D in children causes rickets, while a deficiency in adults causes osteoporosis.
C (vitamin E deficiency) and E (vitamin E toxicity) are incorrect. Vitamin E is an antioxidant that protects membrane-bound polyunsaturated fatty acids and other oxygen-sensitive substances, such as vitamin A and vitamin C, from oxidation. A deficiency of vitamin E is rare. Prolonged use of excessive dosages of vitamin E (> 800 units/d) can be toxic. In otherwise healthy individuals, adverse effects include altered immune response and sexual dysfunction. In patients with vitamin K deficiency or altered thyroid, pituitary, or adrenal hormone metabolism, adverse effects include bleeding.

46. *C* (cytarabine plus idarubicin) is correct. During the early phase of AML, the best therapeutic response is achieved by giving a combination of cytarabine and idarubicin. Cytarabine is a cytosine analogue that acts as a cell cycle–specific antineoplastic agent. When cytarabine is incorporated into DNA in place of cytosine, it creates DNA with an incorrect message sequence. Cytarabine also inhibits DNA polymerase, an enzyme that is necessary for DNA chain elongation. Idarubicin is a synthetic analogue of daunorubicin. Like daunorubicin, it is a cell cycle–nonspecific antineoplastic agent that interferes with the DNA-repairing activity of topoisomerase II. When compared with daunorubicin, idarubicin is better able to penetrate cells and exerts a higher antitumor activity.

A (chlorambucil plus prednisone) and E (prednisone) are incorrect. Prednisone use is contraindicated in patients with AML because it increases the risk of life-threatening infections. Chlorambucil, given alone or in combination with prednisone, is the therapy of choice for chronic lymphatic leukemia (CLL).
B (cladribine plus interferon alfa) and D (hydroxyurea) are incorrect. AML is not treated with cladribine plus interferon alfa or with hydroxyurea. The combination of cladribine (2-chlorodeoxyadenosine) and interferon alfa is highly effective for use in the treatment of hairy cell leukemia. Hydroxyurea is used mainly in the treatment of chronic myelogenous leukemia but also in other hyperproliferative conditions such as psoriasis.

47. *E* (vidarabine) is correct. Dendritic keratitis is quite typical of herpes simplex virus (HSV) infection of the eye. Since vidarabine is effective against both HSV-1 and HSV-2, it is the drug of choice to initiate therapy without delay. Chronic blepharoconjunctivitis is the most common cause of blindness in developed countries. Without rapid and effective therapeutic intervention, blindness occurs in about 15% of patients with the acute form of this disease.

A (betamethasone) is incorrect. The patient is most likely to have an HSV infection of the eye. In patients with viral ocular infections, monotherapy with a corticosteroid would facilitate faster and deeper spreading of the infection. Therefore, corticosteroids should not be used alone. They should only be given after treatment with an effective antiviral agent is initiated.
B (interferon alfa) is incorrect. Studies have shown that interferon alfa is effective in vitro against HSV. However, in the United States, interferon alfa is not available as a topical formulation.
C (ketoconazole) and D (tetracycline) are incorrect. The patient is most likely to have an HSV infection of the eye, so ketoconazole (an antifungal agent) or tetracycline (an antibiotic) would not be indicated. Mycotic infections of the eye are extremely rare and have a slow chronic course. It is not necessary to treat them with the kind of urgency used in treating HSV infections. Bacterial

conjunctivitis is less prone to evolve into dendritic keratitis than are viral infections of the eye. Application of tetracycline would cause an unnecessary delay in employing effective treatment.

48. *A* (aztreonam) is correct. Cephalosporins (such as cefepime and ceftazidime) would not be the drugs of choice for treating the patient, because cross-reactivity to cephalosporins is reported in about 3–7% of patients who have a known history of penicillin hypersensitivity. Aztreonam, which is a monocyclic beta-lactam (monobactam) antibiotic, is usually well tolerated by patients who are allergic to penicillins. Aztreonam is effective against aerobic gram-negative bacteria but has no activity against gram-positive or anaerobic bacteria. The drug is used to treat gram-negative infections of the skin, soft tissue, urinary tract, and lower respiratory tract; intra-abdominal and gynecologic infections; and septicemia.

B (cefepime) and C (ceftazidime) are incorrect. As discussed in Option A, patients who are allergic to penicillin may have cross-reactivity to cephalosporins, so a cephalosporin would not be the drug of choice. Ceftazidime, a parenterally administered third-generation cephalosporin, is extremely active against *Pseudomonas aeruginosa* and has a broader spectrum of activity against aerobic gram-negative bacteria than do first- or second-generation agents. Ceftazidime is used in the empiric treatment of fever in neutropenic patients. It is also used in the treatment of meningitis and infections of the lower respiratory tract, skin, soft tissues, urinary tract, bones, and joints. Cefepime is a fourth-generation cephalosporin. It is comparable to ceftazidime in its coverage against *P. aeruginosa,* and it may be more active than ceftazidime against *Enterobacter* infections because of its enhanced stability against beta-lactamases. The uses of cefepime are similar to those of the third-generation cephalosporins.
D (metronidazole) is incorrect. Metronidazole is an antimicrobial and antiprotozoal drug that is used to treat some protozoal infections and is also effective against anaerobic organisms. It would not be effective in the treatment of the gram-negative organism described in this case.
E (nitrofurantoin) is incorrect. Nitrofurantoin is bacteriostatic and bactericidal against many gram-negative and gram-positive organisms; however, *P. aeruginosa* and many *Proteus* species are resistant to the drug. Nitrofurantoin reaches therapeutic concentrations only in the urine. Because nitrofurantoin is concentrated in the urine, it should not be given to patients with impaired renal function.

49. *C* (olanzapine) is correct. Antipsychotic agents cause several adverse effects on the reproductive system, including amenorrhea and galactorrhea. These effects are due to the ability of the agents to block dopamine's tonic inhibition of prolactin secretion. Some of the newer agents, such as olanzapine and quetiapine, have a low potential for increasing prolactin secretion.

A (chlorpromazine), B (haloperidol), and E (thioridazine) are incorrect. Chlorpromazine, haloperidol, and thioridazine are drugs that are used to treat schizophrenia and other psychotic disorders. Chlorpromazine is an aliphatic phenothiazine; haloperidol is a butyrophenone; and thioridazine is a piperidine phenothiazine. All three drugs have a high propensity for increasing prolactin secretion and would therefore be inappropriate for a patient suffering from amenorrhea and galactorrhea.
D (promethazine) is incorrect. Promethazine is not used to treat schizophrenia. Promethazine is a phenothiazine that acts as a histamine H_1 receptor antagonist. It has anticholinergic, sedative, and antiemetic effects and also has some local anesthetic properties. It is mainly used as an antiemetic and as an agent to prevent motion sickness.

50. *C* (clindamycin) is correct. Patients who undergo nasopharyngeal surgery are at risk for infections caused by *Staphylococcus aureus,* anaerobic bacteria that colonize the mouth, and aerobic gram-negative bacteria. In most cases, the drug of choice to prevent these infections is cefazolin. However, in patients who are allergic to penicillin, clindamycin (alone or in combination with gentamicin) is a suitable alternative. Clindamycin is active against aerobic gram-positive cocci as well as several anaerobic gram-negative and gram-positive bacteria.

A (amoxicillin), B (cefazolin), and E (nafcillin) are incorrect. Amoxicillin, cefazolin, and nafcillin are beta-lactam antibiotics, so their use would be contraindicated in patients who are allergic to penicillin G.
D (metronidazole) is incorrect. Patients who undergo nasopharyngeal surgery are at risk for infections caused by *S. aureus,* anaerobic bacteria that colonize the mouth, and aerobic gram-negative bacteria. Metronidazole is not effective against some of these organisms, so it is not the drug of choice. It is effective against anaerobic bacterial infections, amebiasis, giardiasis, and trichomoniasis.

Index

B

C

D

O

P

T